CUNNINGHAM'S MANUAL OF PRACTICAL ANATOMY

Volume 3

Cunningham's Manual of Practical Anatomy

CUNNINGHAM'S MANUAL OF PRACTICAL ANATOMY

Sixteenth edition

Volume 3 Head, neck and brain

Dr Rachel Koshi MBBS, MS, PhD

Professor of Anatomy
Apollo Institute of Medical Sciences and Research
Chittoor, India

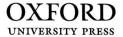
OXFORD
UNIVERSITY PRESS

UNIVERSITY PRESS

Great Clarendon Street, Oxford, OX2 6DP,
United Kingdom

Oxford University Press is a department of the University of Oxford.
It furthers the University's objective of excellence in research, scholarship,
and education by publishing worldwide. Oxford is a registered trade mark of
Oxford University Press in the UK and in certain other countries

Thirteenth edition 1966
Fourteenth edition 1977
Fifteenth edition 1986

Impression: 5

Published in the United States of America by Oxford University Press
198 Madison Avenue, New York, NY 10016, United States of America

British Library Cataloguing in Publication Data
Data available

Library of Congress Control Number: 2016956732

ISBN 978-0-19-874938-7

Printed and bound by Thomson Press India Ltd

I fondly dedicate this book to the late Dr K G Koshi for his encouragement and support when I chose a career in anatomy, and to Dr Mary Jacob, under whose guidance I learned the subject and developed a love for teaching.

Oxford University Press would like to dedicate this book to the memory of the late George John Romanes, Professor of Anatomy at Edinburgh University (1954–1984), who brought his wisdom to previous editions of *Cunningham's*.

Foreword

It gives me great pleasure to pen down the Foreword to the 16th edition of *Cunningham's Manual of Practical Anatomy*. Just as the curriculum of anatomy is incomplete without dissection, so also learning by dissection is incomplete without a manual.

Cunningham's Manual of Practical Anatomy is one of the oldest dissectors, the first edition of which was published as early as 1893. Since then, the manual has been an inseparable companion to students during dissection.

I remember my days as a first MBBS student, the only dissector known in those days was *Cunningham's* manual. The manual helped me to dissect scientifically, step by step, explore the body, see all structures as mentioned, and admire God's highest creation—the human body—so perfectly. As a postgraduate student, I marvelled at the manual and learnt details of structures, in a way as if I had my teacher with me telling me what to do next. The clearly defined steps of dissection, and the comprehensive revision tables at the end, helped me personally to develop a liking for dissection and the subject of anatomy.

Today, as a Professor and Head of Anatomy, teaching anatomy for more than 30 years, I find *Cunningham's* manual extremely useful to all the students dissecting and learning anatomy.

With the explosion of knowledge and ongoing curricular changes, the manual has been revised at frequent intervals. The 16th edition is more student friendly. The language is simplified, so that the book can be comprehended by one and all. The objectives are well defined. The clinical application notes at the end of each chapter are an academic feast to the learners. The lucidly enumerated steps of dissection make a student explore various structures, the layout, and relations and compare them with the simplified labelled illustrations in the manual. This helps in sequential dissection in a scientific way and for knowledge retention. The text also includes multiple choice questions for self-assessment and holistic comprehension.

Keeping the concept of 'Adult Learning Principles' in mind, i.e. adults learn when they 'DO', and with a global movement towards 'competency-based curriculum', students learn anatomy when they dissect; *Cunningham's* manual will help students to dissect on their own, at their own speed and time, and become competent doctors, who can cater to the needs of the society in a much better way.

I recommend this invaluable manual to all the learners who want to master the subject of anatomy.

Dr Pritha S Bhuiyan
Professor and Head, Department of Anatomy
Professor and Coordinator, Department of Medical Education
Seth GS Medical College and KEM Hospital, Parel, Mumbai

Preface to the sixteenth edition

Cunningham's Manual of Practical Anatomy has been the most widely used dissection manual in India for many decades. This edition is extensively revised. The language has been modernized and simplified to appeal to the present-day student. Opening remarks have been added at the start of a chapter, or at the beginning of the description of a region where necessary. This volume on the head and neck, brain, and spinal cord starts with the description of the bones, cavities, organs, muscles, vessels, and nerves of the head and neck. The brain and spinal cord are discussed in the following section. The last section in the volume presents a series of cross-sectional gross anatomy images, as well as computerized tomograms and magnetic resonance images of the head, neck and brain, to enable further understanding of the intimate relationship between the structures described here.

Dissection forms an integral part of learning anatomy, and the practice of dissections enables students to retain and recall anatomical details learnt in the first year of medical college during their clinical practice. To make the dissection process easier and more meaningful, in this edition, each dissection is presented with a heading, and a list of objectives to be accomplished. Many of the details of dissections have been retained from the earlier edition, but are presented as numbered, stepwise easy-to-follow instructions that help students navigate their way through the tissues of the body, and to isolate, define, and study important structures.

This manual contains a number of old and new features that enable students to integrate the anatomy learned in the dissection hall with clinical practice. Numerous X-rays, CTs, and MRIs enable the student to visualize internal structures in the living. Matters of clinical importance when mentioned in the text are highlighted.

A brand new feature of this edition is the presentation of one or more clinical application notes at the end of each chapter. Some of these notes focus attention on the anatomical basis of commonly used physical diagnostic tests such as the corneal and gag reflex. Others deal with the underlying anatomy of clinical conditions such as stroke, otitis media, and radiculopathy. Clinical anatomy of common procedures, such as tracheostomy, are described. Many clinical application notes are in a Q&A format that challenges the student to brainstorm the material covered in the chapter. Multiple-choice questions on each section are included at the end to help students assess their preparedness for the university examination.

It is hoped that this new edition respects the legacy of *Cunningham's* in producing a text and manual that is accurate, student friendly, comprehensive, and interesting, and that it will serve the community of students who are beginning their career in medicine to gain knowledge and appreciation of the anatomy of the human body.

Dr Rachel Koshi

Contributors

Dr J Suganthy, Professor of Anatomy, Christian Medical College, Vellore, India.
Dr Suganthy wrote the MCQs, reviewed manuscripts, and provided help and advice with the artwork.

Dr Aparna Irodi, Professor of Radiology, Christian Medical College and Hospital, Vellore, India.
Dr Irodi kindly researched, identified, and explained the radiology images.

Dr Ivan James Prithishkumar, Professor of Anatomy, Christian Medical College, Vellore, India.
Dr Prithishkumar wrote some of the clinical applications and reviewed the text as a critical reader.

Dr Tripti Meriel Jacob, Associate Professor of Anatomy, Christian Medical College, Vellore, India.
Dr Jacob wrote some of the clinical applications and reviewed the text as a critical reader.

viii

Acknowledgements

Dr Koshi would like to thank the following:

Radiology Department, Christian Medical College, Vellore, India.
The Radiology Department kindly provided the radiology images.

Ms Geraldine Jeffers, Senior Commissioning Editor, and **Karen Moore**, Senior Production Editor, and the wonderful editorial team of Oxford University Press for their assistance.

Reviewers

Oxford University Press would like to thank all those who read draft materials and provided valuable feedback during the writing process:

Dr TS Roy MD, PhD, Professor and Head, Department of Anatomy, All India Institute of Medical Sciences, New Delhi 110029, India.

Dr S Basu Ray, MBBS, MD, NDNB, MNAMS, Professor, Department of Anatomy, All India Institute of Medical Sciences, New Delhi 110029, India.

Dr Sabita Mishra, Professor, Director and Head, Department of Anatomy, Maulana Azad Medical College, New Delhi, India.

Dr Tony George Jacob, MD, DNB, PhD, Assistant Professor, Department of Anatomy, All India Institute of Medical Sciences, New Delhi 110029, India.

Dr CS Ramesh Babu, Associate Professor of Anatomy, Department of Anatomy, Muzaffarnagar Medical College, Muzaffarnagar, India.

Dr Neerja Rani, Assistant Professor, Department of Anatomy, All India Institute of Medical Sciences, New Delhi 110029, India.

Contents

PART 1

Head and neck

CHAPTER 1
Introduction to the head and neck

The section on head and neck deals with the bones, cavities, organs, muscles, vessels, and nerves of the head and neck. It does not include the study of the brain, which is dealt with in a separate section devoted to the brain and spinal cord.

The head and neck section begins with a description of the bones of the region—the cervical vertebrae and skull. The dissectors should study these bones and the bony prominences in the living, as a preliminary to the dissection of the head and neck.

The next few chapters (the scalp and face, anterior triangle, posterior triangle, and back of the neck) complete the superficial dissection of the head and neck. The cranial cavity and deeper structures of the head and neck (the orbit, ear, oral cavity, nasal cavity, pharynx, and larynx) are then dissected and described. The joints of the neck and contents of the vertebral canal are discussed last.

CHAPTER 2
The cervical vertebrae

Introduction

The following brief account of the cervical vertebrae should be studied together with the vertebrae, so that the details mentioned can be confirmed.

There are seven cervical vertebrae [Fig. 2.1]. The third to the sixth are typical. The first and second are modified to permit movements of the head on the neck. The seventh shows some features of a thoracic vertebra. All seven cervical vertebrae have a foramen—the **foramen transversarium**—in the transverse process.

Review the features of a typical vertebra as described in Vol. 2, Chapter 1. The bodies of the cervical vertebrae are smaller and more delicate than those in the thoracic and lumbar regions, as they carry less weight. But they have a larger vertebral foramen to accommodate the cervical swelling of the spinal cord [Fig. 2.2]. In the following descriptions, individual cervical vertebrae are identified as C. 1, C. 2, C. 3, etc., with C. 1 being the first cervical vertebra.

The typical cervical vertebrae

The body of the cervical vertebra is oval in shape, with its long axis transverse [Fig. 2.2]. The superior surface is concave from side to side, and the lateral margins project upwards to articulate with the cutaway inferolateral margins of the body above. The pedicles are short and are directed laterally and backwards from the middle of the posterolateral parts of

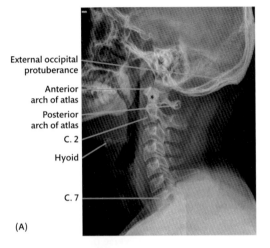

External occipital protuberance
Anterior arch of atlas
Posterior arch of atlas
C. 2
Hyoid
C. 7

(A)

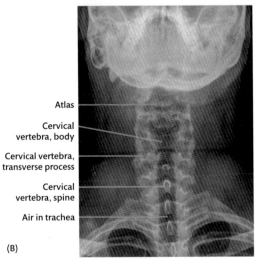

Atlas
Cervical vertebra, body
Cervical vertebra, transverse process
Cervical vertebra, spine
Air in trachea

(B)

Fig. 2.1 (A) Lateral radiograph and (B) anteroposterior (AP) view of the neck. C. 2, C. 7 = second and seventh cervical vertebrae, respectively. * = dens.

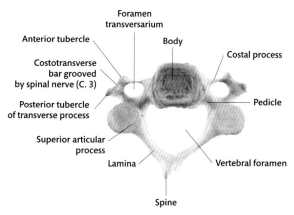

Fig. 2.2 The third cervical vertebra, superior surface.

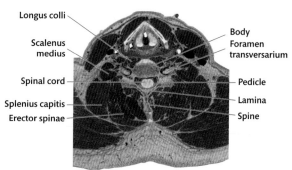

Fig. 2.4 Cervical vertebra, spinal cord, and surrounding muscles seen in a transverse section of the neck.

Image courtesy of the Visible Human Project of the US National Library of Medicine.

the body. They form the posteromedial wall of the foramen transversarium. The laminae are long and rectangular, and almost overlap the adjacent vertebrae in extension. The spines are short and bifid.

The superior and inferior articular processes are short bars of bone at the junction of the pedicle and lamina on each side [Fig. 2.3]. The superior and inferior aspects of the process are obliquely cut to form the articular facets. The superior facets face upwards and backwards, and the inferior facets face downwards and forwards.

The vertebral foramen is large and triangular in shape [Fig. 2.2]. Each transverse process is short and perforated by the foramen transversarium. Anterior to the foramen is a bar of bone—the **costal process**—which projects laterally from the body to the end of the anterior tubercle. The costal process corresponds to the rib and gives attachment to two muscles—the scalenus anterior and longus capitis. Behind the foramen, the true transverse process projects laterally from the junction of the

pedicle and lamina. It ends in the posterior tubercle. This tubercle gives attachment to the scalenus medius and other muscles. A bar of bone—the **costotransverse bar**—unites the anterior and posterior tubercles and completes the foramen transversarium. It is concave superiorly and has the ventral ramus of the corresponding spinal nerve lying on it. The foramen transversarium transmits the vertebral artery (C. 1–C. 6 only), vertebral veins, and sympathetic plexus. Fig. 2.4 is a section through the neck showing the cervical vertebra.

The atypical cervical vertebrae

C. 1 (atlas)

The first cervical vertebra has no body and consists only of two **lateral masses** united by an **anterior** and a **posterior arch** [Fig. 2.5]. (The body

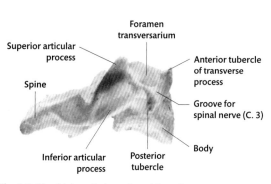

Fig. 2.3 The third cervical vertebra, right surface.

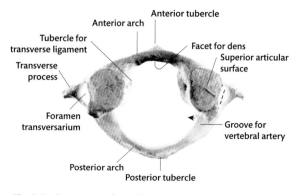

Fig. 2.5 The upper surface of the atlas. The course of the vertebral artery is indicated by a broken line.

of C. 1 is represented by a tooth-like projection from the superior surface of the body of C. 2—the dens.) Each lateral mass has a long, stout transverse process projecting laterally from it. The posterior arch is grooved on its superior surface, behind the lateral mass, by the vertebral artery and the first cervical ventral ramus. The **posterior tubercle** on the posterior arch represents the spine. The superior and inferior **articular facets** lie on the lateral masses anterior to the first and second cervical nerves, respectively. The superior facet is concave and kidney-shaped for articulation with the occipital condyles. The inferior facet is almost circular and slightly concave, and faces downwards and medially. It articulates with the axis. An inward projection from each lateral mass gives attachment to the **transverse ligament of the atlas** which divides the vertebral foramen into a small anterior compartment for the dens, and a larger, oval posterior compartment for the spinal cord and its coverings. The **transverse process** of the atlas is long and thick, and lacks an anterior tubercle. Its **foramen transversarium** is lateral to those of the vertebrae below.

C. 2 (the axis)

The salient feature of the second cervical vertebra is the **dens** [Fig. 2.6]. The dens articulates with, and is held against, the anterior arch of the atlas by the transverse ligament of the atlas. The transverse ligament grooves the posterior surface of the dens.

The thick **pedicle** projects posterolaterally from the side of the body. The **superior articular facet** covers the pedicle, part of the body, and part of the foramen transversarium. It is flatter than the inferior facet of C. 1, with which it articulates. The inferior facet of the axis is typical.

The **laminae** of the axis are thickened for muscle attachments and unite to form a massive **spine**. The transverse process has no anterior tubercle. The **foramen transversarium** turns laterally through 90 degrees under the superior articular facet, so that it is visible from the lateral aspect.

C. 7

The **spine** of the seventh cervical vertebra is long and non-bifid. The **transverse process** does not have an anterior tubercle, and the **foramen transversarium** transmits only veins (not the vertebral artery).

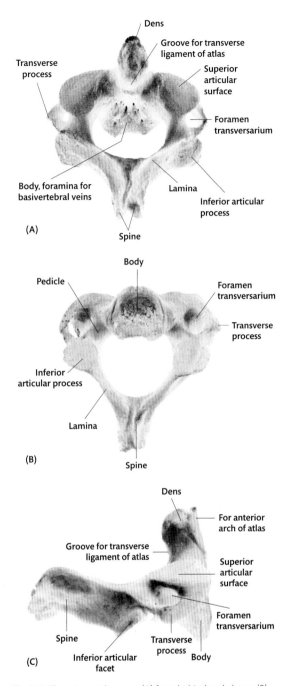

Fig. 2.6 The axis vertebra seen (A) from behind and above, (B) from below, and (C) from the right side.

Surface projections of cervical vertebrae

The **spine of the axis** is palpable at the nape of the neck about 5 cm below the external occipital protuberance.

The **spine of C. 7** (vertebra prominens) is the prominence felt at the root of the neck in the midline.

The **transverse process of C. 1** is palpable through the anterior border of the sternocleidomas-toid immediately below the tip of the mastoid process.

See Clinical Application 2.1 for the practical implications of the anatomy discussed in this chapter.

CLINICAL APPLICATION 2.1 Fracture of cervical vertebrae

A 23-year-old biker sustained severe injuries on the face and multiple injuries to the body in a road traffic accident. He was semi-conscious, but completely unable to move both upper and lower limbs. On examination, he had pain and tenderness of the neck, with radiation of pain from the neck to the shoulder. He was carefully moved from the accident site by trained paramedics.

Study question 1: what diagnosis should you consider? (Answer: fracture of cervical vertebrae with compression of the spinal cord. Cervical vertebral injury usually occurs in high-velocity impact in road traffic accidents, sports, and bullet injury to cervical vertebrae.)

Study question 2: what measures should be undertaken while shifting the patient from the accident site? (Answer: fracture of cervical vertebrae can cause compression of the cervical spinal cord. Hence, the neck should be immobilized during transfer. X-rays or computerized tomography (CT) may need to be done to assess fracture of cervical vertebrae.)

Study question 3: what are the complications of cervical fracture? (Answer: fracture of cervical vertebrae can cause damage of the spinal cord, leading to spinal shock, quadriplegia, or even death.) Spinal shock is caused by a concussion injury to the spinal cord. It manifests as a transient flaccid quadriplegia, with complete loss of reflexes that slowly begin to recover after 24 hours. Recovery is usually complete in spinal shock. Quadriplegia is irreversible, partial, or complete loss of motor and sensory function involving all four limbs.

Study question 4: what is the cause for the radiating pain? (Answer: pain radiating from the neck to the shoulder indicates compression of nerve roots by fractured segments.)

Study question 5: how is cervical fracture treated? (Answer: mild compression fractures may be treated with just a cervical brace. More severe fractures may require surgery and traction.)

CHAPTER 3
The skull

General architecture of the skull

The skeleton of the head is the skull. It is formed by a number of separate bones, almost all of which meet each other at linear fibrous joints—the sutures. Sutures are narrow gaps between adjacent bones, filled with dense fibrous tissue in early life. Bony fusion across the fibrous tissue begins after 30 years of age. The mandible (bone of the lower jaw) articulates with the skull at a synovial joint—the temporomandibular joint—the only movable joint in the skull. The skull without the mandible is the **cranium**. For descriptive purposes, the cranium is divided into the neurocranium and viscerocranium. The neurocranium surrounds the brain and its coverings (meninges) and increases in depth from anterior to posterior. The viscerocranium is the facial skeleton and lies inferior to the shallow, anterior part of the neurocranium.

A number of bony foramina are present in the skull, especially at the base. These give passage to nerves and vessels entering and leaving the skull. You should note the positions of these foramina and relate it to the structures which pass through them as you proceed with the study of the head, neck, and brain.

External features of the skull

Frontal or anterior view of the skull

Examine the frontal or anterior aspect of the skull and identify the bones seen in this view. They are the frontal bone, ethmoid, lacrimal bone, maxilla, zygomatic bone, nasal bone, and mandible [Fig. 3.1A].

The bone of the forehead is the **frontal bone**. It consists of right and left halves which usually fuse together early in life. From the top of the head, the frontal bone curves antero-inferiorly to the superior margins of the orbits and the root of the nose. It also forms portions of the roof of the orbits (the sockets for the eyeballs), the roof of the nasal cavities, and the nasal septum between the two nasal cavities. The **frontal eminence** is the most prominent and convex part of the frontal bone.

The main elements of the facial skeleton are the right and left **maxillae**. The body of each maxilla lies below the orbit, lateral to the nasal cavity. It has the shape of a three-sided pyramid and contains the **maxillary air sinus**. The body has (1) an anterolateral or anterior surface; (2) a posterolateral or infratemporal surface; and (3) a superior or orbital surface. The base is directed medially and forms the lateral wall of the nasal cavity. The apex points laterally and is overlapped by the **zygomatic bone** (cheek bone). The anterior surface projects on the face; the posterolateral surface forms the anterior wall of the infratemporal fossa, and the superior surface forms the floor of the orbit.

The curved alveolar process of the maxilla projects down from the body of the maxilla and bears the sockets for the upper teeth. Medial to the orbit, the maxilla articulates directly with the frontal bone through the **frontal process of the maxilla**. This process forms the lower part of the medial margin of the orbit. It articulates anteriorly with the **nasal bone** and posteriorly with the **lacrimal bone**. The lacrimal bone articulates posteriorly with the orbital plate of the **ethmoid** to form the greater part of the **medial wall of the orbit**. [Further details of the bony orbit are described in Chapter 11.]

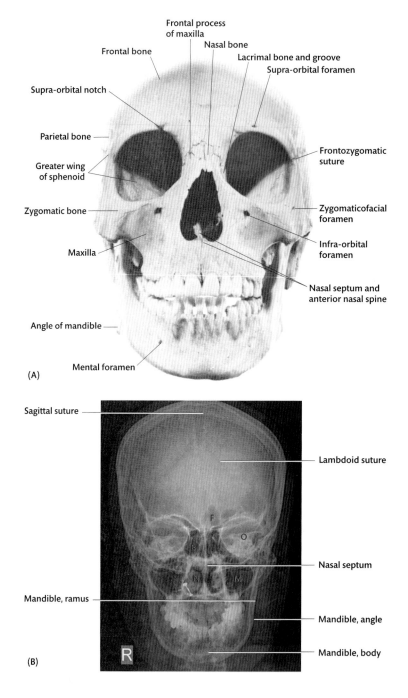

Frontal process
of maxilla
Nasal bone
Frontal bone
Lacrimal bone and groove
Supra-orbital foramen
Supra-orbital notch
Parietal bone
Frontozygomatic
suture
Greater wing
of sphenoid
Zygomatic bone
Zygomaticofacial
foramen
Infra-orbital
foramen
Maxilla
Nasal septum and
anterior nasal spine
Angle of mandible
Mental foramen

(A)

Sagittal suture

Lambdoid suture

Nasal septum

Mandible, ramus

Mandible, angle

Mandible, body

(B)

Fig. 3.1 (A) Anterior view of the skull. The alveolar bone has been worn away from the roots of the anterior teeth in the mandible. (B) Plain X-ray of the skull—anteroposterior view. E = ethmoid air sinus. F = frontal air sinus. M = maxillary air sinus. N = nasal cavity. O = orbit. (A nose pin is seen on the right side.)

The zygomatic bone forms the prominence of the cheek and articulates with the apex of the maxilla. The **frontal process** of the zygomatic bone extends upwards along the lateral margin of the orbit to meet the zygomatic process of the frontal bone. It forms the lateral wall of the orbit with the greater wing of the sphenoid bone. The zygomatic bone between the orbit and anterior surface of the maxilla forms the lateral half of the inferior orbital margin.

The anterior nasal aperture lies in the midline and is pear-shaped. The inferior and lateral margins of the aperture are formed by the maxilla. The superior margin is formed by the two nasal bones, which articulate with each other in the midline. The bony nasal septum seen between the two nasal cavities is formed partly by the perpendicular plate of **ethmoid bone**. The ethmoid bone also forms parts of the lateral wall of the nasal cavities. Inferior to the nasal aperture, the two maxillae are firmly united in the median plane by the articulation of the alveolar processes.

The bone of the lower jaw is the **mandible**. Identify the horizontal **body** of the mandible which bears the alveolar sockets for the lower teeth. The lower border of the body extends laterally to the **angle** of the mandible. The two halves of the mandible are fused together in the adult at the **symphysis menti**. The **mental foramen** lies about 4 cm lateral to the midline between the alveolar border and the lower border of the mandible. In the living, it is felt as a slight depression. Fig. 3.1B is a plain radiograph of the skull, anteroposterior view.

Superior view of the skull

The vault of the skull is formed by the frontal bone in front, the two parietal bones laterally, and the occipital bone at the back. The frontal bones have been described in the anterior view. The two **parietal bones** articulate anteriorly with the frontal bone at the **coronal suture**, and with each other in the midline at the **sagittal suture**. From the sagittal suture, the parietal bones arch downwards and laterally and form the greatest and widest part of the dome of the skull. Paired parietal foramina are seen on either side of the sagittal suture. Posteriorly, the parietal bones articulate with the **squamous part of the occipital bone**, at the **lambdoid suture**. The **parietal eminence** is the most convex and prominent part of the parietal bone [Fig. 3.2].

The meeting point of the coronal and sagittal sutures is the **bregma**. It represents the position of the **anterior fontanelle** in the infant. The meeting point of the sagittal and lambdoid sutures is the **lambda**. It represents the position of the **posterior fontanelle** in the infant [Fig. 3.2].

Posterior view of the skull

Most of the posterior aspect of the skull is made up of the parietal and occipital bones, with a small contribution from the temporal bone. The parietal

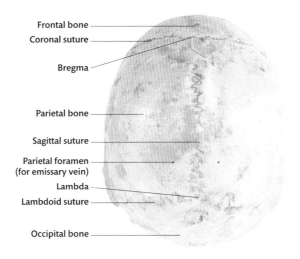

Fig. 3.2 Superior view of the skull.
© tarapong srichaiyos/ Shutterstock.com.

bones make up the superior and lateral aspects. The upper part of the squamous part of the occipital bone lies in the interval between the diverging posterior margins of the parietal bones. The posterior aspect of the mastoid process of the temporal bone is seen inferolaterally. In the lambdoid suture, small bones called sutural bones or wormian bones are often present [Fig. 3.3].

The **external occipital protuberance** is a midline projection seen at the lower part of the posterior view. On either side, bony linear elevations—the **superior nuchal lines**—extend laterally from the external occipital protuberance. Parallel and approximately 1 cm superior to the superior nuchal lines are faint bony ridges—the **highest nuchal lines**.

At the lower end, the lambdoid suture is continuous with the parietomastoid suture between the parietal bone and the mastoid process, and with the occipitomastoid suture between the occipital bone and the mastoid process [Figs. 3.3, 3.4A].

Lateral view of the skull

Start your study of the lateral view of the skull by identifying the parts of the frontal, parietal, occipital, maxilla, and zygomatic bones described in the anterior and superior views [Fig. 3.4A]. Review the zygomatico-frontal suture on the lateral wall of the orbit, and the coronal, lambdoid, parietomastoid, and occipitomastoid sutures.

The **temporal process** of the zygomatic bone forms the broad, anterior part of the **zygomatic**

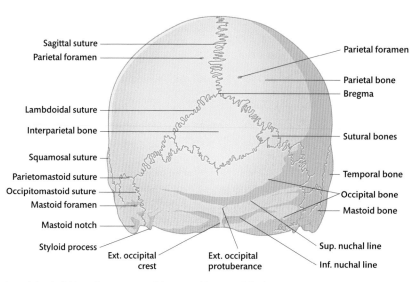

Sagittal suture
Parietal foramen
Lambdoidal suture
Interparietal bone
Squamosal suture
Parietomastoid suture
Occipitomastoid suture
Mastoid foramen
Mastoid notch
Styloid process
Ext. occipital crest
Ext. occipital protuberance

Parietal foramen
Parietal bone
Bregma
Sutural bones
Temporal bone
Occipital bone
Mastoid bone
Sup. nuchal line
Inf. nuchal line

Fig. 3.3 Posterior view of the skull. Note the presence of the sutural bone and the large interparietal bone.

arch lateral to, and below, the orbit. It joins the zygomatic process of the temporal bone to complete the arch.

The **greater wing of the sphenoid** forms the lateral wall of the skull behind the orbit. It articulates anteriorly with the frontal and zygomatic bones, superiorly with the frontal and parietal bones, and posteriorly with the squamous part of the temporal bone. The 'H'-shaped area where the frontal, parietal, temporal, and sphenoid bones meet is called the **pterion**.

Various parts of the **temporal** bone are seen on the lateral surface. The **squamous part of the temporal bone** lies below the inferior margin of the parietal bone. Anteriorly, it articulates with the greater wing of the sphenoid. Superiorly and posteriorly, it articulates with the parietal bone, at the **squamosal suture**. The **zygomatic process** of the temporal bone arises from the postero-inferior aspect of the squamous part. It turns forwards to join the temporal process of the zygomatic bone, to form the zygomatic arch. At the root of the zygomatic process of the temporal bone is the **tubercle**, which is immediately anterior to the head of the mandible when the mouth is shut, but above it when the mouth is open.

Below the root of the zygomatic process, the inferior surface of the squamous part has a large notch—the **mandibular fossa**—for articulation with the head of the mandible. Behind the mandibular fossa is the **tympanic part** of the temporal bone, which forms the anterior, inferior, and

lower part of the posterior wall of a bony canal—the **external acoustic meatus**. Anteriorly, the **tympanic part** of the temporal bone meets the squamous part in the posterior wall of the mandibular fossa at the **squamotympanic fissure**. Posteriorly, the tympanic part of the temporal bone fuses with the mastoid process. Also seen in this view is the **styloid process of the temporal bone**, projecting downwards and forwards from the base of the skull [Fig. 3.5].

The **supramastoid crest** is a blunt ridge which begins immediately above the external acoustic meatus and curves posterosuperiorly. It is continuous superiorly with the **superior** and **inferior temporal lines** which curve forwards, marking the upper limit of the temporal region. (The temporal fossa is limited above by the superior temporal line and below by the zygomatic arch [Fig. 3.4A].)

Below the zygomatic arch is the ramus of the mandible—a wide, flat plate of bone which extends superiorly from the posterior part of the body. It ends superiorly in the **condylar** and **coronoid processes** of the mandible. The condylar process projects upwards from the posterior margin of the ramus and forms the **neck** and **head** of the mandible [Fig. 3.4A]. Fig. 3.4B is a lateral radiograph of the skull.

Disarticulate the mandible to get a fuller appreciation of the lateral view of the cranium.

Behind the maxilla, two plates of bone—the **medial** and **lateral pterygoid plates** or

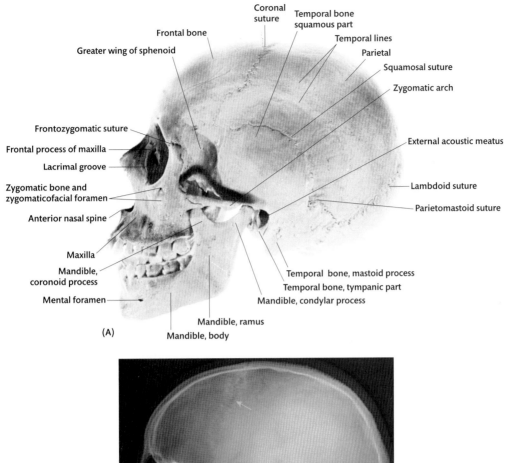

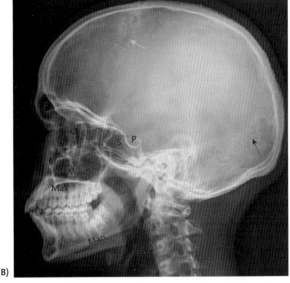

Fig. 3.4 (A) Lateral view of the skull. (B) Lateral radiograph of the skull. F = frontal sinus. M = maxillary sinus. Man = mandible. Max = maxilla. O = orbit. P = pituitary fossa. Ph = pharynx. S = sphenoid sinus. Yellow arrow = coronal suture. Red arrow = lambdoid suture.

laminae—extend downwards and forwards from the base of the sphenoid bone. Inferiorly, the anterior border of the pterygoid plates articulates with the maxilla. Superiorly, the two pterygoid laminae are separated from the maxilla by a narrow fissure—the **pterygomaxillary fissure**. The region lateral to the lateral pterygoid lamina is the **infratemporal fossa** [Fig. 3.5]. (The medial pterygoid plate is not seen in the lateral view.)

Inferior view of the skull

The inferior surface of the skull is described after disarticulating the mandible. It extends from the upper central incisors anteriorly to the external

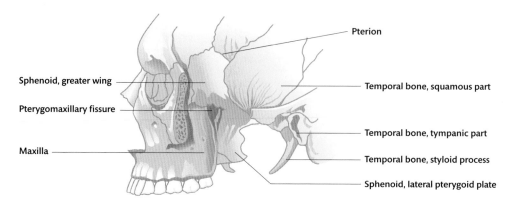

Pterion

Sphenoid, greater wing

Temporal bone, squamous part

Pterygomaxillary fissure

Maxilla

Temporal bone, tympanic part

Temporal bone, styloid process

Sphenoid, lateral pterygoid plate

Fig. 3.5 Lateral view of the cranium. (The mandible and zygomatic arch have been removed.)

occipital protuberance posteriorly. It is important to appreciate that the posterior two-thirds of the skull overlie, and are continuous with, the structures in the neck [Figs. 3.6, 3.7].

From the upper margins of the alveolar processes, the **palatine processes of the maxilla** extend horizontally inwards to meet in the midline. Posteriorly, the palatine processes of the maxilla articulate with the **horizontal plates of the palatine bone** to complete the hard palate. As such, the

anterior two-thirds of the bony palate are formed by the palatine processes of the maxillae, and the posterior one-third by the horizontal plates of the palatine bones. The hard palate separates the nasal cavities from the oral cavity. Lying lateral to the hard palate, and separated from it by the alveolar arch, are the maxillae and zygomatic bones.

Posterior to the hard palate, and close to the midline, is the **pharyngeal part** of the base of the skull. It is formed by the **body of the sphenoid**

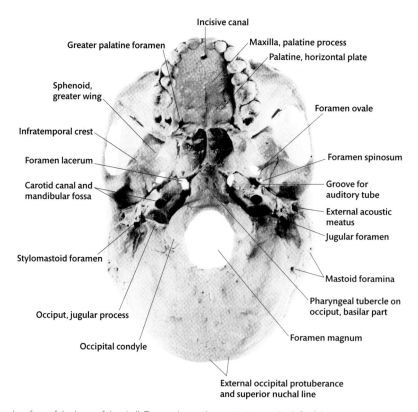

Incisive canal

Greater palatine foramen

Maxilla, palatine process

Palatine, horizontal plate

Sphenoid, greater wing

Foramen ovale

Infratemporal crest

Foramen lacerum

Foramen spinosum

Carotid canal and mandibular fossa

Groove for auditory tube

External acoustic meatus

Jugular foramen

Stylomastoid foramen

Mastoid foramina

Pharyngeal tubercle on occiput, basilar part

Occiput, jugular process

Occipital condyle

Foramen magnum

External occipital protuberance and superior nuchal line

Fig. 3.6 The external surface of the base of the skull. Two molar teeth are missing on the left of the picture, one and a half on the right.

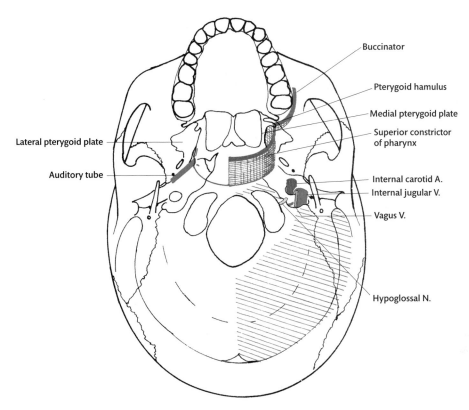

Fig. 3.7 External surface of the base of the skull to show the position of the superior constrictor, buccinator, and auditory tube.

(which is overlapped by the **vomer**) and the **basilar part of the occipital bone**. A small midline prominence on the basilar part of the occipital bone, 1 cm anterior to the foramen magnum, is the **pharyngeal tubercle**. About 1.5 cm from the midline, the two **pterygoid processes** descend from the body of the sphenoid. Each pterygoid process is formed by a **medial** and **lateral pterygoid plate**, which are fused together anteriorly, but separated from each other by the **pterygoid fossa** posteriorly. Inferiorly, the posterior margin of the medial pterygoid plate curves laterally as the **pterygoid hamulus** [Fig. 3.7].

Lateral to the lateral pterygoid plate lies the greater wing of the sphenoid. Traced laterally, this plate of bone turns sharply at the **infratemporal crest** to continue on the lateral surface of the skull. Laterally and posteriorly, the greater wing of the sphenoid articulates with the squamous and petrous parts of the temporal bone. The spine of the sphenoid is a small, sharp bony projection at the posterolateral angle of the greater wing.

A number of important foramina are seen in this region. On the greater wing of the sphenoid are the **foramen ovale** and **foramen spinosum**. The **foramen lacerum** lies at the apex of the petrous part of the temporal bone and is bounded by that bone, the basilar part of the occiput, and the body of the sphenoid. On the inferior aspect of the petrous part of the temporal bone is the **carotid canal**. The **stylomastoid foramen** lies between the styloid and mastoid processes of the temporal bone [Fig. 3.6]. The bony part of the auditory tube lies in the groove between the greater wing of the sphenoid and the petrous temporal bone [Fig. 3.7].

Between the infratemporal crest on the greater wing of the sphenoid and the lateral pterygoid lamina is the **infratemporal fossa**.

Posterior to the pharyngeal area on the base of the skull is the area for attachment to the pre- and post-vertebral muscles of the neck. Identify the large **foramen magnum** which lies in this region [Fig. 3.6]. The foramen magnum is oval and is longer than it is wide. The anterolateral margin of the foramen magnum has an oval, curved articular facet—the **occipital condyle**. The occipital condyles articulate with the superior articular facets of the first cervical vertebra—the atlas [see Fig. 2.5]. Lateral to the condyle is the jugular process of the occipital bone, which articulates with the temporal bone to form the **jugular foramen**. The jugular foramen lies immediately posterior to the carotid canal. The **hypoglossal canal** for the twelfth cranial nerve lies immediately above the occipital condyles.

Posterior to the foramen magnum, the greater part of the inferior surface of the cranium is formed by the occipital bone. This surface is roughened by the attachment of the muscles of the back of the neck. This area is divided transversely by an ill-defined **inferior nuchal line** and is limited posteriorly by the **external occipital protuberance** in the midline and the **superior nuchal line** which extends laterally from it [Fig. 3.6].

Internal features of the skull

Internal features of the vault

The cranial vault or calvaria is oval in shape. The internal surface is deeply concave and is made up of the squamous part of the frontal bone in front, the two parietal bones behind it, and the squamous part of the occipital bone behind. Note the coronal suture between the frontal and parietal bones, the sagittal suture between the two parietal bones, and the lambdoid suture between the occipital and parietal bones [Fig. 3.8].

Internal features of the base of the cranial cavity

The inferior aspect of the cranial cavity supports the brain. It is divided into three distinct fossae—the **anterior**, **middle**, and **posterior** cranial fossae [Fig. 3.9].

Anterior cranial fossa

The floor of the anterior cranial fossa is formed by the orbital plates of the frontal bone which project posteriorly above the orbit. They are separated from each other by the **cribriform plate** of the **ethmoid bone** which lie in the roof of the nasal cavities. In the midline, a bony ridge—the **crista galli**—projects upwards between the two anterior cranial fossae. A small foramen—the **foramen caecum**—lies anterior to the crista galli and transmits an emissary vein. Posteriorly, the anterior cranial fossa is formed by the body of the sphenoid in the midline, and the two lesser wings of the sphenoid laterally. The ethmoid and orbital plates of the frontal bone articulate with the sphenoid to complete the floor of the anterior cranial fossa.

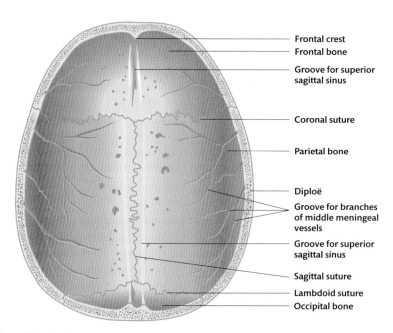

Fig. 3.8 Internal surface of the calvaria.

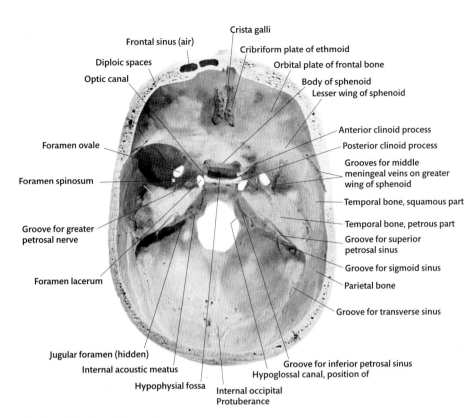

Crista galli
Frontal sinus (air)
Cribriform plate of ethmoid
Diploic spaces
Orbital plate of frontal bone
Optic canal
Body of sphenoid
Lesser wing of sphenoid
Anterior clinoid process
Foramen ovale
Posterior clinoid process
Grooves for middle
meningeal veins on greater
wing of sphenoid
Foramen spinosum
Temporal bone, squamous part
Temporal bone, petrous part
Groove for superior
petrosal sinus
Groove for greater
petrosal nerve
Groove for sigmoid sinus
Parietal bone
Foramen lacerum
Groove for transverse sinus
Jugular foramen (hidden)
Groove for inferior petrosal sinus
Internal acoustic meatus
Hypoglossal canal, position of
Hypophysial fossa
Internal occipital
Protuberance

Fig. 3.9 Internal surface of the base of the skull.

Each lesser wing of the sphenoid has a free curved posterior margin which forms the posterior limit of the anterior cranial fossa and ends medially in an **anterior clinoid process**. The anterior clinoid process lies immediately lateral to the optic canal. Laterally, the tip of each lesser wing fuses with the corresponding greater wing of the sphenoid bone. Between the greater and lesser wings of the sphenoid is the **superior orbital fissure**.

Middle cranial fossa

In the midline, the floor of the **middle cranial fossa** is narrow and formed by the **body of the sphenoid**. The central part of the body is hollowed out to form the **hypophysial fossa** which lodges the pituitary gland [Fig. 3.4B]. The hypophysial fossa is limited posteriorly by a rectangular plate of bone—the **dorsum sellae**. The superolateral corners of the dorsum sellae project upwards as the **posterior clinoid processes**. Anteriorly, the fossa is limited by the **tuberculum sellae**, with the horizontal **sulcus chiasmatis** in front of it. On each side, the sulcus leads into an **optic canal**, which transmits the corresponding optic nerve and ophthalmic artery.

The lateral part of the middle cranial fossa is made up mainly of the greater wing of the sphenoid. Each **greater wing** is roughly rectangular in shape and projects laterally from the body. The anterior part of the greater wing has an upturned portion which articulates superiorly with the lesser wing of the sphenoid and the inferior margins of the frontal and parietal bones. The **foramen rotundum** is present on the greater wing of the sphenoid, close to the body, near the medial end of the superior orbital fissure. More posteriorly are the **foramen ovale** and the **foramen spinosum**. The anterior surface of the **petrous part of the temporal bone** forms the posterior part of the floor of the middle cranial fossa.

The apex of the petrous temporal bone is directed towards the body of the sphenoid. The **foramen lacerum** lies between the apex of the petrous temporal bone and the body of the sphenoid [Fig. 3.9].

Posterior cranial fossa

The posterior cranial fossa is large and deep. In the midline, it is made up of the posterior surface of the dorsum sellae in front, followed by the posterior surface of the body of the sphenoid, the basilar part of the occipital bone, and the squamous part of the occipital bone. The **foramen magnum** separates the basilar and squamous parts of the occipital bone. The sloping cranial surface of the median parts of the sphenoid and occipital bones are together known as the **clivus**.

The lateral margin of the basilar part of the occipital bone is separated from the **petrous part of the temporal bone** by the **petro-occipital fissure**. The **jugular foramen** is a large opening situated at the posterior end of this petro-occipital suture. The **hypoglossal canal** lies medial to the jugular foramen, immediately above the anteromedial margin of the foramen magnum. The posterior surface of the petrous part of the temporal bone forms the anterior limit of the posterior cranial fossa laterally. The **internal acoustic meatus** is present on this surface. The medial surface of the **mastoid part of the temporal bone** forms the lateral wall of the posterior cranial fossa. The squamous part of the occipital bone forms a large part of the floor of the posterior cranial fossa. In the midline, a linear elevation—the internal occipital crest—extends backwards from the foramen magnum and ends in a bony prominence—the **internal occipital protuberance**. Extending laterally from the internal occipital prominence to the mastoid angle of the parietal bone is a groove for the transverse sinus. At the lateral end, the groove for the transverse sinus continues with the groove for the sigmoid sinus on the petrous temporal bone. Four shallow fossae are present—two below the groove for the transverse sinus, and two above it [Fig. 3.9].

See Clinical Applications 3.1 and 3.2 for the practical implications of the anatomy discussed in this chapter.

CLINICAL APPLICATION 3.1 Anterior fontanelle

The fontanelles are fibrous, membranous gaps between the bones of the vault of the cranium. They are present in the infant and are found at the four angles of the parietal bone where ossification is not yet complete. The anterior fontanelle is the largest. It is diamond-shaped and situated at the junction of the sagittal and coronal sutures. It usually closes by 18 months of age.

Palpation of the anterior fontanelle is an important clinical examination in the infant. A tense, bulging fontanelle may indicate raised intracranial pressures due to meningitis or obstruction to flow of cerebrospinal fluid (CSF). A sunken fontanelle is a sign of dehydration. Delayed closure of the anterior fontanelle commonly occurs in achondroplasia, rickets, and hypothyroidism.

CLINICAL APPLICATION 3.2 Fracture of mandible

A 24-year-old male presented with multiple facial lacerations, following a road traffic accident. Examination revealed severe pain and swelling of the lower jaw, intra-oral bleeding, and an inability to open the mouth. Examination revealed deformity of the lower jaw and loss of sensation over the lower lip.

Study question 1: what is the likely diagnosis? (Answer: fracture of the mandible.)

Study question 2: which are the common sites of fracture of the mandible? (Answer: the mandible is the most common facial bone to be fractured in facial trauma. The second is the maxilla. Common sites of fracture of the mandible include: the coronoid process and the body and angle of the mandible. Fractures involving the coronoid process cause swelling over the temporomandibular joint, severe limitation of mouth opening, and deviation of the jaw to the affected side on opening the mouth.)

Study question 3: why is there loss of sensation of the lower lip? (Answer: injury to the mental branch of the inferior alveolar nerve causes paraesthesiae or loss of sensation over the lower lip [Chapter 4].)

Study question 4: how are fractures of the mandible treated? (Answer: the aim of fracture reduction is functional alignment of bone fragments and restoration of normal occlusion. This can be achieved by reduction, followed by immobilization. Reduction and alignment of fractured segments can be done using surgical incisions of the oral mucosa (open reduction) or simple manipulation without any incision (closed reduction). Immobilization can be achieved with the help of plates and screws or wires.)

CHAPTER 4
The scalp and face

Introduction

We begin the study of the head with dissection of the scalp, including the temple, and the face. The chapter also includes the study of the lacrimal apparatus.

Surface anatomy

Begin by identifying the bony and soft tissue landmarks of the head by examining your own head and those of your partners.

Auricle

The external ear lies nearer the back of the head than the front and is at the level of the eye and nose. The main parts of the auricle or external ear—the lobule, helix, antihelix, tragus, antitragus, and intertragic notch—are shown in Fig. 4.1.

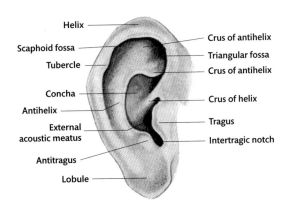

Helix
Scaphoid fossa
Tubercle
Concha
Antihelix
External acoustic meatus
Antitragus
Lobule

Crus of antihelix
Triangular fossa
Crus of antihelix
Crus of helix
Tragus
Intertragic notch

Fig. 4.1 The auricle.

Back and side of the head

The **external occipital** protuberance is the midline bony elevation felt where the back of the head joins the neck. From this protuberance, an indistinct, curved ridge—the **superior nuchal line**—extends laterally on each side between the scalp and the neck. The superior nuchal line passes towards the corresponding **mastoid process**—a rounded bony elevation behind the lower part of the auricle. Press your finger into the surface depression below and in front of the mastoid process. The resistance felt is the transverse process of the atlas. It is covered by the lower part of the parotid salivary gland, the anterior border of the sternocleidomastoid muscle, and the accessory nerve.

At the lateral end of the eyebrow, feel for the anterior end of the **temporal line**. The **parietal and frontal eminences** are the most convex parts of the parietal and frontal bones. The **vertex** is the topmost part of the head.

Face

External nose

The term 'nose' includes the paired nasal cavities which extend posteriorly from the nostrils to the pharynx. The mobile anterior part of the external nose consists of skin and cartilage. The rigid upper part—the bridge of the nose—is formed by the two **nasal bones** and the two **frontal processes of the maxillae** [see Fig. 3.1]. The skin is adherent to the cartilages but is mobile over the bones. The part of the nasal cavity immediately above each nostril is the **vestibule of the nose**. The vestibule is lined by hairy skin, and its lateral wall is expanded to form the **ala** of the nose.

Lips, cheeks, and teeth

The lips and cheeks are composed primarily of muscle and fat. They are covered on the external surface with skin, and lined on the internal surface with mucous membrane. The space that separates the lips and cheeks from the teeth and gums is the **vestibule of the mouth**. A full set of adult **teeth** consists of 32 teeth, 8 in each half of the jaw. From before backwards, these are: two incisors, one canine, two premolars, and three molars. There are 20 teeth in the primary dentition, i.e. five in each half of the jaw: two incisors, one canine, and two molars, also called 'milk' molars. The **oral fissure**, the gap or space between the lips, is opposite the biting edge of the upper teeth. The corner or angle of the mouth is opposite the first premolar tooth. The median groove on the external surface of the upper lip is the **philtrum**. In the midline, the internal surface of each lip is attached to the gum by a fold of mucous membrane—the **frenulum of the lip**.

Mandible

Identify the horizontal **body** of the mandible below the lower lip and cheeks. Follow the lower border of the mandible backwards to its **angle**. The wide, flat plate of bone which extends superiorly from the posterior part of the body is the **ramus** of the mandible. The ramus of the mandible is covered laterally by the masseter muscle, so that only its posterior border is felt easily. The condylar process projects upwards from the posterior margin of the ramus and forms the **neck** and **head** of the mandible. The neck lies immediately anterior to the lobule of the auricle; the head lies anterior to the tragus. Place your fingertip in front of your

own tragus, and open your mouth. The fingertip slips into a shallow depression created when the head of the mandible glides downwards and forwards. Note that the mouth cannot be closed while the finger remains in this fossa. The two halves of the mandible are united in the midline by the **symphysis menti**. The **mental foramen** is felt as a slight depression on the anterior surface of the mandible, about 4 cm from the midline, halfway between the edge of the gum and the lower border of the mandible [Fig. 4.2].

Zygomatic arch

Palpate the zygomatic arch which extends over the interval between the ear and the eye. The narrow posterior part is formed by the zygomatic process of the temporal bone, and the anterior part by the zygomatic bone [see Fig. 3.4].

Orbit

The bony structure of the orbit has been described in part in Chapter 3. Palpate the orbital margins on yourself, and find: (1) the **supra-orbital notch** on the highest point of the superior margin, about 2.5 cm from the midline; and (2) the **frontozygomatic suture** at the supero-lateral angle [see Figs. 3.1, 3.4].

Eyebrow

The hairy skin above the supra-orbital margin is the eyebrow. Over its medial end is a curved ridge of bone—the superciliary arch. This is well formed only in males and is separated from its fellow on the other side by a smooth median area—the **glabella**.

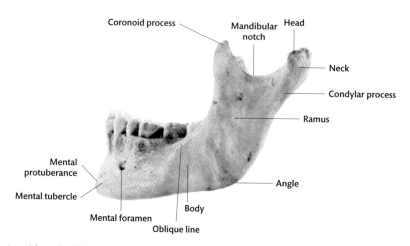

Fig. 4.2 Mandible viewed from the left side.

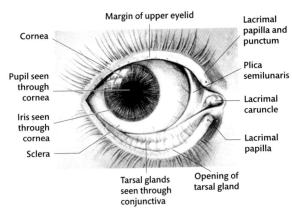

Cornea

Margin of upper eyelid

Lacrimal papilla and punctum

Plica semilunaris

Pupil seen through cornea

Iris seen through cornea

Sclera

Lacrimal caruncle

Lacrimal papilla

Tarsal glands seen through conjunctiva

Opening of tarsal gland

Fig. 4.3 Eyeball and eyelids. Eyelids are slightly everted to show part of the conjunctival sac.

Eye

The white of the eye is the **sclera**. The transparent part of the front of the eye is the **cornea**. The coloured **iris** (usually black or dark brown) is seen through the cornea and has a dark, circular central aperture—the **pupil**. The visible part of the sclera is covered with a moist, transparent membrane—the **conjunctiva**. The conjunctiva passes from the sclera on to the deep surface of the eyelids. The reflection of the conjunctiva on to the eyelids is the **fornix of the conjunctiva**, and the entire conjunctiva encloses the **conjunctival sac**. The sac opens anteriorly between the eyelids through the palpebral fissure [Fig. 4.3].

Eyelids

The eyelids or palpebrae are folds which protect the front of the eye. Each time we blink, the eyelids moisten the exposed surface of the eyeball by spreading lacrimal fluid over it. The upper lid is larger and more mobile than the lower one, and the upper conjunctival fornix is much deeper. When the eyes are closed, the **palpebral fissure** is nearly horizontal and lies opposite the lower margin of the cornea. When the eyes are open, the margins of the eyelids overlap the cornea slightly, the upper eyelid more than the lower.

At the medial angle of the eye is a small, triangular area known as the **lacus lacrimalis**, with a reddish elevation—the **lacrimal caruncle**—near its centre. The lacus carries a few fine hairs which filter the lacrimal fluid passing to the lacrimal canaliculi. Just lateral to the lacus is a small, vertical fold of conjunctiva—the **plica semilunaris** [Fig. 4.3].

The lower eyelid is easily everted by pulling down the skin below it, and the lower fornix is exposed by turning the eyeball upwards. The upper lid is difficult to evert because of the rigid **tarsal plate** buried in it. Once everted, the upper eyelid tends to remain so. Even with the upper eyelid everted, the deep superior fornix is not exposed.

Eyelashes (**cilia**) project from the anterior edge of the free margin of the eyelid. On the deep surface of the eyelids are a number of yellowish, parallel streaks produced by the tarsal glands [Fig. 4.3]. The ducts of these glands open near the posterior edge of the free margin of the eyelids. The free margin of the lids is rounded medially and has a small elevation—the **lacrimal papilla**. Each papilla is surmounted by a tiny aperture—the **lacrimal punctum**. The puncta lead into the lacrimal canaliculus which drains the lacrimal fluid from the conjunctival sac. Note that the puncta face posteriorly into the conjunctival sac, and that the eyelids move medially when the eye is forcibly closed. This action moves the lacrimal fluid towards the puncta at the medial angle of the eye.

Press a fingertip on the skin between the nose and the medial angle of the eye and feel the rounded, horizontal cord—the **medial palpebral ligament**. This ligament connects the upper and lower eyelids (and their muscle the orbicularis oculi) to the medial margin of the orbit. If the eyelids are gently pulled laterally, the medial palpebral ligament is more easily felt and may be seen as a small skin ridge.

Auricle

The auricle is that part of the ear which is seen on either side of the head [Fig. 4.1]. It consists of a thin plate of elastic cartilage covered with skin. (The lobule is devoid of cartilage.)

The cartilage of the auricle is continuous with the cartilage of the external acoustic meatus. The tubular **meatal cartilage** is incomplete above and in front, and its wall is completed by dense fibrous tissue which is continuous with tissue between the tragus and the beginning of the helix.

The muscles of the auricle are supplied by the facial nerve. The skin of the lower part of the auricle is supplied by the great auricular nerve. The upper part of the lateral surface is supplied by the auriculotemporal nerve, and the upper part of the medial surface by the lesser occipital nerve.

The scalp

The scalp extends from the eyebrows in front, to the superior nuchal lines behind. Side to side, it extends between the right and left superior temporal lines. The scalp covers the vault of the skull. It consists of five layers: (1) skin; (2) superficial fascia; (3) **epicranial aponeurosis**; (4) loose connective tissue; and (5) the pericranium [Fig. 4.4]. The epicranial aponeurosis is a flat aponeurotic sheet uniting the frontal and occipital bellies of the occipitofrontalis muscle. The superficial fascia is adherent to the epicranial aponeurosis. The skin is also adherent to the epicranial aponeurosis by dense strands of fibrous tissue which run through the superficial fascia and divide it into a number of separate pockets filled with fat. The blood vessels and nerves of the scalp lie in this superficial layer. Deep to the aponeurosis is a relatively avascular layer of loose areolar tissue which allows the scalp to slide freely on the **pericranium**. The pericranium is the periosteum on the external surface of the skull [Fig. 4.4].

The **temple** is the area bounded by the superior temporal line above and the zygomatic arch below. The skull is thin in this region and covered by the temporalis muscle, the temporal fascia, and a thin extension of the epicranial aponeurosis.

Using the instructions given in Dissection 4.1, dissect the scalp.

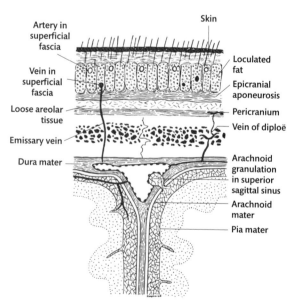

Fig. 4.4 Schematic section through the scalp, skull, meninges, and brain. Note the venous connections through the skull.

Labels: Artery in superficial fascia; Skin; Vein in superficial fascia; Loculated fat; Epicranial aponeurosis; Loose areolar tissue; Pericranium; Vein of diploë; Emissary vein; Dura mater; Arachnoid granulation in superior sagittal sinus; Arachnoid mater; Pia mater

Occipitofrontalis muscle

The occipitofrontalis has the occipital belly on the back of the skull, and the frontal belly anteriorly [Figs. 4.5, 4.8]. The occipital belly arises from the lateral part of the superior nuchal line [see Fig. 4.10]. The occipital bellies are shorter and narrower than the frontal bellies and are widely separated by the aponeurosis.

Each frontal belly lies in the forehead and adjoining part of the scalp. It has no attachment to bone but runs between the skin of the forehead and the epicranial aponeurosis. The medial parts of the frontal bellies lie close together and are attached to the skin of the nose. **Action**: when the frontal belly contracts, it raises the eyebrows and wrinkles the forehead and the skin of the nose. **Nerve supply**: the facial nerve.

Epicranial aponeurosis

The epicranial aponeurosis is attached loosely to the superior temporal lines and firmly to the superior nuchal lines. Between these attachments, it slides freely on the pericranium because of the loose connective tissue deep to it. ➲ Traction injuries of the scalp separate the epicranial aponeurosis from the pericranium. This leads to bleeding from the emissary veins which pass through the loose areolar tissue, and collection of blood in this tissue.

Nerves of the scalp and temple

General features of the nerves

The muscles of the scalp receive motor innervation from the **facial nerve** [Fig. 4.7]. Sensory innervation to the scalp comes from the **trigeminal nerve** and the second and third cervical spinal nerves [Figs. 4.7, 4.9]. Sympathetic innervation to blood vessels and the skin run in the plexuses on the arteries.

Sensory nerves of the scalp

The area behind the imaginary line from the auricle to the vertex is supplied by C. 2 and C. 3, through the large **greater occipital nerve** (C. 2), the **third occipital nerve** (C. 3), and branches of the **great auricular** and **lesser occipital nerves** [Fig. 4.9]. The greater occipital nerve enters the scalp with the occipital artery by piercing the trapezius and the deep fascia, 2.5 cm

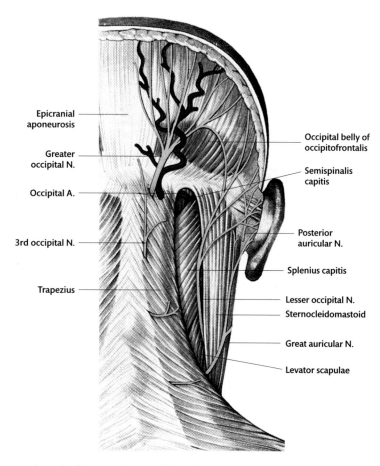

Fig. 4.5 Cutaneous nerves and vessels of the posterior part of the scalp.

DISSECTION 4.1 The scalp

Objectives

I. To reflect the skin of the scalp and trace the vessels and nerves supplying it. **II.** To expose the upper part of the orbicularis oculi and the frontal and occipital bellies of the occipitofrontalis.

Instructions

1. Place a block under the back of the head to raise it to a convenient angle. Make a median incision in the skin of the scalp, from the root of the nose to the external occipital protuberance. Make a coronal incision from the middle of the first incision to the root of each auricle.

2. Continue the coronal incision behind the auricle to the mastoid process, and in front of the auricle to the root of the zygomatic arch. Avoid cutting deep-er than the skin to preserve the vessels, nerves, and muscles in the subcutaneous tissue. Reflect the skin flaps superficial to these structures.

3. Make use of Figs. 4.5, 4.6, and 4.7 to identify the positions of the main structures in the scalp—the greater occipital nerve, lesser occipital nerve, third occipital nerve, great auricular nerve, superficial temporal artery, supra-orbital and supratrochlear arteries and nerves, and temporal branches of the facial nerve—so that they are not damaged.

4. Expose the upper part of the orbicularis oculi [Fig. 4.8].

5. Follow the frontal belly of the occipitofrontalis from below upwards [Fig. 4.8].

6. Find the branches of the supratrochlear and su-pra-orbital vessels and nerves. The supratrochlear vessels and nerve lie about a finger breadth from

the midline, and the supra-orbital another finger breadth further laterally. The supra-orbital nerves and vessels ascend from the supra-orbital notch.

7. Expose the anterior part of the epicranial aponeurosis, and note its extension downwards into the temple.

8. Find two or more **temporal branches of the facial nerve** which cross the zygomatic arch 2 cm or more in front of the auricle [Fig. 4.7]. Trace them upwards to the deep surface of the orbicularis oculi.

9. Find the **superficial temporal artery** [Fig. 4.6] and **veins** and the **auriculotemporal nerve**. These structures cross the root of the zygomatic arch, immediately anterior to the auricle, along with the small branch of the facial nerve to the superior auricular muscles. Trace these structures into the scalp, uncovering this part of the temporal fascia. (The auriculotemporal nerve may be very slender and difficult to find.)

10. Inferior and posterior to the auricle, find the great auricular and lesser occipital nerves [Fig. 4.5], and the posterior auricular vessels and nerve which lie

11. Look for small terminal branches of the **third occipital nerve** in the fascia over the external occipital protuberance [Fig. 4.5].

12. Cut through the dense superficial fascia over the superior nuchal line, 2.5 cm lateral to the external occipital protuberance, and find the occipital vessels and **greater occipital nerve** which pierce the deep fascia here. Trace them superiorly towards the vertex [Fig. 4.5].

13. Lateral to the greater occipital nerve, find the occipital belly of the occipitofrontalis, and expose the posterior part of the epicranial aponeurosis.

14. Make a small incision through the aponeurosis near the vertex. Introduce a blunt probe through it into the loose areolar tissue beneath the aponeurosis, and expose the extent of this tissue by moving the probe in all directions. Note that the aponeurosis is adherent to the periosteum near the temporal and nuchal lines.

immediately behind the root of the auricle. Trace the branches of these nerves.

lateral to the external occipital protuberance. The third occipital nerve pierces the trapezius, 2–3 cm inferior to this [Fig. 4.5]. Anterior to an imaginary line from the ear to the vertex, the sensory supply is from the trigeminal nerve.

The trigeminal nerve is the fifth cranial nerve, named so because it divides into three large nerves—ophthalmic, maxillary, and mandibular. Each of the three divisions supplies sensory branches to the skin of the anterior half of the scalp [Fig. 4.9].

The **ophthalmic nerve** gives rise to two cutaneous branches—the supratrochlear and supra-orbital nerves. The **supratrochlear nerve** emerges at the supra-orbital margin, a finger breadth from the midline. It supplies the paramedian part of the forehead and the medial part of the upper eyelid. The **supra-orbital nerve** emerges more laterally through the supra-orbital notch, supplies the upper eyelid, and then divides into lateral and medial branches. Each branch sends a twig through the bone to the mucous lining of the **frontal sinus** (the cavity in the frontal bone above the nose and orbit). The supratrochlear and supra-orbital nerves together supply the skin of the forehead and of the upper anterior part of the scalp as far as the vertex [Fig. 4.7].

The **maxillary nerve** gives rise to the slender **zygomaticotemporal nerve** which arises from the zygomatic branch of the maxillary nerve in the orbit. It pierces the zygomatic bone and temporal fascia to supply the skin of the anterior part of the temple [Fig. 4.7].

The **auriculotemporal** branch of the **mandibular nerve** emerges from the upper end of the parotid gland, close to the auricle, at the root at the zygomatic arch. It supplies the upper part of the auricle, the external acoustic meatus, and the skin of the side of the head [Fig. 4.7].

Motor nerves of the scalp

The **facial nerve** is the seventh cranial nerve. It supplies the muscles of the scalp and auricle.

The **temporal branches** of the facial nerve emerge from the upper part of the parotid gland, cross the zygomatic arch obliquely, and supply the frontal belly of the occipitofrontalis, the upper part of the orbicularis oculi, and the anterior and superior auricular muscles [Fig. 4.7].

The **posterior auricular nerve** arises from the facial nerve, as it emerges from the stylomastoid foramen. It curves posterosuperiorly below the root of the auricle and runs above the superior nuchal for the forehead which is supplied by the supra-orbital and supratrochlear branches of the internal carotid artery. These arteries run with the supra-orbital and supratrochlear nerves.

Branches from the external carotid artery

The **superficial temporal artery** is a large terminal branch of the external carotid artery. It begins behind the neck of the mandible in, or deep to, the parotid gland. It runs upwards with the auriculotemporal nerve and divides into anterior and posterior branches which run towards the frontal and parietal eminences. The anterior branch is frequently seen through the skin in elderly individuals and is often very tortuous.

Small branches of the superficial temporal artery supply the temple and anterior part of the scalp. The **transverse facial branch** [Fig. 4.6] runs forwards on the masseter muscle, below the zygomatic arch. The **middle temporal branch** crosses the root of the zygomatic arch, pierces the temporal fascia, and runs vertically upwards. The **zygomatico-orbital branch** runs anteriorly above the zygomatic arch between the two layers of the temporal fascia. It anastomoses with branches of the ophthalmic artery.

The small **posterior auricular branch** of the external carotid artery curves posterosuperiorly below and behind the root of the auricle, with the posterior auricular nerve.

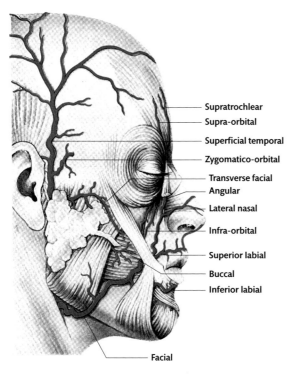

Supratrochlear
Supra-orbital
Superficial temporal
Zygomatico-orbital
Transverse facial
Angular
Lateral nasal
Infra-orbital
Superior labial
Buccal
Inferior labial
Facial

Fig. 4.6 The arteries of the face.

line to supply the occipital belly of the occipitofrontalis and the posterior and superior auricular muscles [Figs. 4.5, 4.7].

Arteries of the scalp and temple

The scalp and temple are mostly supplied by branches of the **external carotid artery**, except

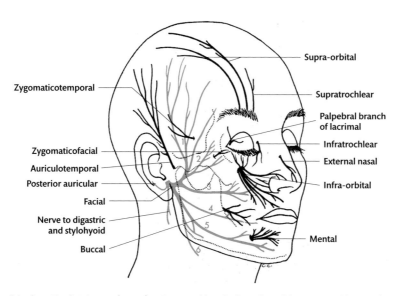

Zygomaticotemporal
Supra-orbital
Supratrochlear
Palpebral branch of lacrimal
Infratrochlear
External nasal
Zygomaticofacial
Auriculotemporal
Infra-orbital
Posterior auricular
Facial
Nerve to digastric and stylohyoid
Buccal
Mental

Fig. 4.7 The nerves of the face. The facial nerve (motor) is shown in blue, the branches of the trigeminal (sensory) in black. 1. Temporal branches of facial. 2 and 3. Zygomatic branches. 4. Buccal branch. 5. Marginal mandibular branch. 6. Cervical branch.

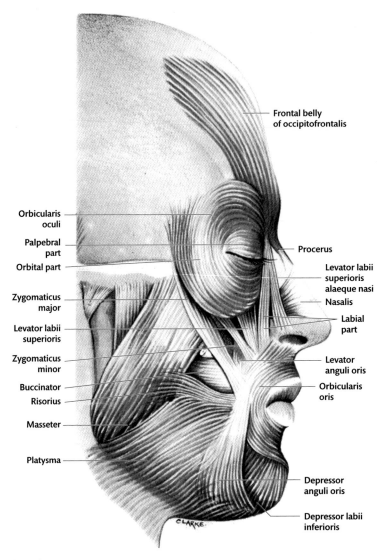

Frontal belly
of occipitofrontalis

Orbicularis
oculi

Palpebral
part

Orbital part

Zygomaticus
major

Levator labii
superioris

Zygomaticus
minor

Buccinator

Risorius

Masseter

Platysma

Procerus

Levator labii
superioris
alaeque nasi

Nasalis

Labial
part

Levator
anguli oris

Orbicularis
oris

Depressor
anguli oris

Depressor labii
inferioris

CLARKE.

Fig. 4.8 The facial muscles and masseter.

The **occipital artery** is a large branch of the external carotid artery. It arises deep to the angle of the mandible and runs posterosuperiorly. It pierces the trapezius with the greater occipital nerve [Fig. 4.5] and supplies the muscles of the neck and the back of the head.

The arteries of the scalp anastomose freely with each other and with those of the opposite side. ◑ As such, wounds of the scalp bleed profusely but heal rapidly. Also, if a large piece of scalp is torn downwards from the skull, it will survive and heal satisfactorily, provided a part of the peripheral attachment containing an artery is intact.

Veins of the scalp and temple

Like the arteries, the veins of the scalp anastomose freely. The main tributaries accompany the arteries

of the scalp, but their proximal parts drain by different routes.

The **supratrochlear** and **supra-orbital veins** unite at the medial angle of the eye to form the **facial vein**. They communicate with veins within the orbit. The **superficial temporal vein** joins the **middle temporal vein** at the root of the zygomatic arch to form the **retromandibular vein**. The **occipital veins** run with the artery in the scalp but leave it to join the suboccipital plexus, deep to the semispinalis capitis muscle at the back of the neck.

Emissary veins pierce the skull and connect the extracranial veins with the venous sinuses within the cranium. Usually one emissary vein passes through each parietal foramen to the superior sagittal sinus, and another through each mastoid

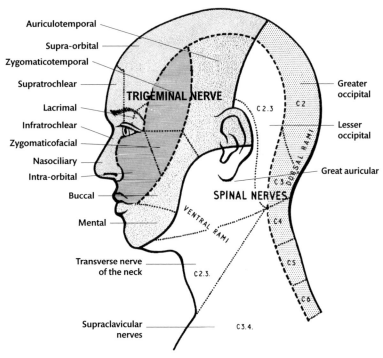

Fig. 4.9 Distribution of cutaneous nerves to the head and neck. The ophthalmic, maxillary, and mandibular divisions of the trigeminal nerve here are indicated by different shading.

foramen to the corresponding sigmoid sinus [see Fig. 3.6]. ⊃ These and other emissary veins, and the communications with the veins in the orbits, form routes along which infection may spread into the skull from the scalp.

Lymph vessels of the scalp and temple

Lymph vessels cannot be demonstrated by dissection. Lymph from the area in front of the ear drains into small **parotid lymph nodes** buried in the surface of the parotid gland. Those from the region behind the ear drain into lymph nodes on the upper end of the trapezius **(occipital nodes)** and the sternocleidomastoid **(retroauricular nodes)**.

Superficial dissection of the face

The face extends from the hairline on the scalp to the chin, and from one auricle to the other. (The forehead is common to the face and the scalp.)

Anterior to an imaginary line from the ear to the vertex, the sensory supply to the face is from the trigeminal nerve, except for the skin over the postero-inferior part of the jaw and the lower part of the auricle. The area over this part of the jaw

and auricle is supplied by the **great auricular** and **lesser occipital nerves** (ventral rami of C. 2 and C. 3 [Fig. 4.9]).

Dissection 4.2 provides instructions on dissection of the face.

Facial muscles

The facial muscles are known collectively as the 'muscles of facial expression'. They are the orbicularis oculi, orbicularis oris, frontal belly of the occipitofrontalis, zygomaticus major, zygomaticus minor, levator labii superioris, levator anguli oris, levator labii superioris alaeque nasi, depressor anguli oris, depressor labii inferioris, mentalis, nasalis, procerus, and risorius. Many of the muscles are named according to their actions, and the actions of others may be inferred from their positions. The muscles of facial expression take origin from the underlying bones [Figs. 4.10, 4.11] and are inserted into the skin of the face. These muscles, including the buccinator, are supplied by the facial nerve [Fig. 4.7].

Orbicularis oculi

The orbicularis oculi has three parts—the orbital part, palpebral part, and lacrimal part.

The scalp and face

Objectives

I. To identify the muscles of facial expression.   **II.** To identify and trace the vessels and nerves of the face.

Instructions

Before you begin, stretch the skin of the eyelids and cheeks by packing the conjunctival sacs and the vestibule of the mouth with cloth or cotton wool soaked in preservative. When the skin of the face is reflected, the attachments of the facial muscles to it are inevitably damaged. This can be minimized by keeping the knife as close to the skin as possible.

1. Make a median incision from the root of the nose to the point of the chin. Make a horizontal incision from the angle of the mouth to the posterior border of the mandible. Reflect the lower flap downwards to the lower border of the mandible, and the upper flap backwards to the auricle.

2. Expose the major facial muscles [Figs. 4.8, 4.10], taking care not to cut through them and damage major branches of the nerves and vessels.

3. Pull the eyelids laterally and identify the medial palpebral ligament; then expose the orbital part of the orbicularis oculi, subsequently following the palpebral part to the margins of the eyelids.

4. Attempt to find the small palpebral branch of the lacrimal nerve entering the lateral part of the upper eyelid through the orbicularis oculi.

5. The orbicularis oris is more difficult to expose because of the large number of facial muscles which fuse with, and help to form it [Fig. 4.8]. At the side of the nose, find the **levator labii superioris alaeque nasi**, with the facial vein lying on its surface.

6. Trace the **facial vein** downwards till it passes deep to the zygomaticus major. Expose that muscle, and then the levator labii superioris, following it upwards to its origin deep to the orbicularis oculi [Fig. 4.8].

7. At the lower border of the mandible, expose the broad, thin sheet of muscle—the **platysma**—which ascends over the mandible from the neck. Note that its posterior fibres curve forwards towards the angle of the mouth to form part of the **risorius muscle** [Fig. 4.8].

8. Find the depressor anguli oris and the depressor labii inferioris [Fig. 4.8].

(The buccinator muscle lies in a deeper plane immediately external to the mucous membrane of the cheek. It is continuous with the lateral part of the orbicularis oris and will be dissected later.)

Orbital part

The fibres of the orbital part arise from the medial palpebral ligament and the adjacent part of the orbital margin [Figs. 4.10, 4.11]. They form complete loops on and around the orbital margin. Muscle fibres sweep superiorly into the forehead (mingling with fibres of the frontalis), laterally into the temple, and inferiorly into the cheek, before returning to their point of origin. A few fibres which arise from the bone superior to the medial palpebral ligament end in the skin of the eyebrow, but the remainder are only loosely attached to the skin [Fig. 4.8].

Palpebral part

The palpebral part of the orbicularis oculi consists of thin fibres which arise from the medial palpebral ligament and form similar loops within the eyelids. They form a continuous layer with the orbital part. A small, partially isolated bundle of muscle fibres— the ciliary bundle—lies in the margin of the eyelid and runs posterior to the roots of the eyelashes.

Lacrimal part

The lacrimal part of the orbicularis oculi is a small sheet of muscle fibres which arises from the posterior margin of the fossa for the lacrimal sac and from the sac itself. It forms slips which pass laterally into the eyelids. **Actions**: a number of different actions are attributed to the orbicularis oculi. (1) The palpebral part, acting alone, closes the eye lightly, as in sleep or blinking. (2) The orbital part screws up the eye to give partial protection from bright light, sun, or wind. (3) The fibres passing to the eyebrows draw them together, as in frowning. (4) The orbital and palpebral parts contract together to close the eye forcibly, protecting it from a blow, and in strong expiratory efforts such as coughing, sneezing, or crying in a child. Tight closure of the eyes during strong expiratory movements prevents over-distension of the orbital veins by compressing the orbital contents. (5) The muscle draws the skin and eyelids medially towards the bony attachments and promotes the flow of

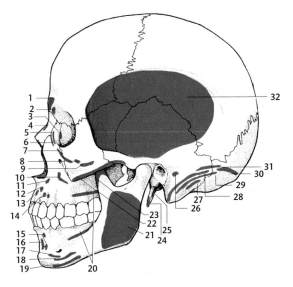

lacrimal fluid towards the lacrimal canaliculi. (6) The lacrimal part probably also dilates the lacrimal sac and promotes the flow of fluid through it. **Nerve supply**: facial nerve—temporal and zygomatic branches.

➲ Paralysis of the orbicularis oculi prevents the eye from being closed. This results in a number of clinical conditions: (1) the exposed cornea becoming dry, sore, and opaque; (2) the lower eyelid falls away from the eyeball, creating a space where tears collect and spill over onto the face; and (3) dirt entering the conjunctival sac is not moved to the caruncular filter and the sac rapidly becomes infected.

Orbicularis oris

The orbicularis oris is the sphincter muscle of the mouth. It is a complex muscle which forms the greater part of the lips. It is composed mainly of interlacing fibres of muscles which converge on the mouth. These muscles include the levator labii superioris, levator labii superioris alaeque nasi, levator anguli oris, zygomaticus major, zygomaticus minor, risorius, depressor labii inferioris, and depressor anguli oris [Fig. 4.12].

29

Fig. 4.10 Lateral view of the skull showing the muscle attachments. 1, 2, and 3. Orbicularis oculi. 4. Procerus. 5. Orbicularis oculi. 6. Levator labii superioris alaeque nasi. 7. Levator labii superioris. 8. Zygomaticus minor. 9. Zygomaticus major. 10. Levator anguli oris. 11 and 12. Nasalis. 13. Depressor septi. 14 and 15. Incisive Mm. 16. Mentalis. 17. Depressor labii inferioris. 18. Depressor anguli oris. 19. Platysma. 20. Buccinator. 21 and 22. Masseter. 23. Temporalis. 24. Styloglossus. 25. Stylohyoid. 26. Auricularis posterior. 27. Longissimus capitis. 28. Sternocleidomastoid. 29. Splenius capitis. 30. Trapezius. 31. Occipitalis. 32. Temporalis.

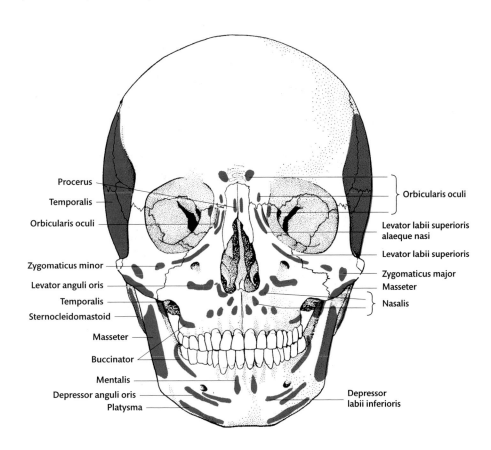

Fig. 4.11 Anterior view of the skull showing muscle attachments.

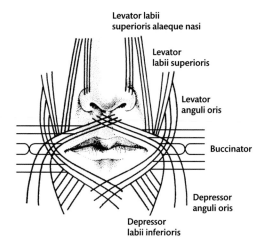

Levator labii
superioris alaeque nasi

Levator
labii superioris

Levator
anguli oris

Buccinator

Depressor
anguli oris

Depressor
labii inferioris

Fig. 4.12 Schematic diagram of the orbicularis oris muscle.

The fibres of the various muscles converging on the mouth mingle and sweep in curves through the lips. The **buccinator** [p. 33] passes horizontally forwards in the cheek [Figs. 4.8, 4.10, 4.11, 4.12]. Its middle fibres interlace near the corner of the mouth to form a marginal bundle and enter the lips. The upper and lower fibres enter the corresponding lip and interdigitate with fibres of the opposite muscle in the midline.

Actions: they confer a wide variety of movements on the lips. They elevate the upper lip, depress the lower lip, and evert or retract both the lips. They act as sphincters at the oral fissure. **Nerve supply**: facial nerve, upper and lower buccal branches.

➲ Paralysis of one-half of the orbicularis oris prevents proper closure of the mouth and affects movements of the lips on that side. Speech is slurred. Food and fluids collect in the vestibule or fall out of the mouth. The lips are pulled towards the normal side by the unopposed action of those muscles. When the patient attempts to blow against resistance, the cheek and lips are blown out and air escapes on the paralysed side.

Dissection 4.3 provides instructions on deep dissection of the vessels and nerves of the face.

DISSECTION 4.3 Vessels and nerves of the face

Objectives

I. To find and trace the facial artery and vein.   **II.** To find and trace the parotid duct.   **III.** To find and trace the branches of the facial nerve.   **IV.** To find and trace the infra-orbital and auriculotemporal nerves.

Instructions

1. Detach the risorius, and reflect it with the remains of the platysma towards the corner of the mouth. Avoid injury to the underlying vessels and nerves.

2. Find the cut end of the great auricular nerve, and trace it upwards over the lower part of the parotid gland.

3. Expose the facial artery and vein at the antero-inferior angle of the masseter, but do not trace them further at the moment [Fig. 4.6].

4. Cut through the fascial covering of the **parotid gland** immediately in front of the auricle from the zygomatic arch to the angle of the mandible. Dissect the fascia carefully forwards to the margins of the gland, looking for the nerves, the vessels, and the duct of the gland which emerge at the anterior border.

5. The **parotid duct** appears at the anterior border of the parotid, about a finger breadth below the zygomatic arch. It is large [Fig. 4.6] and readily palpated in the living by rolling it against the anterior border of the tightened masseter.

6. Above the duct, find: (1) a small detached part of the parotid gland—the **accessory parotid**; (2) the transverse facial artery and vein [Fig. 4.6]; and (3) the zygomatic branches of the facial nerve [Fig. 4.7].

7. Find the **branches of the facial nerve** emerging from the anterior border of the parotid gland, and trace them forwards. This is difficult because they communicate with each other and with the branches of the trigeminal nerve in the face. (The facial nerve is motor to the muscles of the face; the trigeminal nerve is sensory.)

8. Identify the muscles of facial expression: the zygomaticus major, zygomaticus minor, levator labii superioris, and depressor anguli oris.

9. Follow the upper zygomatic branches of the facial nerve. They pass deep to the lateral part of the orbicularis oculi. At this point, the **zygomaticofacial nerve** (sensory) may be found emerging from the zygomatic bone.

10. Trace the lower zygomatic branches of the facial nerve forward, inferior to the orbit and deep to the

zygomatic muscles. Find their communications with the **infra-orbital nerve** (sensory).

11. Trace the branches of the infra-orbital nerve.

12. Cut through the zygomaticus major and minor and levator labii superioris at their origins, and turn them downwards to expose the facial artery and vein. Trace these vessels and their branches.

13. Find the **buccal branch of the facial nerve** at the anterior border of the parotid gland. Trace it forwards through the fat of the cheek to the buccinator muscle.

14. Attempt to find the communications between the buccal branch of the facial nerve and the buccal (sensory) branch of the trigeminal nerve. Follow the buccal branch of the trigeminal nerve posteriorly, till it disappears deep to the ramus of the mandible.

15. Trace the marginal mandibular branch of the facial nerve forwards from the lower border of the parotid gland to the depressor anguli oris. Cut through the depressor anguli oris, and trace the communication of the nerve with the **mental nerve** (sensory) which emerges through the mental foramen. Follow the branches of the mental nerve to the chin and lower lip.

16. At the upper border of the parotid gland, identify: (1) the superficial temporal artery and veins; (2) the **auriculotemporal nerve** close to the auricle; and (3) the temporal branches of the facial nerve anterior to the vessels.

17. At the lower border of the gland, identify again: (1) the anterior and posterior branches of the retro-mandibular vein; and (2) the cervical branch of the facial nerve.

18. Trace the facial vein downwards, till it joins the anterior branch of the retromandibular vein [see Fig. 5.4].

Arteries of the face

The face has a rich arterial supply. The facial and transverse facial arteries anastomose freely with the smaller arteries which accompany the branches of the trigeminal nerve into the face, and with the arteries of the opposite side, especially in the lips. ➲ As such, wounds of the face bleed a lot but also heal rapidly.

Transverse facial artery

The transverse facial artery arises from the superficial temporal artery under cover of the parotid gland. It emerges near the upper end of the gland and runs forwards over the masseter below the zygomatic arch [Fig. 4.6].

Facial artery

The facial artery is a branch of the external carotid artery. It is the main artery of the face. It enters the face by turning around the lower border of the mandible and piercing the deep fascia at the antero-inferior angle of masseter. (It can be palpated against the mandible at this point.) It runs antero-superiorly to a point 1.5 cm lateral to the angle of the mouth, and then ascends more vertically to end near the medial angle of the eye [Fig. 4.6]. It has a sinuous course on the face.

The facial artery gives large branches to the chin, lips (**inferior labial** and **superior labial**), and nose (**lateral nasal**), and smaller branches to the adjacent muscles. An important anastomosis is present at the medial angle of the eye between the facial vessels and those of the orbit. Through this arterial anastomosis, blood from the external carotid artery can reach the internal carotid artery in the skull. Similarly, venous blood from the face can drain into the orbit and skull.

Veins of the face

The face is drained by veins that accompany the arteries that supply it. The veins of the face anastomose freely with each other.

Facial vein

The facial vein is formed by the union of the supra-orbital and supratrochlear veins at the medial angle of the eye. The initial segment of the vein (near the angle of the eye) is also known as the **angular vein**. It runs postero-inferiorly, behind and in the same plane as the artery, but takes a straighter course, close to the anterior border of the masseter. It lies close to the artery again on the surface of the mandible. The vein then descends into the neck, pierces the deep fascia, and receives the anterior branch of the retromandibular vein. In the neck, it crosses the carotid arteries and drains into the internal jugular vein.

The facial vein receives tributaries which correspond to the branches of the facial artery. On the surface of the buccinator, it gives off the **deep facial vein**, which passes medial to the masseter to join the **pterygoid plexus of veins**.

Nerves of the face

Sensory nerves of the face

The great auricular nerve and trigeminal nerve supply sensory innervation to the face [Fig. 4.9]. The trigeminal nerve is the main sensory nerve of the face. It gives rise to three nerves—ophthalmic, maxillary, and mandibular—each of which supplies cutaneous branches to one of three roughly concentric areas of the face [Figs. 4.7, 4.9]. The trigeminal cutaneous area abuts on that supplied by the ventral and dorsal rami of the second cervical nerve. The first cervical nerve does not supply skin.

Great auricular nerve

The skin over the parotid gland and the angle of the mandible are supplied by the **great auricular nerve** (ventral rami of C. 2, C. 3) [Fig. 4.9].

Ophthalmic nerve

The ophthalmic division of the trigeminal nerve supplies the area of skin between the angle of the eye and the vertex of the head [Figs. 4.7, 4.9] through the lacrimal, frontal, and nasociliary branches. These branches pass through the orbit and give rise to five nerves on the face.

1. The **palpebral branch of the lacrimal** nerve supplies the lateral part of the upper eyelid.
2 and 3. The **supra-orbital** and **supratrochlear** branches of the frontal nerve supply the forehead and anterior scalp.
3. The **infratrochlear** branch of the nasociliary nerve supplies the medial parts of the eyelids and the root of the nose.
4. The **external nasal** nerve emerges between the nasal bone and the lateral nasal cartilage [see Fig. 4.16] and supplies the skin of the lower half of the dorsum of the nose. It is a branch of the **anterior ethmoidal nerve** which arises from the nasocili-

ary nerve in the orbit, and enters the nasal cavity through the cribriform plate of the ethmoid.

Maxillary nerve

The maxillary division of the trigeminal nerve supplies an area of skin inferior and lateral to the eye by three branches [Figs. 4.7, 4.9].

1. The **infra-orbital nerve** emerges from the infra-orbital foramen under cover of the orbicularis oculi and levator labii superioris. It gives the **labial**, **palpebral**, and **nasal branches** which supply the skin and mucous membrane of the upper lip, the lower eyelid, the skin between them, and the skin on the side of the nose. These nerves form a **plexus** with the zygomatic branches of the facial nerve. Such plexuses are not the site of union of nerve fibres, but merely places where the nerve fibres run together, so that sensory nerves from the muscles of the face can enter the trigeminal nerve.
2. The **zygomaticofacial nerve** supplies the skin over the bony part of the cheek. It passes from the orbit through the zygomatic bone on to its facial surface [Fig. 4.7].
3. The **zygomaticotemporal nerve** also pierces the zygomatic bone and emerges from its temporal surface. It passes through the temporal fascia and supplies the skin over the anterior part of the temple.

Mandibular nerve

The mandibular division of the trigeminal nerve supplies an area of skin posterior and inferior to the previous areas, by three branches [Figs. 4.7, 4.9].

1. The **auriculotemporal nerve** emerges from the upper border of the parotid gland beside the auricle. It supplies the upper part of the auricle, the external acoustic meatus, and the skin of the side of the head [Fig. 4.7].
2. The **buccal nerve** passes antero-inferiorly, deep to the masseter and the ramus of the mandible. It supplies the skin over the buccinator and sends branches through it to the mucosa of the mouth [Fig. 4.7].
3. The **mental nerve** is a branch of the inferior alveolar nerve. It appears on the face through the mental foramen of the mandible. It divides into branches deep to the depressor anguli oris. These branches supply the skin and mucous membrane of the lower lip, and the skin over the mandible from the symphysis to the anterior border of the masseter [Fig. 4.7].

Motor nerves of the face

The facial nerve is the motor nerve to the muscles of facial expression. It has five terminal branches, or groups of branches—temporal, zygomatic, buccal, marginal mandibular, cervical—which emerge from the parotid gland [Fig. 4.7].

1. The **temporal branches** have been described in the scalp.
2. Small **zygomatic branches** run across the zygomatic arch to supply the orbicularis oculi. Larger branches run forwards below the arch to supply the muscles of the nose—the nasalis and levator labii superioris alaeque nasi—and those between the eye and the mouth—the zygomaticus major, zygomaticus minor, and levator labii superioris.
3. The **buccal** branches run towards the angle of the mouth and supply the muscles of the cheek—the buccinator.
4. The **marginal mandibular** branches run forwards along the mandible and usually curve down into the neck, before running with the inferior labial branch of the facial artery to supply the muscles of the lower lip—the depressor labii inferioris, depressor anguli oris, and mentalis.
5. The **cervical branch** leaves the lower border of the parotid gland and runs forwards and downwards into the neck, to supply the platysma and communicate with the transverse nerve of the neck [Fig. 4.7].

Dissection 4.4 provides instructions on dissection of the buccinator.

DISSECTION 4.4 Buccinator

Objective

I. To expose and study the buccinator.

Instructions

1. Expose the levator anguli oris and the buccinator.
2. Remove the buccal fat from the buccinator, avoiding injury to the buccal nerve. Note the small buccal glands that lie in the fat.
3. Remove the fascia covering the buccinator. Define its attachments to the maxilla and mandible, and trace its fibres towards the angle of the mouth.

The bulk of the cheek and lips is formed by muscles. The muscles are covered externally by skin, and internally by the mucous membrane of the mouth. In addition, the cheek and lips contain buccal and labial salivary glands, few lymph nodes, fascia enclosing the buccinator, and the buccal pad of fat.

Buccinator

The **buccinator** muscle is made up of horizontal fibres which take origin from the outer surfaces of the maxilla and mandible opposite the sockets of the molar teeth, and the **pterygomandibular raphe** [Fig. 4.10]. The pterygomandibular raphe is formed by the interlacing tendinous fibres of the buccinator and the superior constrictor muscle of the pharynx where these muscles meet edge to edge [Fig. 4.8; see also Fig. 6.5]. (The superior constrictor will be seen later when the pharynx is dissected.)

Anteriorly, fibres of the buccinator converge on the corner of the mouth and blend with the orbicularis oris to form a large part of it [Fig. 4.12]. The upper and lower fibres pass directly into the corresponding lips. But the middle fibres decussate (cross each other) near the angle of the mouth, so that the upper fibres enter the lower lip and vice versa. Some of the posterior fibres pass almost vertically downwards from the maxilla to the mandible.

Nerve supply: the buccal branch of the facial nerve. **Actions**: the buccinator is used during mastication to press the cheek against the teeth and prevent food from collecting in the vestibule of the mouth. It also compresses the blown-out cheek (as when blowing a balloon) and raises the intra-oral pressure [Fig. 4.8; see also Figs. 6.5, 17.6].

Buccopharyngeal fascia

The buccopharyngeal fascia covers the external surface of the buccinator and continues backwards over the constrictor muscles of the pharynx. The **parotid duct** pierces the buccopharyngeal fascia and the buccinator, and opens into the vestibule of the mouth, opposite the upper second molar tooth. The fascia and muscle are also pierced by the nerves and vessels of the mucous membrane.

Molar glands and buccal lymph nodes

Four to five small molar mucous salivary glands lie on the buccopharyngeal fascia around the parotid duct. Their ducts follow the parotid duct to the vestibule of the mouth. The buccal lymph nodes are found on the buccopharyngeal fascia.

Buccal pad of fat

An encapsulated mass of fat—the buccal pad of fat—lies on the buccopharyngeal fascia. It is traversed by the buccal nerve and the parotid duct. It adds bulk to the cheek to help to resist the external pressure during sucking. This pad is relatively large in infants when the cheeks are not supported by teeth, and accounts for the fullness of the cheeks in that age group.

Levator anguli oris

The levator anguli oris takes origin from the maxilla, just above the fossa overlying the root of the canine and below the infra-orbital foramen. The origin lies deep to the orbicularis oculi, the levator labii superioris, and the zygomatic muscles. It runs to the angle of the mouth and merges with the fibres of the orbicularis oris. It also sends some fibres into the lower lip [Figs. 4.8, 4.10, 4.11].

Mentalis

This small muscle arises from the outer wall of the canine socket of the mandible. Its slips converge to be inserted into the skin of the chin [Figs. 4.10, 4.11].

Labial and buccal glands

These are small, closely set mucous salivary glands that lie in the submucosa of the lips and cheek. They are palpable as small nodules when the tongue is pressed against them. Their ducts open into the vestibule of the mouth.

Eyelids

The eyelids or palpebrae consist of the following layers:

1. Skin and superficial fascia.
2. Orbicularis oculi.
3. Tarsi and palpebral fascia.
4. Conjunctiva [Fig. 4.13].

DISSECTION 4.5 Palpebral fascia and tarsi

Objective

I. To identify the medial palpebral ligament, palpebral fascia, and tarsal plates.

Instructions

1. Separate the palpebral part of the orbicularis oculi from the remainder of the muscle by a circular incision.

2. Turn the palpebral part towards the palpebral fissure. Avoid injury to the palpebral fascia, vessels, and nerves.

3. Deep to the muscles, identify the medial palpebral ligament at the medial angle of the eye, and the palpebral fascia and tarsi elsewhere.

The skin of the eyelids is very thin. The superficial fascia is thin, loose, and devoid of fat. It allows the skin to move freely over the lid and can become greatly swollen with fluid or blood after an injury.

Using the instructions given in Dissection 4.5, identify the palpebral fascia and tarsi.

Tarsal plates

The tarsal plates and the palpebral fascia together form a continuous layer of the eyelid known as the **orbital septum** [Figs. 4.13, 4.14].

The tarsi are two thin plates of condensed fibrous tissue in the eyelids. They stiffen the eyelids and extend up to the free margin. The **inferior tarsus** is narrow and is attached to the inferior orbital margin by the palpebral fascia. The **superior tarsus** is much larger and can be felt if the upper lid is pinched sideways between the finger and thumb. The deep surface is adherent to the palpebral conjunctiva. The palpebral fascia is attached to its anterior surface some distance below its upper border. The tendon of the **levator palpebrae superioris** (a muscle of the upper eyelid) is attached to the deep surface of the palpebral fascia and the superior tarsus [Figs. 4.13, 4.14]. The lower edge of the superior tarsus is adherent to the skin of the margin of the upper eyelid.

The **tarsal glands** lie in furrows on the deep surfaces of the tarsi. They appear as closely placed, parallel yellow streaks running at right angles to the margin of the lid. Their ducts open on the margin of the eyelid behind the eyelashes.

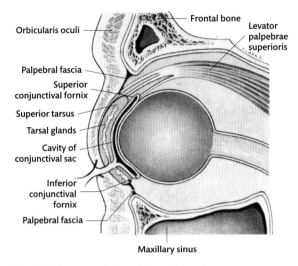

Fig. 4.13 Structure of the eyelids seen in section.

The **ciliary glands** are arranged in several rows immediately behind the roots of the eyelashes. Their ducts open on the margin close to the lashes. (They are too small to be seen by dissection.) ➲ When infected, they produce a red swelling of the margin of the eyelid known as a 'stye'.

The **palpebral fascia** is a thin fibrous membrane which connects the tarsi to the orbital margins. Medially, it passes posterior to the lacrimal sac to be attached to the bone. In the lower eyelid, it is attached to the inferior margin of the inferior tarsus. In the upper eyelid, it is attached to the anterior surface of the superior tarsus, close to the superior margin. The palpebral fascia is pierced by nerves and vessels which pass from the orbit to the exterior [Figs. 4.13, 4.14].

Palpebral ligaments

The **medial** palpebral ligament is a strong fibrous band that connects the superior and inferior tarsi with the medial margin of the orbit. It lies under the skin, anterior to the lacrimal sac, and gives origin to fibres of the orbicularis oculi [Fig. 4.14].

The **lateral** palpebral ligament is a slender fibrous band which lies posterior to the palpebral fascia and connects the lateral ends of the two tarsi to a small tubercle on the lateral orbital margin [Fig. 4.14].

Levator palpebrae superioris

The levator palpebrae superioris takes origin from the posterior part of the orbit. Anteriorly, it forms a tendon which expands into a wide, thin sheet, enters the upper eyelid and merges with the deep surface of the palpebral fascia. A few fibres of the tendon pass through the orbicularis oculi to be inserted into the skin, and others are attached to the front of the superior tarsus. Through a fascial sheath, the tendon is also attached to the superior fornix of the conjunctiva, which is raised with the eyelid by the levator [Fig. 4.13].

Vessels and nerves of eyelids

The **arteries** of the eyelids are derived from the ophthalmic artery. They pierce the palpebral fascia to enter the eyelids and anastomose with each other to form arches near the margins of the lids. These arterial arches lie between the tarsus and the orbicularis oculi.

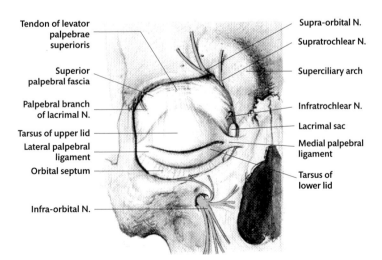

Fig. 4.14 Dissection of the right eyelid. The orbicularis oculi has been removed.

The **veins** of the eyelids run medially and end in the supratrochlear and facial veins.

The motor nerves to the orbicularis oculi come from the temporal and upper zygomatic branches of the facial nerve. The sensory supply to the upper lid is from the palpebral branch of the lacrimal nerve and branches of the supra-orbital, supratrochlear, and infratrochlear nerves. The lower lid is supplied by the infra-orbital and infratrochlear nerves.

The lacrimal apparatus

The lacrimal apparatus consists of the lacrimal gland, lacrimal canaliculi, lacrimal sac, and nasolacrimal duct [Fig. 4.15]. The lacrimal gland produces lacrimal fluid which enters the superolateral part of the conjunctival sac. In the conjunctival sac, it flows over the conjunctiva towards the medial angle of the eye, aided by the contraction of the orbicularis oculi [Fig. 4.3]. From the medial angle, the lacrimal fluid traverses the lacrimal canaliculi, lacrimal sac, and nasolacrimal duct to drain into the nose [Figs. 4.3, 4.15].

Using the instructions given in Dissection 4.6, explore the lacrimal apparatus.

Lacrimal gland

The lacrimal gland [Fig. 4.15; see Fig. 11.4] lies mainly in the superolateral corner of the anterior part of the orbit. A small part of it—the **palpebral process**—extends into the upper eyelid lateral to the tarsus, between the conjunctiva and the palpebral fascia. When the eyelid is everted, it may be seen as a bulge in the conjunctiva. The **ducts** of the lacrimal gland (ten or less) are short and thin. They open into the conjunctival sac near the superior fornix. Small **accessory lacrimal glands** lie near the conjunctival fornices. They can be effective in moistening the conjunctiva if the lacrimal gland is removed.

Conjunctiva

The conjunctiva lines the deep surfaces of the eyelids—the **palpebral conjunctiva**—and covers the exposed surface of the eyeball—the **bulbar conjunctiva**. At the corneoscleral junction, the bulbar conjunctiva becomes continuous with the anterior epithelium of the cornea. The **conjunctival fornices** are produced where the thick, vascular palpebral part of the conjunctiva is reflected from the eyelids on to the eyeball. On the eyeball,

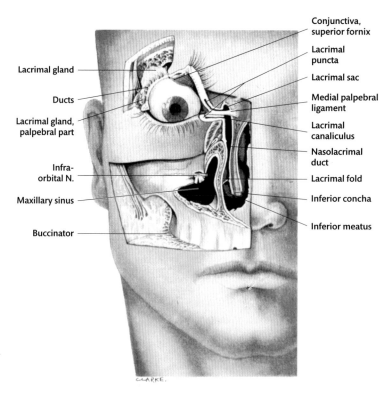

Fig. 4.15 Dissection of the lacrimal apparatus.

DISSECTION 4.6 Lacrimal apparatus

Objectives

I. To expose the lacrimal gland. **II.** To explore the lacrimal puncta, lacrimal canaliculi, lacrimal sac, and nasolacrimal duct.

Instructions

1. Cut through the superolateral part of the palpebral fascia, and expose the lacrimal gland.

2. Raise the gland, and find its ducts by moving the points of a fine forceps up and down in the loose tissue below the gland.

3. Find the lacrimal papillae at the medial ends of the eyelids, and attempt to pass a fine bristle into the lacrimal canaliculi through the puncta.

4. Identify the medial palpebral ligament and the lacrimal sac which lies posterior to it.

5. Note the lacrimal part of the orbicularis oculi passing around the lateral side of the sac.

6. Make an opening into the sac. Pass a probe into it and explore its extent.

7. Then pass the probe downwards into the nose through the nasolacrimal duct. Confirm its orifice in the nasal cavity.

the conjunctiva is thin and transparent and is loosely attached to the sclera. The space bounded by the bulbar and palpebral conjunctivae is known as the conjunctival sac. The conjunctival sac is no more than a capillary interval moistened by lacrimal fluid. It opens to the exterior through the **palpebral fissure** and drains into the lacrimal sac through the canaliculi [Fig. 4.15].

Lacrimal canaliculi

The lacrimal canaliculi are two thin tubes about 1 cm in length. Each begins at a tiny hole (the **lacrimal punctum**) on the summit of a lacrimal papilla. It runs medially in the margin of the eyelid and opens into the lacrimal sac posterior to the medial palpebral ligament [Fig. 4.15].

Lacrimal sac

The lacrimal sac lies posterior to the medial palpebral ligament in the lacrimal groove. It is approximately 1 cm long and 0.5 cm wide. The upper

end of the sac is closed. Its lower end is continuous with the nasolacrimal duct [Fig. 4.15].

Nasolacrimal duct

The nasolacrimal duct is 1.5 cm long and 0.5 cm wide. It begins at the anteromedial part of the floor of the orbit as a continuation of the lacrimal sac, and descends in a bony canal to the inferior meatus of the nasal cavity. The mucous membrane at the medial side of its opening is raised up as the **lacrimal fold**. This fold acts as a flap valve which prevents air and secretions from being blown up the nasolacrimal duct when the intranasal pressure is raised, e.g. in blowing the nose or sneezing [Fig. 4.15; see Fig. 19.7].

Cartilages of the nose

Use Fig. 4.16 to study the names and relations of the cartilages of the nose.

See Clinical Applications 4.1, 4.2, and 4.3 for the practical implications of the anatomy discussed in this chapter.

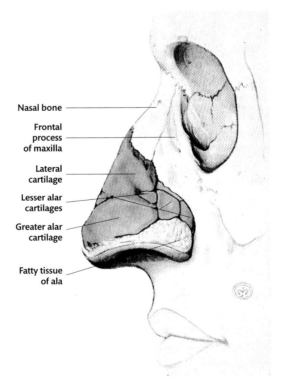

Nasal bone

Frontal process of maxilla

Lateral cartilage

Lesser alar cartilages

Greater alar cartilage

Fatty tissue of ala

Fig. 4.16 Cartilages of the external nose.

CLINICAL APPLICATION 4.1 Scalp–applied anatomy

Common skin conditions like dandruff, dermatitis, and psoriasis involve the skin of the scalp. The abundant hair follicles make this a common site for sebaceous cysts and also infestations like pediculosis (lice).

The connective tissue in the superficial fascia (second layer) of the scalp contains numerous blood vessels and nerves. The dense fibres in this layer attach to the walls of the blood vessels and prevent vasoconstriction following lacerations of the scalp. As a result, wounds of the scalp bleed heavily.

The connective tissue layer that lies deep to the epicranial aponeurosis is of interest for several reasons.

Study question 1: explain why bleeding from this space often presents as a black eye. (Answer: the frontal belly of the occipitofrontalis has no bony attachments, and so the loose areolar tissue of the scalp is continuous with the space between the skeletal muscle and the tarsal plate of the eyelid. As such, blood can track from the scalp into the eyelid.)

Study question 2: explain how infections in the loose areolar tissue space of the scalp can potentially spread into the cranial cavity. (Answer: numerous emissary veins connect veins of the scalp to intracranial venous sinuses and traverse the loose areolar tissue space. Emissary veins are valveless and can carry infections into the cranial cavity and cause meningitis and dural venous thrombosis. For this reason, the loose areolar tissue of the scalp is also called the dangerous layer of the scalp.)

Cephalhaematoma is a sub-periosteal bleed beneath the periosteum of the parietal (rarely occipital) bone during childbirth. This is the result of rupture of minute periosteal arteries, leading to a localized swelling over the parietal bone, not extending beyond its bony margins.

Caput succedaneum is a more diffuse oedema of the subcutaneous tissue of the entire scalp, due to prolonged compression of the fetal head against the bony pelvis of the mother during labour.

CLINICAL APPLICATION 4.2 Sensory nerve blocks in the face

Individual branches of the trigeminal nerve can be blocked using anaesthetic agents for doing surgical procedures in the face. The connective tissue around a sensory nerve is injected with an anaesthetic agent, which then temporarily stops transmission of pain. Knowledge of the course and area supplied by the nerve is essential for achieving proper anaesthesia.

1. Supra-orbital and supratrochlear nerve blocks to anaesthetize the forehead and anterior scalp are done by infiltrating the nerve at the supra-orbital margin.

2. Infra-orbital nerve block to anaesthetize the midface region is done by infiltrating the nerve at the infra-orbital foramen, either intraorally or through the skin of the face.

3. Posterior superior alveolar nerve blocks to anaesthetize the maxillary molar teeth are done by infiltrating the nerve at the maxillary tuberosity.

4. Anterior superior alveolar nerve block to anaesthetize the upper canine and incisors is done by infiltrating the nerve where the mucobuccal fold meets the apex of the canine tooth.

5. Inferior alveolar nerve block to anaesthetize all the mandibular teeth is done by infiltrating the nerve at the lingula of the mandible.

6. Mental nerve block to anaesthetize the lower lip and skin of the chin is done by infiltrating the nerve as it emerges from the mental foramen.

7. Lingual nerve block to anaesthetize the anterior two-thirds of the tongue is done by infiltrating the nerve next to the second mandibular molar tooth.

CLINICAL APPLICATION 4.3 Lacrimal fluid

Under ordinary conditions, the lacrimal fluid flows downwards over the eyeball, and most of it evaporates. The remaining is carried medially by the frequent involuntary contractions of the orbicularis oculi which move the eyelids and the lacrimal fluid medially, due to the attachment of the muscle to the medial palpebral ligament. Excessive secretion by the lacrimal gland, due to irritation of the conjunctiva or in response to strong emotions, floods the conjunctiva and the lacrimal fluid overflows as tears. When the orbicularis oculi is paralysed, the eyes remain open, the lacrimal fluid is not spread, and the cornea becomes dry. Tears pool in the sagging, paralysed lower lid and spill over onto the face.

CHAPTER 5
The posterior triangle of the neck

Introduction to the neck

The **side of the neck** is limited inferiorly by the clavicle, and superiorly by the lower border of the mandible, the mastoid process of the temporal bone, and the superior nuchal line of the occipital bone. It extends from the midline in front to the anterior border of the trapezius at the back. The sternocleidomastoid muscle runs obliquely across the side of the neck and divides it into **anterior** and **posterior triangles** [Figs. 5.1, 5.2].

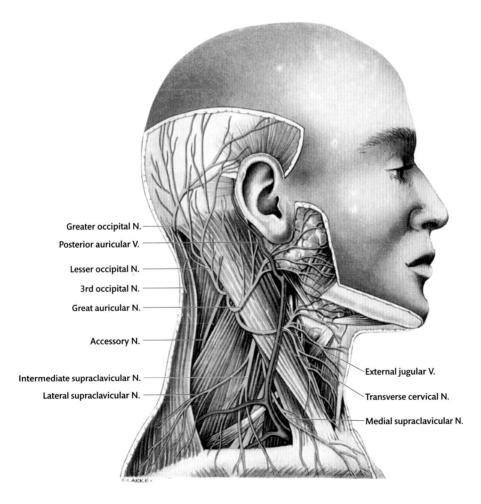

Greater occipital N.
Posterior auricular V.
Lesser occipital N.
3rd occipital N.
Great auricular N.
Accessory N.
Intermediate supraclavicular N.
Lateral supraclavicular N.
External jugular V.
Transverse cervical N.
Medial supraclavicular N.

Fig. 5.1 Cutaneous branches of the cervical plexus.

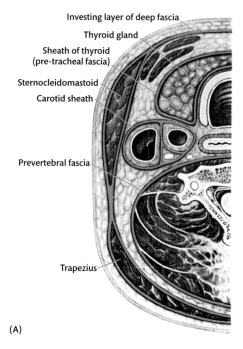

(A)

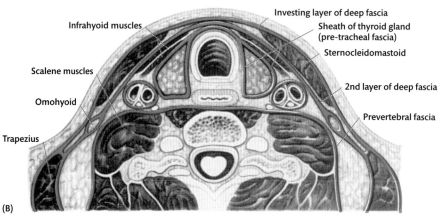

(B)

Fig. 5.2 (A) Cervical fascia (blue) in transverse section at the level of the thyroid isthmus. (B) Cervical fascia (blue) in transverse section of the lower part of the neck.

(Chapter 7 on the back of the neck deals with the structures under cover of the trapezius and includes the erector spinae, muscles of the suboccipital region, other back muscles, and their blood vessels and nerves.)

Surface anatomy of the posterior triangle of the neck

The upper 3–4 cervical vertebrae are overlapped anteriorly by the facial skeleton. As such, the cervical vertebrae extend to a much higher level than the chin. The first cervical vertebra lies at the level

of the tip of the mastoid process—the same level as the hard palate. The second lies at the level of the oral cavity, and the third lies at the level of the symphysis menti [see Fig. 2.1].

The **sternocleidomastoid muscle** extends from the manubrium sternum and the medial third of the clavicle to the mastoid process of the temporal bone behind the ear. It raises a low ridge diagonally across the side of the neck. This ridge is made prominent when the face is turned towards the opposite side. The **external jugular vein** is seen crossing the surface of the sternocleidomastoid, almost vertically from a point behind the angle of the mandible to the clavicle [Fig. 5.1].

The **lesser supraclavicular fossa** is a shallow depression between the sternal and clavicular parts of the sternocleidomastoid. It is above the medial part of the clavicle and overlies the internal jugular vein. The **greater supraclavicular fossa** is a larger depression above the intermediate third of the clavicle, between the lower parts of the trapezius and sternocleidomastoid. It overlies the cervical part of the brachial plexus and the third part of the subclavian artery. It is made obvious when the shoulders are shrugged.

General arrangement of neck structures

The major structures of the neck are surrounded by the **investing layer of the deep fascia**. This fascia encloses the trapezius and sternocleidomastoid muscles and forms the superficial covering of the posterior triangle. Deep to this layer of fascia are two compartments. (1) The larger posterior compartment consists of the vertebral column and the muscles which immediately surround it. This compartment is enclosed in a sleeve of fascia which passes anterior to the vertebral bodies and is known as the **prevertebral fascia**. Laterally, this fascia covers the muscles which form the floor of the posterior triangle, and the erector spinae muscles. (2) The smaller anterior compartment contains the pharynx, larynx, oesophagus, trachea, and their associated muscles. These structures are covered anteriorly by the **pretracheal fascia**. This compartment also contains the vertical neurovascular bundle of the neck. The ventral rami of the **cervical nerves** emerge from the vertebral canal between the muscles attached to the anterior and posterior tubercles of the transverse processes [Fig. 5.2]. Since these nerves arise within the prevertebral fascia, they may either carry a sheath of this fascia outwards with them—the fascia of the cervico-axillary canal [see Fig. 5.7]—or continue to remain within the fascia (the phrenic nerve).

The posterior triangle

Boundaries and contents of the posterior triangle

The boundaries of the posterior triangle are the posterior margin of the sternocleidomastoid, the

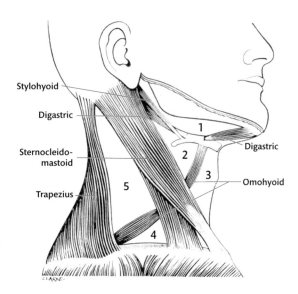

Fig. 5.3 The triangles of the neck. Anterior triangle: 1. Digastric triangle; 2. Carotid triangle; 3. Muscular triangle. Posterior triangle: 4. Subclavian triangle; 5. Occipital triangle.

anterior margin of the trapezius, and the intermediate third of the clavicle [Fig. 5.3].

The investing layer of the deep fascia forms the roof of the triangle and is pierced by the external jugular vein, the cutaneous branches of the cervical plexus, and lymph vessels passing from the superficial structures to the nodes in the triangle.

The floor of the triangle is formed from above downwards by the splenius capitis, levator scapulae, and scalenus medius, covered by the prevertebral fascia [Fig. 5.4].

Using the instructions given in Dissection 5.1, reflect the skin of the posterior triangle and begin tracing the cutaneous nerves and veins.

Deep fascia of the posterior triangle

The **roof** of the posterior triangle is formed by the investing layer of the deep cervical fascia. The **floor** is formed by the prevertebral fascia.

In the posterior triangle, the investing layer of the deep fascia extends from the intermediate third of the clavicle to the superior nuchal line. It is a thin sheet which splits inferiorly into superficial and deep layers. The superficial layer fuses with the clavicle. The deep layer splits to enclose the posterior belly of the omohyoid muscle [Figs. 5.2B, 5.4], passes deep to the clavicle, and is attached to its lower surface. It holds the inferior belly of the omohyoid in place. The space between the two layers of fascia extends medially deep to

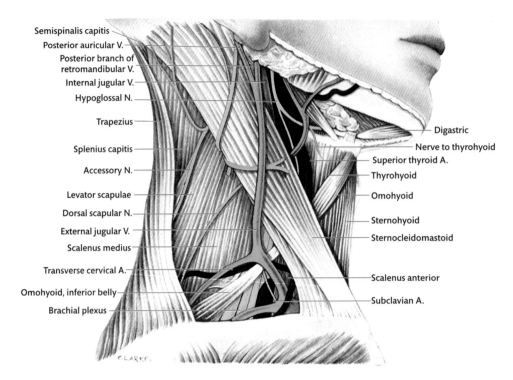

Semispinalis capitis
Posterior auricular V.
Posterior branch of retromandibular V.
Internal jugular V.
Hypoglossal N.
Trapezius
Splenius capitis
Accessory N.
Levator scapulae
Dorsal scapular N.
External jugular V.
Scalenus medius
Transverse cervical A.
Omohyoid, inferior belly
Brachial plexus

Digastric
Nerve to thyrohyoid
Superior thyroid A.
Thyrohyoid
Omohyoid
Sternohyoid
Sternocleidomastoid
Scalenus anterior
Subclavian A.

CLARKE.

Fig. 5.4 Lateral view of the superficial structures in the neck.

DISSECTION 5.1 Skin reflection and cutaneous nerves and veins of the posterior triangle-1

Objectives

I. To reflect the skin of the posterior triangle. **II.** To identify and trace the great auricular nerve, lesser occipital nerve, transverse cutaneous nerve of the neck, and supraclavicular nerves. III. To identify and trace the external jugular vein [Fig. 5.1].

Instructions

1. Reflect the skin of the posterior triangle. Avoid damage to the supraclavicular nerves, which lie deep to the platysma in the lower part of the triangle, and to the accessory nerve which is in the investing layer of the deep fascia in the upper part of the triangle.

2. Make an incision through the skin along the middle of the sternocleidomastoid muscle from the mastoid process to the sternal end of the clavicle. Do not cut into the superficial fascia, or the great auricular nerve, transverse nerve of the neck, and the external jugular vein will be damaged.

3. Extend the incision along the clavicle to its acromial end, and reflect the flap of skin back to the anterior border of the trapezius.

4. Turn the platysma upwards and forwards from the clavicle, superficial to the supraclavicular nerves and the **external jugular vein**. Find this vein, and trace it upwards till it is joined by the posterior auricular vein, and downwards till it pierces the deep fascia.

5. Find the three cutaneous nerves which pierce the deep fascia at the middle of the posterior border of the sternocleidomastoid. (1) The **lesser occipital nerve** runs upwards along the posterior border of the sternocleidomastoid. (2) The **great auricular nerve** crosses the sternocleidomastoid obliquely towards the auricle. (3) The **transverse nerve of the neck** passes horizontally forwards across the sternocleidomastoid.

6. Find the medial, intermediate, and lateral **supraclavicular nerves**, either individually or by finding one branch and tracing it back to the trunk.

the sternocleidomastoid behind the clavicle, and contains the terminal parts of the external jugular and transverse cervical veins and the suprascapular vessels. The **accessory nerve** enters the triangle at the posterior border of the sternocleidomastoid and runs postero-inferiorly across the triangle embedded in the investing fascia [Fig. 5.4]. The fascia is pierced by: (1) cutaneous branches of the cervical plexus; (2) the external jugular vein; and (3) small cutaneous arteries.

The **prevertebral fascia** covers the muscles on the floor of the posterior triangle—the levator scapulae, scalenus anterior, medius, and posterior. It passes in front of the cervical vertebrae and prevertebral muscles [Fig. 5.2].

Dissection 5.2 continues the study of the cutaneous nerves and veins of the posterior triangle.

Cutaneous branches of the cervical plexus

The cervical plexus is formed by the ventral rami of the upper four cervical nerves. It lies in the upper part of the neck, deep to the internal jugular vein and the sternocleidomastoid muscle. Its cutaneous branches emerge at the middle of the posterior border of the sternocleidomastoid. [see Fig. 4.9; Figs. 5.4, 5.5].

Lesser occipital nerve (C. 2)

The lesser occipital nerve ascends on the posterior border of the sternocleidomastoid, giving small branches to the skin of the neck. It pierces the deep fascia and sends branches to the upper part of the cranial surface of the auricle and the skin over the mastoid process. It may communicate with the greater occipital nerve [Fig. 5.1].

Great auricular nerve (C. 2, 3)

The great auricular nerve turns around the posterior border of the sternocleidomastoid, pierces the deep fascia, and runs towards the parotid gland behind and parallel to the external jugular vein. The **posterior branch** supplies the skin on both surfaces of the auricle and on the mastoid process. The **anterior branch** supplies the skin over the angle of the mandible and the parotid gland, and communicates with the facial and auriculotemporal nerves in that gland [Fig. 5.1].

Transverse nerve of the neck (C. 2, 3)

The transverse nerve of the neck passes forwards towards the anterior triangle of the neck on the superficial surface of the sternocleidomastoid. Its upper and lower branches supply most of the skin on the side and front of the neck. The upper branch communicates with the cervical branch of the facial nerve [Fig. 5.1].

Supraclavicular nerves (C. 3, 4)

The medial, intermediate, and lateral supraclavicular nerves arise as a single trunk. Diverging as they

---

DISSECTION 5.2 Cutaneous nerves and veins of the posterior triangle-2

Objectives

I. To identify and trace the nerve to the subclavius, and the accessory nerve. **II.** To identify and trace the transverse cervical and suprascapular veins.

Instructions

1. Follow the supraclavicular nerves to their common trunk.

2. Cut through the investing fascia above the clavicle and along the posterior border of the sternocleidomastoid to expose its deeper layer.

3. Find the external jugular, transverse cervical, and suprascapular veins in the space between the two layers, and trace the veins to their termination.

4. Find the **nerve to the subclavius** on the lateral side of the external jugular vein, and trace it in both directions. It may give an accessory branch to the phrenic nerve.

5. Find the entry of the anterior jugular vein into the external jugular vein, and the **suprascapular artery** deep to the clavicle. Trace the artery and its vein deep to the trapezius by pushing the fat out of the way. They run towards the scapular notch beside the attachment of the inferior belly of the omohyoid.

6. Follow the cutaneous nerves emerging at the middle of the posterior border of the sternocleidomastoid. Take care not to damage the accessory nerve where the lesser occipital nerve hooks round it.

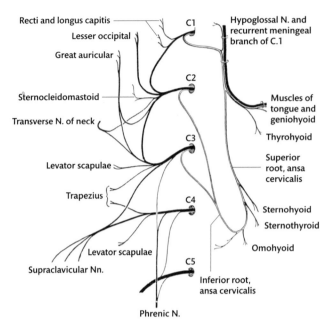

Fig. 5.5 Cervical plexus and ansa cervicalis. C. 1–C. 5, ventral rami of the upper five cervical nerves. Note that the nerves to the genio-hyoid and thyrohyoid muscles and the superior root of the ansa are derived from the first cervical ventral ramus (although they appear to arise from the hypoglossal nerve).

descend, they send small branches to the skin of the neck and pierce the deep fascia a little above the clavicle. The nerves pass over the corresponding thirds of the clavicle and supply the skin on the front of the chest, down to the level of the sternal angle, and over the upper half of the deltoid muscle [Fig. 5.1].

External jugular vein

The external jugular vein varies greatly in size and is often conspicuous in the neck. It begins by the union of the posterior branch of the retromandibular vein and the posterior auricular vein on the surface of the sternocleidomastoid, behind the angle of the mandible. It passes vertically downwards in the superficial fascia, deep to the platysma [Fig. 5.4]. It pierces the investing layer of the deep fascia at the posterior border of the sternocleidomastoid, 2–3 cm above the clavicle. In the posterior triangle, it descends beside the sternocleidomastoid and crosses the lower roots of the brachial plexus and the third part of the subclavian artery. It drains into the subclavian vein behind the clavicle. It receives the transverse cervical, suprascapular, and anterior jugular veins. It drains into the subclavian vein behind the clavicle.

Dissection 5.3 provides instructions on dissection of the posterior triangle.

Accessory nerve (eleventh cranial)

The accessory nerve in the posterior triangle consists of nerve fibres which arise in the cervical part of the spinal cord. These fibres, the **spinal part**, enter the cranium through the foramen magnum. In the cranial cavity, they join with the nerve fibres arising from the medulla oblongata (**cranial part**), and together they exit from the skull through the jugular foramen.

The spinal part immediately separates from the cranial part of the nerve [see Fig. 9.12]. It passes postero-inferiorly across the transverse process of the atlas, supplies the sternocleidomastoid muscle, and pierces its deeper part. It emerges from the posterior border of the sternocleidomastoid a little above its middle, runs in the investing layer of the deep fascia covering the posterior triangle, and passes deep to the trapezius about 5 cm above the clavicle. It is the only motor supply to the sternocleidomastoid and trapezius. The branches from the cervical plexus (C. 2, 3, 4) are sensory [Fig. 5.4].

Dissection 5.4 provides instructions on deep dissection of the posterior triangle.

DISSECTION 5.3 Posterior triangle

Objectives

I. To identify and clean the inferior belly of the omohyoid. **II.** To trace the accessory nerve and branches of the third and fourth cervical nerves to the trapezius. **III.** To clean the brachial plexus, and identify and trace the branches in the posterior triangle. **IV.** To expose the subclavian vessels.

Instructions

1. Remove the fat and fascia from the posterior triangle, starting at the apex where the occipital artery crosses it.

2. Find the accessory nerve [Fig. 5.4] at the posterior border of the sternocleidomastoid, and follow it and the branches from the third and fourth cervical nerves near it, to the trapezius. Branches of the same nerves may be found entering the levator scapulae.

3. Remove the fascia from the inferior belly of the omohyoid, and turn the muscle forwards to expose the nerve entering its deep surface near the sternocleidomastoid.

4. Expose the upper part of the brachial plexus, and trace it backwards to its roots. Avoid damage to the nerves arising from the roots. (1) The **suprascapular nerve** runs postero-inferiorly immediately above the plexus, under cover of the omohyoid. (2) Slightly above the supraclavicular nerve, the thin **dorsal scapular nerve** (C. 5) runs postero-inferiorly deep to the trapezius. (3) The three roots of the **long thoracic nerve** arise from the back of the roots of the plexus (C. 5, 6, 7) and descend behind it. The upper two pierce the scalenus medius muscle. Find the long thoracic nerve in the axilla, and trace it up to the three roots of origin.

5. Find the superficial cervical artery at the upper border of the omohyoid. Follow it across the posterior triangle and back towards its origin by removing the deeper layer of the investing fascia.

6. Follow the nerve to the subclavius to its termination.

7. Expose the subclavian vessels and the brachial plexus posterior to them.

DISSECTION 5.4 Deep dissection of the posterior triangle

Objective

I. To expose the scalenus anterior and the vessels and nerves in relation to it.

Instructions

1. Cut through the clavicular attachment of the sternocleidomastoid, and reflect this part of the muscle forwards.

2. Remove the underlying fatty tissue to expose the scalenus anterior in front of the brachial plexus.

3. Define the borders of the scalenus anterior, and expose the omohyoid muscle, the superficial cervical artery, the anterior and internal jugular veins, and the phrenic nerve anterior to it.

4. Depress the clavicle, and expose the subclavian vein.

Scalenus anterior

The scalenus anterior arises from the anterior tubercles of the third to sixth cervical transverse processes and is inserted into the scalene tubercle on the medial margin of the first rib, posterior to the subclavian vein. It lies anterior to the ventral rami of the fourth to eighth cervical nerves, the cervical pleura, and the subclavian artery. Anteriorly, the phrenic nerve and internal jugular vein descend obliquely in front of the muscle from its lateral to medial borders. The muscle is also crossed more horizontally by the superficial cervical and suprascapular vessels and the anterior jugular vein [Fig. 5.6; see Figs. 9.9, 9.17, 10.1].

Nerve supply: the ventral rami of adjacent nerves. **Action**: it raises the first rib (inspiration) and produces lateral flexion of the neck.

Omohyoid, inferior belly

The inferior belly of the omohyoid is a slender muscle which arises from the transverse scapular

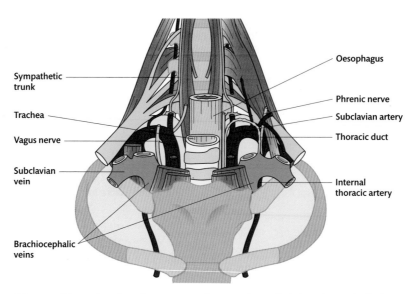

Sympathetic trunk

Trachea

Vagus nerve

Subclavian vein

Brachiocephalic veins

Oesophagus

Phrenic nerve

Subclavian artery

Thoracic duct

Internal thoracic artery

Fig. 5.6 Dissection of the root of the neck to show the structures adjacent to the cervical pleura (green shading).

ligament and the adjacent part of the scapula [see Fig. 3.16, Vol. 1]. It runs anterosuperiorly across the posterior triangle, a short distance superior to the clavicle. It joins the tendon which links it to the superior belly of the omohyoid, deep to the sternocleidomastoid.

Nerve supply: a branch of the ansa cervicalis [p. 60]. **Action**: it helps to steady or depress the hyoid bone in speaking and swallowing.

Subclavian artery, third part

The right subclavian artery arises from the brachiocephalic trunk, posterior to the right sternoclavicular joint. The left arises from the arch of the aorta and enters the neck behind the left sternoclavicular joint. In the root of the neck, both arteries arch laterally in front of the cervical pleura and continue as the axillary artery at the outer border of the first rib. The scalenus anterior lies in front of the artery at its highest part and divides it into three parts—a first part medial to the scalenus anterior, a second part behind it, and a third part lateral to it. The first and second parts of the artery are described in Chapter 9.

The third part of the subclavian artery begins about a finger breadth above the clavicle. It descends across the cervical pleura and lies in the subclavian groove of the first rib, anterior to the lower trunk of the brachial plexus and scalenus medius. It ends at the outer border of the first rib, behind the middle of the clavicle. The suprascapular artery and the external jugular vein and its tributaries lie

in front of the artery, between it and the clavicle [Fig. 5.6].

Subclavian vein

The subclavian vein is the continuation of the axillary vein from the outer border of the first rib. It passes medially, antero-inferior to the third part of the subclavian artery and the scalenus anterior. It unites with the internal jugular vein behind the sternoclavicular joint to form the brachiocephalic vein. The external jugular vein is the only tributary of the subclavian vein. It joins the subclavian vein at the lateral border of the scalenus anterior. The subclavian vein has a valve near its junction with the brachiocephalic vein [Fig. 5.6].

Suprascapular and superficial cervical vessels

The suprascapular and superficial cervical arteries arise from the **thyrocervical trunk**—a short branch of the first part of the subclavian artery. (The inferior thyroid artery is the other branch of the thyrocervical trunk.)

The **superficial cervical artery** runs laterally, anterior to the scalenus anterior, phrenic nerve, upper and middle trunks of the brachial plexus, and the suprascapular nerve, to the anterior border of the levator scapulae [Fig. 5.4].

The **suprascapular artery** passes inferolaterally behind the clavicle, in front of the scalenus anterior and the subclavian artery. It joins the suprascapular nerve at the postero-inferior angle of the posterior triangle and descends with it to the scapular notch [see Fig. 4.2, Vol. 1].

The corresponding veins end in the external jugular vein.

The brachial plexus

The **supraclavicular part** of the brachial plexus lies in the lower part of the posterior triangle. It continues behind the clavicle into the axilla as the **infraclavicular part**.

The brachial plexus is formed by the union of the ventral rami of C. 5–T. 1, at the lateral border of the scalenus anterior, deep to the lower third of the sternocleidomastoid. It ends in the axilla by dividing into the nerves of the upper limb. The supraclavicular (cervical) part of the brachial plexus consists of the roots, trunks, and divisions [Fig. 5.7].

Using the instructions given in Dissection 5.5, dissect the supraclavicular part of the brachial plexus.

Roots of the brachial plexus

The roots of the brachial plexus are the ventral rami of the lower four cervical and first thoracic nerves (C. 5–T. 1). In addition, the plexus receives a variable contribution from the fourth cervical and second thoracic nerves as well.

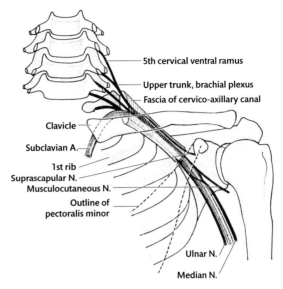

Fig. 5.7 Brachial plexus and axillary artery in the cervico-axillary canal.

Trunks of the brachial plexus

The fifth and sixth cervical ventral rami (with a small contribution from the fourth) unite to form the upper trunk. The seventh cervical ventral ramus continues as the middle trunk. The eighth cervical and first thoracic ventral rami (with a small contribution from the second thoracic ventral ramus) unite to form the lower trunk [Fig. 5.7].

DISSECTION 5.5 Supraclavicular part of the brachial plexus

Objective

I. To expose the roots and trunks of the brachial plexus.

Instructions

The brachial plexus should be dissected in conjunction with the dissection of the axilla. To expose the brachial plexus in its full extent, the clavicle should be divided between drill holes placed in its intermediate third. This allows the shoulder to fall back and opens the cervico-axillary canal. Subsequently, the clavicle should be wired together through the drill holes to replace the parts in their normal relationships.

1. Clean the fascia overlying the scalenus anterior and medius, and find the C. 5, C. 6, C. 7, C. 8, and T. 1 roots of the brachial plexus.

2. Trace C. 5 and C. 6 laterally to the formation of the upper trunk.

3. Note that C. 7 continues as the middle trunk.

4. Trace C. 8 and T. 1 laterally to the formation of the lower trunk.

5. Find the long thoracic nerve on the medial wall of the axilla, and trace it back to its origin from the roots.

6. Find and trace the nerve to the subclavius and the suprascapular nerve to the upper trunk.

7. Trace the phrenic nerve from where it has been identified on the scalenus anterior to the roots.

Divisions of the brachial plexus

Each trunk splits into an anterior and a posterior division. The three posterior divisions unite to form the **posterior cord**. The anterior divisions of the upper and middle trunks unite to form the **lateral cord**. The anterior division of the lower trunk forms the **medial cord**.

Relations of the brachial plexus

The **supraclavicular part** of the brachial plexus lies on the scalenus medius. The lower trunk lies on the superior surface of the first rib, posterior to the subclavian artery [Fig. 5.6]. The roots of the long thoracic nerve are posterior to the plexus. The external jugular vein, the inferior belly of the omohyoid, and the suprascapular and superficial cervical vessels are anterior to it.

Brachial plexus branches in the neck

All the roots of the brachial plexus receive **grey rami communicantes** from the sympathetic trunk. The upper two roots receive from the middle cervical ganglion, and the others from the cervico-thoracic ganglion.

Most of the branches in the neck are muscular and pass to the upper limb. Small nerves also pass to the scalene muscles, the longus colli [see Fig. 3.21, Vol. 1; see Fig. 10.1], and the phrenic nerve.

The **dorsal scapular nerve** passes backwards from the fifth cervical ventral ramus through the scalenus medius. It runs inferolaterally, anterior to the levator scapulae and the two rhomboids, supplying all three.

The thin **nerve to the subclavius** arises where the fifth and sixth cervical ventral rami unite. It descends across the brachial plexus and subclavian vessels, and enters the posterior surface of the subclavius. It often sends a branch to the **phrenic nerve** which may replace the phrenic contribution of C. 5.

The **suprascapular nerve** arises from the junction of the fifth and sixth cervical ventral rami. It runs postero-inferiorly on the scalenus medius, lateral to the plexus. It descends with the suprascapular vessels over the scapula and supplies the supraspinatus, infraspinatus, and the shoulder joint.

The **long thoracic nerve** arises by a series of branches from the upper three roots of the plexus. It descends on the surface of the scalenus medius and enters the axilla over the serratus anterior on the first rib.

See Clinical Applications 5.1 and 5.2 for the practical implications of the anatomy discussed in this chapter.

CLINICAL APPLICATION 5.1 External jugular vein laceration

A young man sustained a cut on the right side of his neck in a street fight and was found bleeding heavily on the road. He was rushed to a hospital. On arrival in the emergency unit, he was bleeding heavily from the site of injury, and was cyanotic and dyspnoeic. On examination, it was found that his external jugular vein had been lacerated.

Study question 1: how and where is the external jugular vein formed? And how and where does it terminate? (Answer: the external jugular vein begins by the union of the posterior branch of the retromandibular and posterior auricular veins on the surface of the sternocleidomastoid. It ends by draining into the subclavian vein in the posterior triangle.)

Study question 2: name the layer of the deep cervical fascia pierced by the vein before its termination. (Answer: investing layer of the deep fascia.)

The tight attachment of the fascia to the wall of the vein causes the wound to be pulled open. The negative intrathoracic pressure causes air to enter into the vein, leading to an air embolus.

Study question 3: from your knowledge of anatomy, in which chamber of the heart would the air embolus in the external jugular vein enter? (Answer: the embolus will go through the external jugular vein, subclavian vein, right brachiocephalic vein, and superior vena cava into the right atrium. The air embolus in the right atrium accounts for the cyanosis and dyspnoea.)

Study question 4: speculate on what steps could be taken to prevent a fatal air embolism in this case. (Answer: pressure on the vein will help control the bleeding and prevent air from entering into it.)

CLINICAL APPLICATION 5.2 Scalenus anterior syndrome

A 43-year-old painter presented with a history of pain and tingling sensation in the medial aspect of his forearm and hand, especially while lifting his arm above his shoulder to paint a wall.

Study question 1: what is the likely diagnosis? (Answer: compression of the lower part of the brachial plexus. The scalene triangle is formed by the scalenus anterior anteriorly, the scalenus medius posteriorly, and the first rib inferiorly, and contains the brachial plexus and subclavian artery. Compression of the brachial plexus in the scalene triangle is a probable diagnosis.)

Study question 2: what factors often lead to compression of the contents? (Answer: any clinical conditions which decrease the space within the scalene triangle can cause compression. Common conditions include hypertrophied scalenus anterior muscle, cervical rib, and fibromuscular bands between the two scalene muscles.)

Study question 3: what are the symptoms that arise due to compression? (Answer: compression of the lower trunk of the brachial plexus causes pain, numbness, or tingling sensation of the medial aspect of the forearm and arm. Compression of the subclavian artery can cause ischaemia, leading to pain and blanching of the hand.)

Study question 4: how is the diagnosis of the scalenus anterior syndrome confirmed? (Answer: several manoeuvres can be done to precipitate symptoms and confirm the diagnosis of the scalenus anterior syndrome. The Wright's test stimulates change in the radial pulse with hyperabduction of the arm. A fall in the radial pulse on hyperabduction of the arm indicates compression of the subclavian artery above the shoulder joint. More conclusive results are obtained by X-ray, magnetic resonance imaging, and subclavian Doppler sonography).

CHAPTER 6
The anterior triangle of the neck

Introduction

The anterior triangle of the neck is the area bound by the midline, the mandible, and the sternocleid-omastoid muscle [Figs. 6.1, 6.2].

Surface anatomy

Draw a finger down the anterior median line of your neck from the chin to the sternum, and iden-tify, in sequence: (1) the body of the hyoid bone

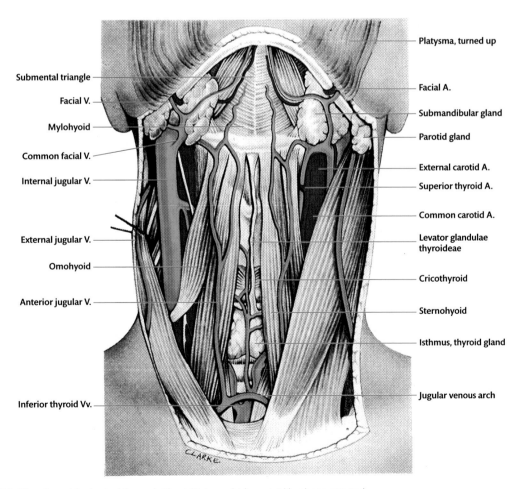

Submental triangle
Facial V.
Mylohyoid
Common facial V.
Internal jugular V.
External jugular V.
Omohyoid
Anterior jugular V.
Inferior thyroid Vv.

Platysma, turned up
Facial A.
Submandibular gland
Parotid gland
External carotid A.
Superior thyroid A.
Common carotid A.
Levator glandulae thyroideae
Cricothyroid
Sternohyoid
Isthmus, thyroid gland
Jugular venous arch

CLARKE

Fig. 6.1 Dissection of the front of the neck. The right sternocleidomastoid has been retracted.

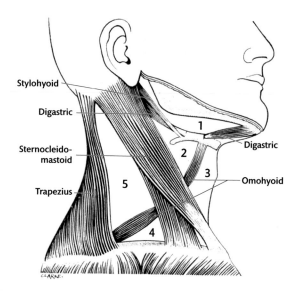

Stylohyoid

Digastric

Sternocleido-
mastoid

Trapezius

Digastric

Omohyoid

Fig. 6.2 The triangles of the neck. Anterior triangle: 1. Digastric triangle; 2. Carotid triangle; 3. Muscular triangle. Posterior triangle: 4. Subclavian triangle; 5. Occipital triangle.

cartilage; and (4) the rings of the trachea which are partly masked by the isthmus of the thyroid gland.

Grasp the front of the U-shaped **hyoid bone** between the finger and thumb. Trace it backwards to the greater horns. The tips of the greater horn may be overlapped by the sternocleidomastoid muscles. Trace the superior border of the **thyroid cartilage** posteriorly from its midline notch. Note that it ends in a projection—the superior horn—immediately anterior to the sternocleidomastoid. The **isthmus of the thyroid gland** [Fig. 6.1] forms a soft mass on the second, third, and fourth tracheal rings and slips upwards past the palpating finger when you swallow.

Press the tip of your fingers into the side of your neck from the mastoid process downwards. The deep bony resistances felt are the **transverse processes of the cervical vertebrae**. Only the transverse process of the first cervical vertebra can be felt clearly, immediately antero-inferior to the tip of the mastoid process. The fourth is at the level of the upper border of the thyroid cartilage. The sixth is at the level of the cricoid cartilage.

Using the instructions given in Dissection 6.1, open the anterior triangle and study its superficial content.

approximately 1 cm below, and 6 cm behind, the chin; (2) the **laryngeal prominence**, the sharp protuberance of the anterior border of the thyroid cartilage; (3) the rounded arch of the **cricoid**

DISSECTION 6.1 Skin reflection of the anterior triangle

Objectives

I. To reflect the skin over the anterior triangle. **II.** To expose the platysma. **III.** To identify and trace the vessels and nerves in the superficial tissue. **IV.** To explore the suprasternal space.

Instructions

1. Make a midline skin incision from the chin to the sternum, and reflect the flap of skin inferolaterally. Do not cut deep, but remain superficial to the fibres of the platysma in the posterosuperior part.

2. Reflect the platysma upwards, keeping close to its deep surface and dividing any nerves which enter it.

3. Find the branches of the transverse cervical nerve [see Fig. 5.1] as they cross the sternocleidomastoid, and follow them anteriorly to their termination.

4. Identify the cervical branch of the facial nerve as it leaves the lower border of the parotid gland, and trace it antero-inferiorly.

5. Find the **anterior jugular vein** near the midline. Trace it inferiorly till it pierces the deep fascia about 2 cm above the sternum.

6. Expose the deep fascia of the anterior triangle.

7. Make a transverse incision through the first layer of the deep fascia immediately above the sternum, and extend the incision 4 cm upwards along the anterior border of the sternocleidomastoid. Reflect this fascia to open the **suprasternal space** between the first (superficial) and second (deep) layers of the fascia.

8. Trace the anterior jugular vein and the deeper layer of the fascia laterally deep to the sternocleidomastoid. Follow the fascia upwards till it fuses with the first layer (midway between the sternum and the thyroid cartilage). Follow it downwards to its fusion with the back of the sternum.

Superficial fascia

The superficial fascia in this region contains a variable amount of fat. It is only loosely connected to the skin and deep fascia, so the skin is freely movable. The superficial fascia contains the anterior jugular veins, the decussating fibres of the platysma, and a few small **submental lymph nodes**. These nodes lie on the deep fascia and drain lymph from the anterior part of the floor of the mouth.

Platysma

This thin sheet of muscle lies in the superficial fascia, superficial to the cutaneous branches of the cervical plexus and the external jugular vein. It extends down from the face to the upper part of the chest over the superior part of the anterior triangle and the antero-inferior part of the posterior triangle [see Fig. 3.11, Vol. 1].

The platysma takes origin from the skin and fascia over the upper parts of the pectoralis major and deltoid. The anterior fibres are attached to either the lower border of the anterior part of the mandible or meet with the fibres of the opposite side below the chin. The posterior fibres curve upwards over the mandible to the skin of the lower face and mingle with the muscles of the lips, helping to form the risorius [see Fig. 4.8].

Nerve supply: the cervical branch of the facial nerve. **Action**: it pulls down the corner of the mouth, elevates the skin over the upper part of the chest, and tenses the skin of the neck. It contracts most obviously in strenuous inspiratory effort and may prevent compression of the airway by the skin.

Cervical branch of the facial nerve

The **cervical branch of the facial nerve** emerges from the lower border of the parotid gland and pierces the deep fascia. Branches arising from it spread on the deep surface of the platysma to supply it. Some fibres go over the border of the mandible to supply the muscles of the lower lip.

Anterior jugular vein

The anterior jugular vein is usually the smallest of the three jugular veins—the internal, external, and anterior jugular veins. It varies inversely in width with the external jugular vein. It begins below the chin and descends in the superficial fascia, about 1 cm from the midline [Fig. 6.1]. Approximately

53

2 cm above the sternum, it pierces the first layer of the deep fascia, runs laterally in the suprasternal space, passes deep to the sternocleidomastoid, and joins the external jugular vein. It is united to its fellow in the suprasternal space through the **jugular arch**, which may be large, and forms an important anterior relation to the trachea and thyroid gland.

The two anterior jugular veins may be replaced by a single median vein, or the anterior and external jugular veins may be partly or completely replaced by a single vein which descends along the anterior border of the sternocleidomastoid to the jugular arch. [Fig. 6.1].

Dissection 6.2 provides instructions on cleaning the sternocleidomastoid and identifying the accessory nerve.

Sternocleidomastoid

This important landmark muscle of the neck is easily seen in the living. When contracted, it stands out as a well-defined ridge between the anterior and posterior triangles [Fig. 6.2].

The sternocleidomastoid originates by two heads: a rounded, tendinous **sternal head** from the upper part of the anterior surface of the manubrium sternum, and a thin, fleshy **clavicular head** from the upper surface of the medial third of the clavicle. The sternal head ascends across the medial part of the sternoclavicular joint. It widens rapidly and overlaps the clavicular head a short distance above the clavicle. The two heads fuse with each other about halfway up the neck. The thick, anterior border of the sternocleidomastoid is inserted into the anterior surface of the mastoid process. The posterior part is thin and aponeurotic, and is attached to the lateral surface of the mastoid process and the lateral half of the superior nuchal line. The deep part of the sternocleidomastoid is pierced by the accessory nerve. It receives its main blood supply from the occipital and superior thyroid arteries.

Nerve supply: the accessory nerve is the motor nerve to the muscle. The ventral ramus of the second cervical nerve is sensory. **Actions**: acting alone, the sternocleidomastoid tilts the head to its own side and rotates the head, so that the face is turned towards the opposite side. Acting together, the two muscles flex the neck. In forced inspiration, the two muscles act together and raise the sternum when neck flexion is prevented by the extensors.

◑ Damage of the spinal part of the accessory nerve paralyses the sternocleidomastoid, causing the neck to be flexed to the opposite side and the face turned to the paralysed side by the unopposed action of the normal sternocleidomastoid. This condition is known as **wry neck**.

Deep fascia of the neck

Review the details of the three layers of the deep fascia described in Chapter 5. In the midline, the **investing layer** of the cervical deep fascia is attached to the mandible, hyoid bone, and sternum. Superiorly, it encloses the anterior bellies of the digastric muscles. Inferiorly, it encloses the **suprasternal space** which contains the jugular arch, the sternal head of the sternocleidomastoid, the lowest parts of the anterior jugular veins, and an occasional lymph node [Fig. 6.3]. The deeper **pre-tracheal fascia** descends from the thyroid and cricoid cartilages to invest the **thyroid gland** and cover the front and side of the trachea. It fuses with the back of the pericardium in the thorax [Fig. 6.3].

Dissection 6.3 describes the dissection of the midline structures of the neck.

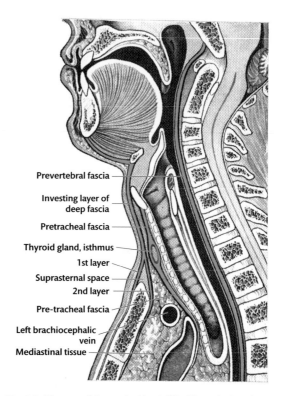

Prevertebral fascia
Investing layer of deep fascia
Pretracheal fascia
Thyroid gland, isthmus
1st layer
Suprasternal space
2nd layer
Pre-tracheal fascia
Left brachiocephalic vein
Mediastinal tissue

Fig. 6.3 Diagram of the cervical fascia (blue) in sagittal section.

Suprahyoid region

The **submental triangle** in the midline is bound by the hyoid bone and the anterior bellies of the digastric muscles. The roof of the triangle is formed by the muscular floor of the mouth, i.e. the mylohyoid muscles. The submental lymph nodes lie in the superficial fascia of the triangle [Fig. 6.1].

Infrahyoid region

A number of midline structures lie between the infrahyoid muscles of the two sides [Fig. 6.1]. From above downwards, these are:

1. The **thyrohyoid ligament** which unites the upper border of the thyroid cartilage and the upper border of the hyoid bone. It passes deep to the hyoid bone and is separated from it by a bursa. The bursa permits the upper edge of the thyroid cartilage to ascend inside the concavity of the hyoid bone during swallowing.
2. The **laryngeal prominence** is formed by the thyroid cartilage. The cartilage is notched on its superior margin.

DISSECTION 6.3 Midline structures of the neck

Objective

I. To clean and identify the midline structures in the front of the neck.

Instructions

1. Remove the deep fascia from the anterior bellies of the digastric muscles and from the area between them. This exposes parts of the two mylohyoid muscles which are inserted into a median raphe.

2. Continue the removal of this fascia below the hyoid. This exposes the infrahyoid muscles between the hyoid and the sternum on each side of the midline.

3. Separate these muscles in the midline to expose the pre-tracheal fascia.

4. Below the isthmus of the thyroid gland [Fig. 6.1], remove this fascia to expose the trachea and the inferior thyroid veins. The small thyroidea ima artery may be seen ascending to the thyroid in this region.

5. At the upper border of the isthmus, look for the slender fibromuscular band—the **levator glandulae thyroideae**—which may be present between the isthmus and the hyoid bone.

6. Remove the pre-tracheal fascia from the isthmus.

7. Find the **cricothyroid ligament** between the median parts of the cricoid and thyroid cartilages. The small cricothyroid muscle covers it on each side.

8. Find the **median thyrohyoid ligament** between the thyroid cartilage and hyoid bone, and the anastomosis of the infrahyoid arteries on it. Follow the ligament upwards behind the body of the hyoid bone.

---

3. The **cricothyroid ligament** attaches the thyroid cartilage to the arch of the cricoid cartilage. On the side of the ligament, the **cricothyroid muscle** radiates posterosuperiorly from the cricoid to the thyroid cartilage. The cricothyroids are important muscles of speech and the only intrinsic laryngeal muscles to be located on the external surface of the larynx.

4. The **isthmus of the thyroid gland** usually lies on the second to fourth tracheal rings and has a rich vascular anastomosis on its surface. Occasionally, a small lobe—the **pyramidal lobe**—projects upwards from it and may give rise to a slender slip of fibromuscular tissue—the **levator glandulae thyroideae**—which attaches it to the hyoid bone. The levator glandulae thyroideae is the embryological remnant of the tubular downgrowth from the tongue—the **thyroglossal duct**.

5. Below the isthmus of the thyroid gland is the trachea with the **jugular arch** and the **inferior thyroid veins** anterior to it. Occasionally, the left brachiocephalic vein and the brachiocephalic artery extend high enough to appear in front of the trachea at the root of the neck.

Subdivisions of the anterior triangle

In addition to the submental triangle, the anterior triangle may be divided into three subsidiary triangles: the carotid, muscular, and digastric triangles [Fig. 6.2].

Dissection 6.4 provides instructions to dissect the digastric triangle.

Digastric triangle

The digastric triangle is part of the submandibular region (Chapter 16). It is bound by the anterior belly of the digastric in front, the posterior belly of the digastric and stylohyoid behind, and the lower border of the mandible above. Its roof is formed by the mylohyoid and hyoglossus muscles [Figs. 6.1, 6.2, 6.4, 6.5].

A number of important structures lie in the digastric triangle. The lower (superficial) part of the **submandibular gland** almost fills the triangle. The **submandibular lymph nodes** lie on the surface of the gland, especially along the lower border of the mandible. These nodes drain lymph from the side of the tongue, teeth, lips, and cheek to the deep cervical lymph nodes beneath the sternocleidomastoid.

The **facial vein** pierces the deep fascia covering the triangle at the lower border of the mandible. It crosses the submandibular gland, unites with the anterior branch of the retromandibular vein, and drains into the internal jugular vein. The **facial artery** curves round the lower border of the mandible, gives off the submental artery, and pierces

DISSECTION 6.4 Digastric triangle

Objective

I. To identify the boundaries and contents of the digastric triangle [Fig. 6.4].

Instructions

1. Identify the facial artery and vein at the lower border of the mandible.

2. Cut the deep fascia from the mandible, and turn it downwards, exposing part of the submandibular gland.

3. Identify the anterior and posterior bellies of the digastric muscle at the lower border of the gland.

4. Follow the facial vein postero-inferiorly, superficial to the gland and the posterior belly of the digastric.

5. At the lower border of the mandible, find the **submental branch of the facial artery**. Trace it forwards by pushing the submandibular gland aside and removing the fat and lymph nodes beside it. (The artery runs with the mylohyoid nerve

which supplies the mylohyoid and the anterior belly of the digastric.)

6. Pull the submandibular gland laterally to expose the intermediate tendon of the digastric, the fascial sling which attaches it to the hyoid, and the stylohyoid muscle. The stylohyoid muscle splits to enfold the intermediate tendon of the digastric and lies on the upper surface of the posterior belly of the digastric.

7. Follow the stylohyoid and the posterior belly of the digastric as far as the angle of the mandible.

8. Pull the submandibular gland backwards to expose the posterior border of the mylohyoid.

9. Find the hypoglossal nerve and one of the veins of the tongue passing above the free border of the mylohyoid.

10. Identify the hyoglossus, a thin sheet of muscle deep to the hypoglossal nerve [see Fig. 6.6].

11. Remove the fascia from the rest of the mylohyoid and from the hyoglossus.

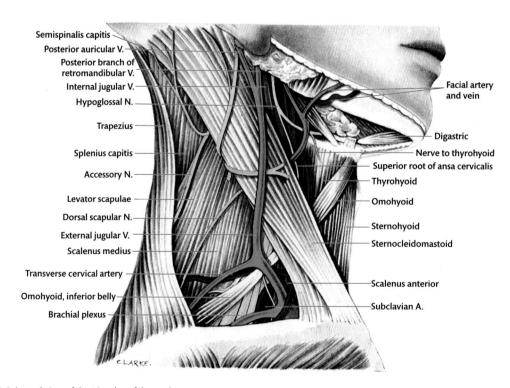

Fig. 6.4 Lateral view of the triangles of the neck.

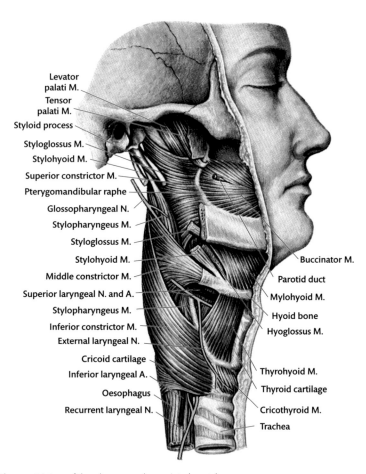

Fig. 6.5 Lateral view of the constrictors of the pharynx and associated muscles.

the deep fascia. The **submental artery** passes forwards with the corresponding vein and the mylohyoid nerve [Fig. 6.1].

The **mylohyoid nerve** lies on the inferior surface of the mylohyoid near the mandible. It supplies the mylohyoid and the anterior belly of the digastric. The **hypoglossal nerve** lies in a deeper plane, passes above the mylohyoid, and lies on the hyoglossus. The **intermediate tendon of the digastric** lies on the hyoglossus, immediately above the hyoid bone, and is held to the bone by a loop of fascia which forms a pulley for it. This arrangement permits anteroposterior movements of the hyoid when it is elevated by digastric muscles [Fig. 6.1].

Carotid triangle

The carotid triangle is bound by the sternocleidomastoid behind, the posterior belly of the digastric superiorly, and the superior belly of the omohyoid inferiorly [Fig. 6.2]. It contains the vertical

neurovascular bundle of the neck—the common carotid and external and internal carotid arteries, internal jugular vein, and vagus nerve—covered by the sternocleidomastoid. The floor of the triangle is formed by the hyoglossus and thyrohyoid muscles anteriorly and by the middle and inferior constrictor muscles of the pharynx posteriorly [Figs. 6.4, 6.5].

Dissection 6.5 provides instructions to dissect the carotid triangle.

Carotid sheath

The **carotid sheath** is a fascial sheath enclosing the internal jugular vein, the common and internal carotid arteries, the vagus nerve, and the superior and inferior roots of the ansa cervicalis [see Fig. 5.2A]. The sympathetic trunk is on the posteromedial wall of the sheath, and many **lymph nodes** lie on its superficial surface.

The common carotid artery divides at the level of the upper border of the thyroid cartilage into the internal and external carotid arteries. The internal

DISSECTION 6.5 Carotid triangle

Objective

I. To study the boundaries and contents of the carotid triangle [Fig. 6.4].

Instructions

1. Remove the fat and fascia from the area between the posterior belly of the digastric and the superior belly of the omohyoid [Fig. 6.2].

2. Expose the internal jugular vein laterally, the common and internal carotid arteries medial to it, and the external carotid artery anteromedial to the internal carotid artery.

3. Find the facial and lingual veins entering the internal jugular vein in the upper part of the triangle, and the superior thyroid vein entering it in the lower part.

4. Between the vein and the internal carotid artery, find the **hypoglossal nerve**. Follow it forwards across the external carotid artery, and find the following branches in the carotid triangle: (1) the superior root of the ansa cervicalis, given off where the nerve hooks round the occipital artery to enter the triangle; and (2) the branch to the thyrohyoid muscle given off as the hypoglossal leaves the carotid triangle [Fig. 6.4].

5. Remove the superficial part of the carotid sheath which surrounds the internal jugular vein, carotid arteries, and vagus nerve. Avoid injury to the superior root of the **ansa cervicalis** anterior to the vein and to its inferior root lateral to the vein. (The inferior root of the ansa cervicalis arises from the second and third cervical ventral rami. The two roots unite to form a loop—the ansa cervicalis—at a lower level.)

6. Expose the **external carotid artery** and its branches [Figs. 6.6, 6.7]. The superior thyroid is the lowest branch in the carotid triangle [Fig. 6.7]. The lingual, facial, and occipital arteries arise in the upper part of the triangle; the occipital artery arises opposite the facial artery [Fig. 6.7].

7. Find the internal laryngeal nerve in the interval between the hyoid bone and thyroid cartilage [Fig. 6.6]. Trace it posterosuperiorly, deep to the carotid arteries, to the parent stem, the superior laryngeal branch of the vagus. From the superior laryngeal nerve, follow the slender external laryngeal nerve downwards, deep to the superior thyroid artery [Fig. 6.5].

8. Expose the part of the hyoglossus which lies in the carotid triangle immediately above the hyoid bone. Note the hypoglossal nerve on its surface, and the **lingual artery** lying deep to it. The lingual artery lies on the middle constrictor of the pharynx [Fig. 6.5], which separates it from the mucous membrane of the pharynx.

9. Raise the posterior belly of the digastric to expose the middle constrictor at the hyoid bone [Fig. 6.5].

10. Find the thyrohyoid muscle in the floor of the carotid triangle.

11. Push the superior thyroid and carotid arteries posteriorly, and remove the fat surrounding the external laryngeal nerve. This exposes a part of the inferior constrictor muscle which passes backwards from the side of the thyroid cartilage.

12. Separate the internal and common carotid arteries from the internal jugular vein, and expose the vagus nerve in the posterior part of the carotid sheath between them. Pull the arteries anteromedially, and find the sympathetic trunk posteromedial to the sheath.

jugular vein descends vertically, first with the internal and then the common carotid artery medial to it.

External carotid artery

The external carotid artery begins at the upper border of the thyroid cartilage as a branch of the common carotid artery. It ascends along the side of the pharynx, anteromedial to the internal carotid artery. It gives off the following branches in the carotid triangle [Fig. 6.7]. (The full extent of the external carotid artery, and finer details of its branches, are described with the deeper dissection of the neck—Chapter 9.)

1. The **superior thyroid artery** curves antero-inferiorly and disappears deep to the omohyoid. It gives off the infrahyoid, sternocleidomastoid, and superior laryngeal branches in the triangle. The superior laryngeal artery enters the larynx with the internal laryngeal nerve.

2. The **ascending pharyngeal artery** arises from the lowest part of the external carotid artery. It

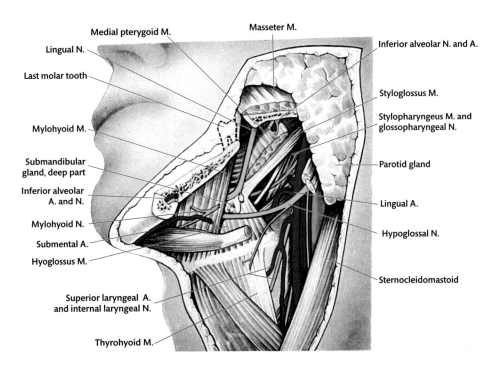

Fig. 6.6 Deep dissection of the submandibular region.

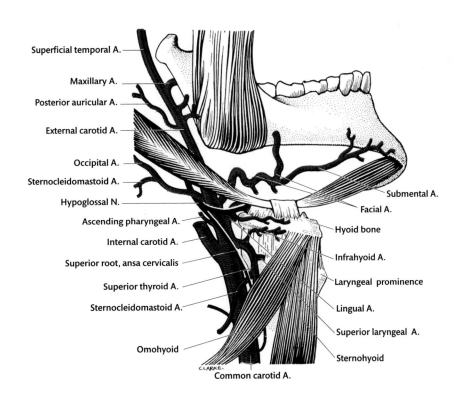

Fig. 6.7 External carotid artery and its branches. The mandible has been tilted upwards.

ascends deep to the internal carotid artery on the lateral side of the pharynx.

3. The **lingual artery** arises behind the tip of the greater horn of the hyoid bone. It runs forwards on the middle constrictor of the pharynx, hooks above the tip of the greater horn, and passes medial to the hyoglossus.

4. The **facial artery** arises above the lingual artery and leaves the triangle by looping upwards deep to the posterior belly of the digastric.

5. The **occipital artery** runs posterosuperiorly along the lower border of the posterior belly of the digastric.

Veins in the carotid triangle

The **facial vein** enters the carotid triangle superficial to the posterior belly of the digastric. It unites with the anterior branch of the retromandibular vein, as it crosses the carotid arteries, and drains into the internal jugular vein [Fig. 6.4]. It may receive the lingual and superior thyroid veins.

The **lingual vein** is formed at the posterior border of the hyoglossus by the union of veins which run with the lingual artery and the hypoglossal nerve. It crosses the carotid arteries and drains into either the internal jugular or the facial vein.

The **superior thyroid vein** drains into either the internal jugular or the facial vein.

Nerves in the carotid triangle

The **accessory nerve** runs postero-inferiorly across the upper angle of the triangle, either superficial or deep to the internal jugular vein.

The **hypoglossal nerve** (which supplies the muscles of the tongue) appears at the lower border of the posterior belly of the digastric, curves forwards on the carotid arteries at the root of the occipital artery and the curve of the lingual artery, and leaves the triangle by passing deep to the posterior belly of the digastric. In the carotid triangle, the hypoglossal nerve gives off the **superior root of the ansa cervicalis** (which descends on the internal and common carotid arteries) and the thyrohyoid branch which passes forwards to that muscle. Both branches are composed of fibres of the ventral ramus of the first cervical nerve, which join the hypoglossal close to the skull [Figs. 6.4, 6.6, 6.7]. Further details of the hypoglossal nerve are given in Chapters 9 and 16.

Ansa cervicalis

The ansa cervicalis is formed by two roots which unite with each other to form a loop. The slender **inferior root of the ansa cervicalis** arises from the ventral rami of the second and third cervical nerves behind the internal jugular vein. It curves forwards, usually on the lateral surface of the vein, and passes down on the common carotid artery. Here it joins the superior root from the hypoglossal nerve. The loop lies at the level of the lower part of the larynx.

The ansa cervicalis consists of nerve fibres from the cervical ventral rami of C. 1, C. 2, and C. 3. It supplies the **infrahyoid muscles**—sternohyoid, sternothyroid, and omohyoid. The thyrohyoid and geniohyoid are supplied by C. 1 fibres which run along with the hypoglossal nerve [see Fig. 16.3]. (In this way, the hypoglossal nerve forms a secondary plexus with the first three cervical ventral rami.) Together they supply a ventral strip of muscle from the tongue to the sternum.

Muscular triangle

This is a triangular space bound by the sternocleidomastoid inferolaterally, the superior belly of the omohyoid superolaterally, and the midline anteriorly. It contains the infrahyoid muscles and the midline structures of the neck [Figs. 6.1, 6.2].

Dissection 6.6 provides instructions to dissect the muscular triangle.

DISSECTION 6.6 Muscular triangle

Objective

I. To study the boundaries and contents of the muscular triangle.

Instructions

1. Pull back the sternal head of the sternocleidomastoid to expose the anterior jugular vein deep to it.

2. Find the intermediate tendon of the omohyoid, and raise the superior belly to expose its nerve. Trace this nerve to the ansa cervicalis, and expose the entire ansa and its branches.

3. Remove the fascia from the infrahyoid muscles, but retain their nerves.

4. Define the attachments of the sternohyoid. To define the sternal attachment, pass the handle of a knife down between it and the sternum. Then divide the muscle low down, and reflect it upwards to the hyoid. This exposes the sternothyroid, thyrohyoid, and their attachments.

Infrahyoid muscles

The infrahyoid muscles—sternohyoid, sternothyroid, thyrohyoid, and omohyoid—form two layers of ribbon-like muscles extending from the sternum to the hyoid bone [Fig. 6.1]. The deeper muscle layer (sternothyroid and thyrohyoid) is interrupted at the thyroid cartilage. The muscles lie on the trachea, thyroid gland, larynx, and thyrohyoid membrane. The thin fascia which encloses them is thickened around the intermediate tendon of the omohyoid and holds it down to the sternum and clavicle.

The **sternohyoid** lies superficial to the sternothyroid and thyrohyoid. It extends from the posterior surface of the manubrium and the medial end of the clavicle to the lower border of the hyoid bone adjacent to the midline [Fig. 6.1].

The superior belly of the **omohyoid** is attached to the inferior surface of the body and the greater horn of the hyoid, immediately lateral to the sternohyoid [Fig. 6.1]. Inferiorly, it continues with the inferior belly of the omohyoid at the intermediate tendon. The intermediate tendon lies on the internal jugular vein under the sternocleidomastoid, at the level of the cricoid cartilage. The inferior belly of the omohyoid extends from the intermediate tendon to the scapular notch [see Fig. 4.2, Vol. 1].

The **sternothyroid** is shorter and wider, and is situated deep to the sternohyoid. It arises from the sternum and first costal cartilage below the attachment of the sternohyoid. It ascends to the oblique line on the lateral surface of the thyroid cartilage [see Fig. 20.2], superficial to the attachment of the pre-tracheal fascia and the cricothyroid muscle. It is anterior to the large vessels of the thorax at the root of the neck, and to the thyroid gland.

The **thyrohyoid** seems like the upward continuation of the sternothyroid. It extends from the oblique line on the thyroid cartilage to the lower border of the greater horn of the hyoid bone [Fig. 6.5]. It is deep to the omohyoid and sternohyoid, and covers the entry of the internal laryngeal nerve to the larynx.

Nerve supply: the ventral rami of the first three cervical nerves supply the omohyoid, sternohyoid, and sternothyroid muscles through the ansa cervicalis. The thyrohyoid nerve, C. 1 fibres which run with the hypoglossal, supplies the thyrohyoid. **Actions**: the infrahyoid muscles move the larynx and hyoid bone in speech and swallowing. They can: (1) depress the hyoid bone or, when acting with the suprahyoid muscles, fix the hyoid to form a stable base for the tongue; (2) draw the larynx towards the hyoid (thyrohyoid), as in the early phase of swallowing; and (3) depress the larynx, leaving the hyoid in position (sternothyroid), as in the last phase of swallowing.

See Clinical Application 6.1 for the practical implications of the anatomy discussed in this chapter.

CLINICAL APPLICATION 6.1 Carotid artery stenosis

A 75-year-old woman was brought to the hospital by relatives, with a history of disorientation and memory loss. On examination, the woman was well oriented in time and space, and could recall events that occurred in the distant past, as well as events that occurred earlier that day. She, however, recounted that she had no clear recollection of events that happened 2 days ago—the day the relatives reported disorientation. The physician made a tentative diagnosis of transient ischaemic attack and ordered a colour Doppler study.

Study question 1: what is a transient ischaemic attack? (Answer: a sudden, focal loss of neurological function which disappears within 24 hours is a transient ischaemic attack.)

Study question 2: from your knowledge of anatomy, involvement of which vessel could have caused this ischaemia? (Answer: internal carotid artery or vertebral artery. However, disorientation and memory loss is more likely to occur with involvement of the internal carotid artery.)

Colour Doppler of the neck vessels showed stenosis (narrowing) of the internal carotid artery in the neck by an atherosclerotic plaque. A carotid endarterectomy was performed to remove the plaque, and the patient had an uneventful recovery.

Study question 3: what important structures lie close to the internal carotid artery in the neck? (Answer: cranial nerves IX, X, XI, and XII, and the laryngeal and pharyngeal branches of X and XI lie close to the internal carotid artery in the neck. They are bound to the artery by the carotid sheath.)

CHAPTER 7
The back

Introduction to the back

This chapter describes the muscles, vessels, and nerves of the posterior aspect of the trunk, with special attention to the back of the neck. The contents of the vertebral column are discussed separately in Chapter 21.

Back of the neck

Begin the study of this region by reviewing the surface anatomy of the back [Vol. 1, p. 43]. The investing layer of the deep fascia encloses the trapezius and is attached at the midline to the external occipital protuberance, ligamentum nuchae, and spine of the seventh cervical vertebra.

Dissection 7.1 gives instructions on skin reflection and identification of cutaneous nerves of the back.

General arrangement of muscles of the back

The muscles of the back are classified into two groups: the **extrinsic** and **intrinsic** muscles. The extrinsic muscles are posterior (superficial) to the intrinsic muscles and act on the upper limb and rib cage. The muscles acting on the upper limb

---

DISSECTION 7.1 Skin reflection and identification of cutaneous nerves of the back

Objectives

I. To reflect the skin on the back of the neck. **II.** To identify and trace the posterior auricular, greater occipital, and third occipital nerves.

Instructions

1. Make a vertical midline incision through the skin from the external occipital protuberance to the seventh cervical spine. Make a horizontal incision laterally from the lower end of the first incision. Reflect the skin flap, and examine the posterior triangle from behind.

2. Expose the occipital belly of the occipitofrontalis, with the occipital branch of the **posterior auricular nerve** (branch of the facial nerve) running across it near its attachment [Fig. 7.1].

3. Find a branch of the occipital artery on the back of the scalp, and a branch of the greater occipital nerve beside it. Trace both downwards to the main stem of the nerve and artery. The **greater occipital nerve** pierces the deep fascia 2–3 cm lateral to the external occipital protuberance with the occipital artery [Fig. 7.1].

4. The **third occipital nerve** lies in the superficial fascia, medial to the greater occipital nerve. Find and follow it in both directions. Like the cutaneous branches of the other cervical dorsal rami, it pierces the trapezius and the deep fascia close to the midline.

5. Remove the superficial and deep fascia from the surface of the trapezius.

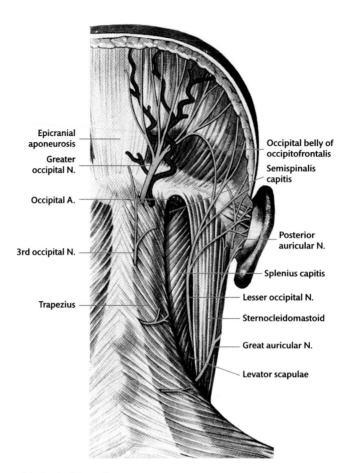

Epicranial aponeurosis

Greater occipital N.

Occipital A.

3rd occipital N.

Trapezius

Occipital belly of occipitofrontalis

Semispinalis capitis

Posterior auricular N.

Splenius capitis

Lesser occipital N.

Sternocleidomastoid

Great auricular N.

Levator scapulae

Fig. 7.1 Superficial structures of the back of the neck.

are the trapezius, latissimus dorsi, levator scapulae, and rhomboids major and minor. The muscles acting on the rib cage are the serratus posterior superior and serratus posterior inferior.

The intrinsic muscles of the back are confined to the back and are supplied by the dorsal rami of the spinal nerves. They include the splenius, erector spinae, semispinalis, and muscles of the suboccipital triangle. They are arranged in layers [Table 7.1]. The interspinales are short muscles which extend between adjacent spinous processes, and the intertransversarii extend between adjacent transverse processes. Detailed dissection and description of all the muscles of the back is beyond the scope of this book.

Extrinsic muscles

The upper limb muscles on the back are described in Vol. 1, Chapter 4. The cervical parts of the trapezius, levator scapulae, and serratus posterior superior and inferior are described here.

Table 7.1 Intrinsic muscles of the back

Layer	Muscles
Superficial layer	Splenius
Intermediate layer (erector spinae)	i. Spinalis
	ii. Longissimus
	iii. Iliocostalis
Deep layer (spinotransverse group)	i. Rotators
	ii. Multifidus
	iii. Semispinalis

Trapezius

The trapezius arises from the medial third of the superior nuchal line, external occipital protuberance, ligamentum nuchae, spines of the seventh cervical, and all the thoracic vertebrae. At the cervicothoracic junction, it arises from an aponeurosis which spreads laterally into the muscle [see Fig. 4.4, Vol. 1].

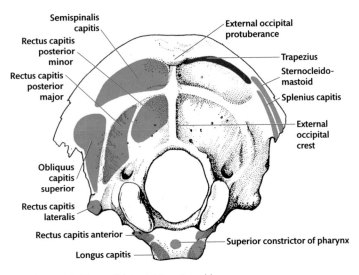

Fig. 7.2 Muscle attachments to the occipital bone. Origin, red; insertions, blue.

The upper fibres run downwards and laterally, and are inserted into the lateral third of the clavicle. They form the slope of the shoulder. The middle fibres run horizontally to the medial edge of the acromion and the lateral part of the superior margin of the crest of the spine of the scapula. The lower fibres run upwards and laterally to the superior margin of the crest of the spine of the scapula [Figs. 7.1, 7.2].

Nerve supply: motor fibres are from the spinal accessory nerve—the eleventh cranial nerve. Sensory fibres are from the third and fourth cervical nerves. **Actions:** the middle fibres pull the scapula medially, bracing the shoulder backwards. The upper fibres elevate the scapula. The lower fibres depress the medial part of the scapula. Acting together, the upper and lower parts rotate the scapula laterally, turning the glenoid cavity upwards, as in raising the arm above the head. The trapezius also extends the head on the neck.

Using the instructions given in Dissection 7.2, complete the superficial dissection of the neck.

Levator scapulae

The levator scapulae arise from the transverse processes of the upper four cervical vertebrae. It descends as two or more slips and is inserted into the medial border of the scapula from the upper angle to the spine of the scapula [see Fig. 4.4, Vol. 1].

Nerve supply: ventral rami of the third and fourth cervical nerves and the dorsal scapular nerve. **Actions**: elevation and medial rotation of

---

DISSECTION 7.2 Superficial dissection of the back of the neck

Objectives

I. To reflect the trapezius and trace the vessels and nerves deep to it. **II.** To reflect the levator scapulae and trace the vessels and nerves deep to it.

Instructions

1. Reflect the trapezius laterally by separating it from the superior nuchal line and dividing it vertically 1 cm from the vertebral spines.

2. Find the accessory nerve on its deep surface with the branches from the third and fourth cervical nerves. Find the superficial cervical artery which runs with the accessory nerve.

3. Define the attachments of the levator scapulae, and follow the deep cervical artery and the dorsal scapular nerve on its deep surface.

---

the scapula. It also helps to hold the scapula steady in movements of the upper limb.

Serratus posterior muscles

The serratus posterior muscles are exposed when the trapezius, latissimus dorsi, and rhomboid muscles are removed and the scapula is pulled laterally. They are thin musculo-aponeurotic sheets on the back of the thorax.

The serratus posterior superior runs inferolaterally from the seventh cervical and upper two or three thoracic spines to the second to fifth ribs.

The serratus posterior inferior passes superolaterally from the lumbar fascia and the lower two thoracic spines to the last four ribs.

Nerve supply: the serratus posterior superior receives branches from the second to fourth intercostal nerves. The serratus posterior inferior receives branches from the lower intercostal and subcostal nerves. **Actions**: both muscles are inspiratory muscles; the superior elevates the upper ribs, and the inferior holds down the lower ribs against the pull of the diaphragm.

Intrinsic muscles

Using the instructions given in Dissection 7.3, identify some of the intrinsic muscles.

Superficial layer–splenius

The splenius is most superficially placed among the intrinsic muscles of the back. It covers the deeper muscles of the neck like a blanket. It arises from the lower part of the ligamentum nuchae, the spines of the seventh cervical and upper six thoracic vertebrae. The muscle fibres run superolaterally, and the lower fibres—the **splenius cervicis**—are inserted into the transverse processes of the upper two or three cervical vertebrae, deep to the levator scapulae. The upper fibres—the **splenius capitis**—are inserted into the lower part of the mastoid process and the lateral part of the superior nuchal line, deep to the sternocleidomastoid [Figs. 7.1, 7.2, 7.3, 7.4].

Nerve supply: the dorsal rami of the cervical nerves which pierce it. **Actions**: acting together, the muscles of both sides extend the neck and the head on it. Acting on one side only, the splenius turns the face to the same side.

Intermediate layer–erector spinae and thoracolumbar fascia

Thoracolumbar fascia

The thoracolumbar fascia is a strong aponeurotic layer which extends from the ilium and dorsal surface of the sacrum to the upper thoracic region. It binds down the erector spinae group of muscles and is particularly thick in the lumbar and sacral regions [Vol. 2, Chapter 10].

The thoracic part of this fascia is relatively thin and transparent. It extends from the tip of the spine of the vertebrae and supraspinous ligaments to the angles of the ribs. Superiorly, the fascia passes deep to the serratus posterior superior and fades out into the neck. Inferiorly, it is continuous with the posterior layer of the lumbar part, deep to the serratus posterior inferior [Fig. 7.5].

Erector spinae

The major part of the erector spinae muscle takes origin from the sacrum and ascends into the lumbar, thoracic, and cervical regions [Fig. 7.3]. It fills the space between the spines and transverse processes of the vertebrae and splits into three vertical columns of muscles. From lateral to medial, the three columns are: the **iliocostalis**, **longissimus**,

---

DISSECTION 7.3 Intrinsic muscles of the back-1

Objective

I. To identify the splenius, erector spinae, semispinalis, and longissimus [Fig. 7.3].

Instructions

1. Reflect the serratus posterior superior, and find the nerves entering its deep surface.

2. Remove the thoracic part of the thoracolumbar fascia to expose the longitudinal erector spinae muscles, with the splenius curving superolaterally across it above the mid-thoracic region.

3. Define the attachments of the splenius, and find the nerves piercing it. Then separate the splenius from the vertebral spines, and turn it superolaterally.

4. Remove the thoracic part of the thoracolumbar fascia to expose the erector spinae muscles.

5. Examine the semispinalis (part of the spinotransverse group of muscles) and longissimus muscles (part of the erector spinae).

6. Identify the part of the obliquus capitis superior which is exposed.

7. Detach the sternocleidomastoid from the superior nuchal line, and expose the insertion of the splenius capitis.

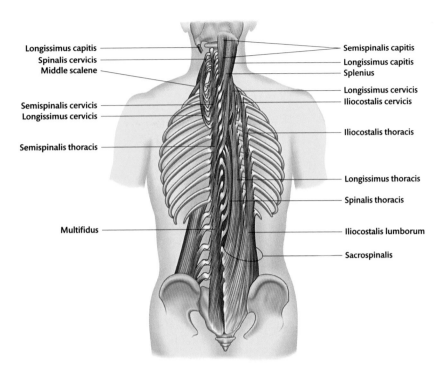

Longissimus capitis
Spinalis cervicis
Middle scalene

Semispinalis cervicis
Longissimus cervicis

Semispinalis thoracis

Multifidus

Semispinalis capitis
Longissimus capitis
Splenius
Longissimus cervicis
Iliocostalis cervicis

Iliocostalis thoracis

Longissimus thoracis
Spinalis thoracis

Iliocostalis lumborum
Sacrospinalis

Fig. 7.3 Intrinsic muscles of the back.

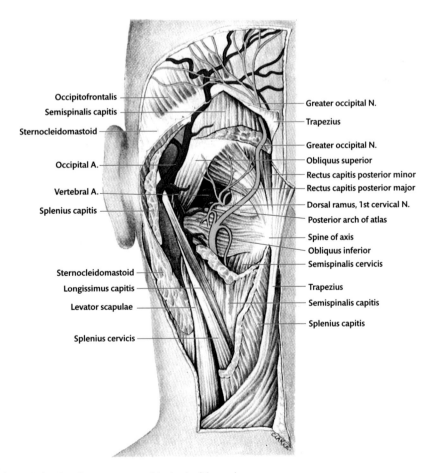

Occipitofrontalis
Semispinalis capitis
Sternocleidomastoid

Occipital A.

Vertebral A.
Splenius capitis

Sternocleidomastoid
Longissimus capitis
Levator scapulae

Splenius cervicis

Greater occipital N.
Trapezius
Greater occipital N.
Obliquus superior
Rectus capitis posterior minor
Rectus capitis posterior major
Dorsal ramus, 1st cervical N.
Posterior arch of atlas
Spine of axis
Obliquus inferior
Semispinalis cervicis
Trapezius
Semispinalis capitis
Splenius capitis

Fig. 7.4 The suboccipital region. Deep structures of the back of the neck.

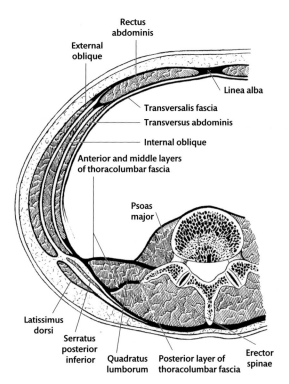

Rectus abdominis

External oblique

Linea alba

Transversalis fascia

Transversus abdominis

Internal oblique

Anterior and middle layers of thoracolumbar fascia

Psoas major

Latissimus dorsi

Serratus posterior inferior

Quadratus lumborum

Posterior layer of thoracolumbar fascia

Erector spinae

Fig. 7.5 Diagram of a section through the abdominal wall at the level of the second lumbar vertebra to show the arrangement of the thoracolumbar fascia.

and **spinalis**. The iliocostalis is inserted into the lower ribs and cervical transverse processes. The longissimus is inserted into the cervical transverse processes and the mastoid process. The spinalis is inserted into the spinous process. At the insertion into the spine and transverse process, fresh slips arise from the same situations and continue

upwards. The longissimus cervicis and capitis are described in further detail below.

Deep layer

Deep to the erector spinae are the muscles which connect the sacrum with the transverse processes, laminae, and spines. They are known as the **spinotransverse muscles** and include the **semispinalis**, **multifidus**, and **rotatores** [Fig. 7.3]. The semispinalis cervicis and capitis are described in further detail [p. 69].

Nerve supply: dorsal rami of spinal nerves. **Actions**: these muscles act on the vertebral column to bring about: (1) extension; (2) rotation; and (3) lateral flexion. In addition, they help to balance the vertebral column on the pelvis and maintain erect posture during all movements.

Using the instructions given in Dissection 7.4, dissect the semispinalis, longissimus, and suboccipital muscles.

Longissimus

This slender muscle is part of the erector spinae. In the neck, it lies under cover of the splenius, immediately posterior to the transverse processes [Fig. 7.3]. It has two parts—the **longissimus cervicis** and **longissimus capitis**. The longissimus takes origin from the upper thoracic transverse processes. The longissimus capitis is inserted to the back of the mastoid process under cover of the splenius and sternocleidomastoid. The longissimus cervicis lies anterior to the longissimus capitis. It

---

DISSECTION 7.4 Intrinsic muscles of the back-2

Objectives

I. To expose the semispinalis and longissimus and study their attachments.   **II.** To identify and trace the occipital and deep cervical arteries.   **III.** To identify the suboccipital muscles.

Instructions

1. Remove the fascia from the semispinalis capitis and from the longissimus. (Do not disturb the nerves which pierce the semispinalis close to the midline.)

2. Determine the attachments of these muscles.

3. Reflect the longissimus capitis from the skull, and follow the occipital artery deep to the mastoid process over the obliquus capitis superior.

4. Trace the obliquus capitis superior to the transverse process of the atlas and to the skull [Fig. 7.4].

5. Detach the semispinalis capitis from the occipital bone, and turn it laterally, preserving the nerves which pierce it.

6. Identify the suboccipital muscles and semispinalis cervicis, with the dorsal rami running over them.

7. Identify the **deep cervical artery** ascending on the semispinalis capitis to anastomose with the occipital artery. (If a branch from the first cervical dorsal ramus enters the semispinalis capitis, it should be retained by cutting out a piece of the muscle with the nerve, as this makes the dissection of that ramus much easier.)

8. Define the attachments of the semispinalis cervicis.

is inserted into the posterior surfaces of the cervical transverse processes of C. 2–C. 7 vertebrae.

Occipital artery

The occipital artery arises from the external carotid artery in the front of the neck. It runs posterosuperiorly deep to the posterior belly of the digastric. It grooves the skull deep to the mastoid notch and the insertion of the posterior belly of the digastric. It then passes posteriorly immediately deep to the muscles attached to the superior nuchal line, crosses the apex of the posterior triangle, and pierces the trapezius 2–3 cm from the midline with the greater occipital nerve. It ramifies on the back of the head, supplying the posterior half of the scalp [Fig. 7.1].

Branches: in the back, the artery gives off mainly (1) muscular branches. In addition, it gives: (2) a mastoid branch which enters the mastoid foramen to supply the bone and dura mater; and (3) a descending branch which passes deep to the semispinalis capitis and anastomoses with the deep cervical branch of the subclavian artery.

Semispinalis capitis

This long muscle is part of the deep layer. It produces the rounded ridge on either side of the median furrow in the back of the neck, even though it is deep to the trapezius and splenius. It has the same origin as the longissimus capitis—the upper thoracic transverse processes—and is inserted into the medial half of the area between the superior and inferior nuchal lines [Figs. 7.2, 7.3, 7.4].

Nerve supply: dorsal rami of the upper cervical nerves. **Action**: it extends the neck and the head on the neck.

Semispinalis cervicis

This bulky muscle lies deep to the semispinalis capitis and has the same origin—the upper thoracic transverse procceses. It passes superomedially to the spines of the second to fifth cervical vertebrae, principally the second—a feature which partly accounts for the size of the spine of the axis.

Ligamentum nuchae

The ligamentum nuchae is a median fibrous septum between the muscles of the back of the neck. It is a continuation of the supraspinous and interspinous ligaments uniting the cervical vertebrae. It extends from the spine of the seventh cervical vertebra to the external occipital protuberance and crest. Anteriorly, it is attached to the posterior tubercle of the atlas and the spines of the other cervical vertebrae [Fig. 7.6].

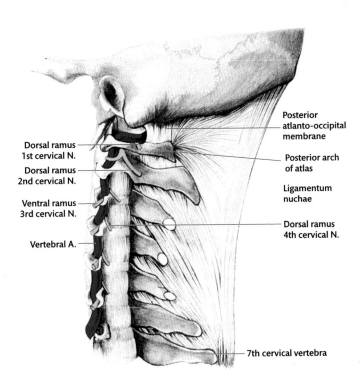

Fig. 7.6 Dissection of the ligamentum nuchae and of the vertebral artery in the neck. The neck is slightly flexed.

Deep cervical artery

The deep cervical artery arises from the costocervical trunk of the subclavian artery. It passes into the back of the neck between the seventh cervical transverse process and the neck of the first rib. It ascends deep to the semispinalis capitis and anastomoses with the descending branch of the occipital artery [see Fig. 9.8].

Suboccipital triangle

This small intermuscular triangle is formed by the **rectus capitis posterior major** superomedially, the **obliquus capitis inferior** inferiorly, and the **obliquus capitis superior** superolaterally. The **rectus capitis posterior minor** lies medial to the major. These muscles hold the skull to the axis and atlas. The triangle is roofed over by the semispinalis capitis and crossed by the greater occipital nerve, which hooks around the lower border of the obliquus capitis inferior. The floor of the triangle is formed by the posterior atlanto-occipital membrane and the posterior arch of the atlas, with the first cervical nerve and the vertebral artery lying on it. The dorsal ramus of the first cervical nerve enters the triangle. The triangle contains the suboccipital plexus of veins which drain to the vertebral and deep cervical veins [Fig. 7.4].

Using the instructions given in Dissection 7.5, dissect the suboccipital triangle.

Dorsal ramus of the first cervical (suboccipital) nerve

The dorsal ramus of the first cervical nerve emerges from the vertebral canal between the posterior arch of the atlas and the vertebral artery. It gives branches to the muscles of the suboccipital triangle—rectus capitis posterior major, rectus capitis posterior minor, obliquus capitis superior, obliquus capitis inferior, and semispinalis capitis—and a communicating branch to the greater occipital nerve [Fig. 7.4].

Vertebral artery

The third part of the vertebral artery leaves the foramen transversarium of the atlas and hooks posteromedially on the posterior surface of the lateral mass of the atlas. It grooves the lateral mass and the lateral part of the posterior arch of the atlas. It passes anterior to the thickened lateral edge of the

DISSECTION 7.5 Suboccipital triangle

Objectives

I. To identify the dorsal ramus of the first cervical nerve.
II. To expose the muscles of the suboccipital triangle.

Instructions

1. Identify the dorsal ramus of the first cervical nerve, as it emerges between the vertebral artery and the posterior arch of the atlas. (The suboccipital triangle is difficult to dissect because of the dense fibrous tissue in it. If the branch of the dorsal ramus of the first cervical nerve to the semispinalis capitis has been retained, it can be followed to the ramus and the other branches traced from there. Alternatively, a communicating branch to the greater occipital nerve or the branch to one of the muscles of the triangle may be found and followed.)

2. Remove the fascia from the triangle and the surrounding muscles.

posterior atlanto-occipital membrane and enters the vertebral canal [Figs. 7.4, 7.6; see Figs. 8.15, 9.8].

Suboccipital plexus of veins

The suboccipital plexus of veins lies in and around the suboccipital triangle. It forms a route of communication between the occipital veins, the internal vertebral venous plexuses [see Fig. 13.8, Vol. 2], an emissary vein from the sigmoid sinus, muscular veins, the deep cervical vein, and the plexus of veins around the vertebral artery. As it unites many different veins, it provides a number of alternative routes for venous drainage when any of the venous channels are blocked.

Suboccipital muscles

The following four muscles attach the atlas and axis to the occiput and stabilize the head on the cervical vertebra. The first three form the boundaries of the suboccipital triangle.

The **rectus capitis posterior major** passes superolaterally from its origin on the spine of the axis to the lateral half of the area below the inferior nuchal line on the occiput [Figs. 7.2, 7.4].

The **obliquus capitis inferior** takes origin from the spine of the axis and is inserted into the transverse process of the atlas [Figs. 7.2, 7.4].

The **obliquus capitis superior** runs posterosuperiorly from its origin on the transverse process of the atlas and to the lateral half of the area between the superior and inferior nuchal lines [Figs. 7.2, 7.4].

The **rectus capitis posterior minor** passes from its origin on the tubercle of the posterior arch of the atlas to the insertion on the medial part of the area below the inferior nuchal line, under cover of the rectus capitis posterior major [Figs. 7.2, 7.4].

Nerve supply: the dorsal ramus of C. 1. **Action**: the main function of these muscles is to stabilize the head on the atlas and axis, by acting as ligaments of variable length and tension.

Dorsal rami of spinal nerves

The dorsal rami of the spinal nerves are the nerves of the back. They supply the intervertebral joints, ligaments and muscles of the back (but not the muscles of the upper limb which extend over the back), and the overlying skin.

The general arrangement and distribution of the dorsal rami follow the pattern shown in Fig. 7.7, with the following exceptions.

1. The first cervical, fourth and fifth sacral, and coccygeal nerves do not divide into medial and lateral branches.
2. The dorsal rami of the first and last two cervical (sometimes C. 5 and 6, or C. 6 and 7) and the last two lumbar nerves do not have cutaneous branches.
3. Above the mid-thoracic region, the cutaneous branches arise from the medial branches of the dorsal rami and emerge close to the midline (2–3 cm). Below the mid-thoracic region, the cutaneous branches arise from the lateral branches and emerge 8–9 cm from the midline (in line with the angles of the ribs) [see Fig. 4.4, Vol. 1]. The cutaneous branches of the small dorsal rami of the sacral nerves emerge on an imaginary line between the posterior superior iliac spine and the tip of the coccyx.
4. The cutaneous branches of some dorsal rami are large and supply an extended area of skin. The dorsal rami of C. 2 (greater occipital nerve) supplies a large part of the scalp. Those of T. 1 and 2 extend laterally over the scapula. Those of L. 1, 2, and 3 extend over the buttock to the level of the greater trochanter. It is almost as if the territory of these nerves were pulled out by the growing head and limbs.
5. The upper cervical dorsal rami and the sacral dorsal rami form simple looped plexuses. The cervical plexus is deep to the semispinalis capitis, and the sacral plexus is deep to the gluteus maximus.

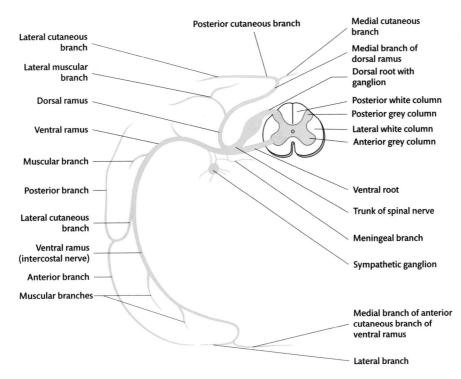

Fig. 7.7 Diagram of a typical spinal nerve.

Lateral cutaneous branch
Lateral muscular branch
Dorsal ramus
Ventral ramus
Muscular branch
Posterior branch
Lateral cutaneous branch
Ventral ramus (intercostal nerve)
Anterior branch
Muscular branches

Posterior cutaneous branch

Medial cutaneous branch
Medial branch of dorsal ramus
Dorsal root with ganglion
Posterior white column
Posterior grey column
Lateral white column
Anterior grey column
Ventral root
Trunk of spinal nerve
Meningeal branch
Sympathetic ganglion
Medial branch of anterior cutaneous branch of ventral ramus
Lateral branch

Greater occipital nerve

The **greater occipital nerve** is the cutaneous branch of the dorsal ramus of C. 2. It is the thickest cutaneous nerve in the body. It emerges below the middle of the obliquus capitis inferior, curves superomedially across the suboccipital triangle, and pierces the semispinalis capitis. It ascends on the semispinalis capitis, pierces the trapezius 2–3 cm lateral to the external occipital protuberance, and spreads out on the back of the scalp, reaching as far as the vertex. Though it is mainly cutaneous, it also supplies the semispinalis capitis [see Fig. 4.9; Figs. 7.1, 7.4].

Third occipital nerve

The third occipital nerve is the small cutaneous branch of the dorsal ramus of C. 3. It pierces the semispinalis capitis and trapezius, and supplies the skin at the back of the neck up to the external occipital protuberance [Fig. 7.1].

Arteries of the back

Arteries of the cervical region

The main arterial supply to the cervical region comes from the **deep cervical** branch of the costocervical trunk of the subclavian artery. It anastomoses with the descending branch of the **occipital artery** deep to the semispinalis capitis, and with the **superficial cervical artery**. In addition, small branches of the vertebral artery supply the muscles of the back of the neck.

In the thorax, the posterior branches of the **intercostal arteries** supply the muscles and skin of the back, together with branches from the deep cervical artery.

Posterior branches of the lumbar arteries supply the back in the lumbar region.

Veins of the back

The veins follow the corresponding arteries. They drain into the vertebral and deep cervical veins in the neck, and to the intercostal and lumbar veins in the thoracic and lumbar regions. These veins are also linked to the posterior vertebral and internal vertebral venous plexuses.

The extensive **posterior vertebral venous plexus** lies posterior to the vertebral arches. It drains the veins of the back into the vessels indicated above.

See Clinical Application 7.1 for the practical implications of the anatomy discussed in this chapter.

CLINICAL APPLICATION 7.1 Occipital neuralgia

Occipital neuralgia is a form of headache characterized by severe pain that begins in the upper neck and back of the head. This pain is typically one-sided and can be throbbing, aching, or sharp and stabbing. It is in the distribution of the occipital nerves.

Study question 1: name the sensory nerves which supply the upper part of the neck and back of the head, and give their root values. (Answer: greater occipital nerve; dorsal ramus of C. 2. Third occipital nerve; dorsal ramus of C. 3. A portion of the back of the head near the auricle is supplied by the lesser occipital nerve; ventral ramus of C. 2.) The cause of occipital neuralgia is poorly understood. It is thought to result from irritation or inflammation of the C. 2 fibres by arthritis of the atlanto-axial joint, or entrapment of the nerve in muscles or surrounding fascia.

CHAPTER 8
The cranial cavity

Introduction

In this chapter, the soft tissue structures seen on the interior of the cranium after removing the brain are described. The sutural ligaments and endosteum of the skull are also described.

Start the study of this region by removing the skull cap, as described in Dissection 8.1.

Skull cap or calvaria

Sutural ligaments

The periosteum on the external surface of the skull is continuous with the endosteal layer of the dura mater on the internal surface, through sutural ligaments at the sutures. These ligaments hold the

---

DISSECTION 8.1 Removal of the skull cap

Objective

I. To remove the skull cap in preparation to expose the brain.

Instructions

1. Support the head on a block, and make a sagittal cut through the epicranial aponeurosis from the root of the nose to the external occipital protuberance. Pull each half of the scalp laterally, and detach it from the temporal lines.

2. Strip the periosteum (**pericranium**) from the external surface of the vault of the skull down to a level of the upper attachment of the temporalis muscle [see Fig. 4.10]. (At the **sutures**, it will be necessary to cut through the periosteum which is continuous through the sutures with the dura lining the interior of the skull.)

3. Turn the scalp, periosteum, and upper parts of the temporalis muscles down over the auricles.

4. To remove the skull cap, or **calvaria**, first make a horizontal mark on the skull by encircling it with a piece of string. The line should pass no more than 1 cm above the orbital margins and external occipital protuberance.

5. Using a saw, cut along this line, but avoid cutting deeper than the marrow cavity. (You will know when you reach the marrow cavity as the sawdust will turn red.) The outer table of the skull has now been divided. In the temporal region, the skull is very thin and there may be no **marrow cavity** (**diploë**), so proceed with caution.

6. Introduce a blunt chisel into the saw cut, and split the inner table by a series of short, sharp taps with a hammer. Even when the inner table is broken, the calvaria will not lift free because it is firmly adherent to the underlying dura mater.

7. Introduce the thick part of the chisel into the cut, and force the skull cap upwards. The dura will tear away from the skull, taking the vessels of the skull with them.

8. Examine the calvaria.

bones together and allow growth between them. Starting at the third to fourth decades of life, the adjacent skull bones unite by ossification of the sutural ligaments—a process known as **synostosis**. This process begins at the internal surface [see Figs. 3.2, 3.8].

The meninges

The entire central nervous system (the brain and spinal cord) is enclosed in three membranes or meninges—the dura mater, the arachnoid, and the pia mater. The membranes are separated from each other by two spaces—the subdural and subarachnoid spaces [Fig. 8.1].

Dura mater

This outermost layer of meninges is a thick fibrous layer. In the cranium, the dura mater has an inner or **meningeal layer**, and an outer or **endosteal layer**. The meningeal layer covers the brain, and the endosteal layer is adherent to the surrounding bone.

When the skull cap is detached, the outer surface of the endosteal layer is exposed. It is rough because of the fine fibrous and vascular processes which pass between this layer and the bones. Torn blood vessels are most numerous, close to the midline where one of the largest intracranial venous channels—the superior sagittal sinus—lies deep to the endocranium. If a blunt instrument is pressed

on the sinus, blood oozes from the numerous small veins which have been ruptured. The endosteal layer is more firmly attached to the base of the cranial cavity than to the vault, with the degree of adhesion varying with age and from individual to individual.

A number of branching vessels ascend on the outer surface of the dura mater towards the vertex. These are the branches of the **middle meningeal artery**. The corresponding veins lie on the external surface of the artery. They groove the inner table of the skull and stand out on the surface of the dura. These vessels supply the skull (particularly the red bone marrow in its diploë) and the dura mater which is fused to its internal surface. The meningeal vessels do not supply the pia-arachnoid or the brain itself.

The two layers of the dura are firmly adherent to each other, except: (1) where the meningeal layer forms rigid folds or partitions between the major parts of the brain (these folds incompletely subdivide the cranial cavity and support the brain); and (2) where the venous sinuses of the dura mater lie between the endosteal and meningeal layers [Fig. 8.2]. At the foramen magnum, the spinal dura fuses with the meningeal layer of the cranial dura.

The internal surface of the dura mater is smooth and glistening. It is separated from the equally smooth external surface of the arachnoid by a capillary interval—the **subdural space**. This space encloses the brain and spinal cord, except at a few points. It is absent where structures pierce the meninges to enter or leave the brain and spinal cord, and where arachnoid villi [p. 76] are present. The space allows movement between the dura and the structures it encloses.

The arachnoid and subarachnoid space

The arachnoid and pia mater lie inside the dura mater and develop from a single mass of loose connective tissue immediately surrounding the central nervous system. The two layers are separated by the subarachnoid space. The arachnoid mater is applied to the inner surface of the dura mater, and the pia mater is applied to the outer surface of the central nervous system [Fig. 8.1]. Cerebrospinal fluid (CSF) from the cavities of the brain circulates in the subarachnoid space. Strands of tissue—the **trabeculae**—extend between the arachnoid and the pia. In places where the arachnoid and pia are close together, the trabeculae are numerous so that

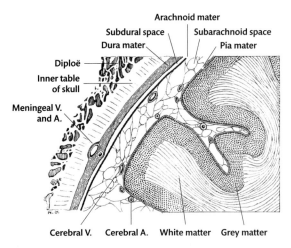

Arachnoid mater
Subdural space   Subarachnoid space
Dura mater   Pia mater
Diploë
Inner table of skull
Meningeal V. and A.

Cerebral V.   Cerebral A.   White matter   Grey matter

Fig. 8.1 Diagrammatic section to show the relation of the meninges to the skull and brain. Note that the meningeal vessels lie on the external surface of the dura mater, are in the endocranium, while the cerebral vessels lie in the subarachnoid space.

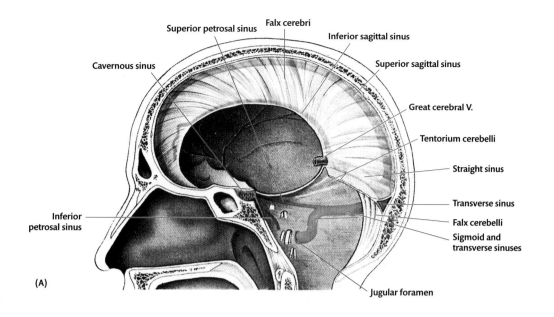

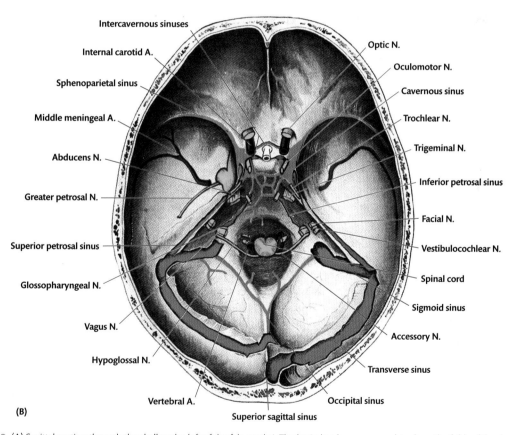

Fig. 8.2 (A) Sagittal section through the skull to the left of the falx cerebri. The brain has been removed to show the folds of the dura mater which incompletely partition the cranial cavity. (B) Dissection of the floor of the cranial cavity after removal of the brain.

the subarachnoid space forms a fluid-filled sponge protecting the brain. Where the meningeal layers are more widely separated, the trabeculae are usually fewer and a simple fluid-filled space results. Such larger subarachnoid spaces are known as **cisterns**.

The **arachnoid** is a thin, transparent, avascular membrane, with trabeculae passing to the pia

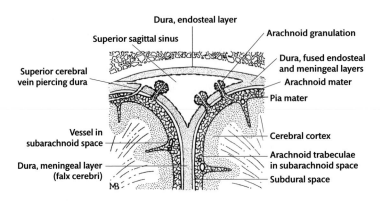

Fig. 8.3 Diagrammatic transverse section through the superior sagittal sinus and surrounding brain.

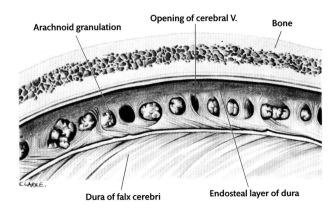

Fig. 8.4 Median section through the skull and superior sagittal sinus. Note the arachnoid granulations protruding into the sinus.

mater from its deep surface. In a few places, notably at the superior sagittal sinus, the arachnoid pierces the dura as a number of finger-like or cauliflower-shaped projections. The finger-like projections are **arachnoid villi**; the more bulbous ones are **arachnoid granulations** [Figs. 8.3, 8.4]. At the tip of the arachnoid villi are perforations through which the subarachnoid space communicates with the venous sinus [p. 77]. Like the dura, the arachnoid extends along the nerves which arise from the central nervous system for a short distance, before becoming continuous with the **epineurium**.

Pia mater

The pia mater is a vascular membrane which covers the surface of the central nervous system and follows most of the irregularities of the surface [Fig. 8.1]. The pia mater is thicker than the arachnoid, especially on the spinal cord and the medulla oblongata of the brain. The blood vessels of the central nervous system lie on the external surface of the pia mater. Their branches carry a sleeve of the pia mater and an extension of the subarachnoid space with them for a short distance into the central nervous system. This space is the **perivascular space**. Also, each rootlet of nerves entering or leaving the brain carries an extension of the pia mater as it crosses the subarachnoid space. These extensions become continuous with the perineurium of the nerves. Another modification of the pia mater—the **ligamentum denticulatum** of the spinal cord—is described in Chapter 21.

Cerebrospinal fluid

CSF is produced by the **choroid plexuses** in the cavities of the brain (the ventricles). The CSF leaves the ventricular system from the fourth ventricle and enters the subarachnoid space.

Using the instructions given in Dissection 8.2, open the superior sagittal sinus.

DISSECTION 8.2 Exploration of the superior sagittal sinus

Objective

I. To open the superior sagittal sinus.

Instructions

1. Make a median sagittal incision through the endocranium, and open the superior sagittal sinus as far as possible.

Structure of dural venous sinuses

Dural venous sinuses are venous channels lined with endothelium. Use Figs. 8.2A and B to identify the superior and inferior sagittal sinuses, straight sinus, transverse sinuses, sigmoid sinuses, and cavernous sinuses. Most of the sinuses lie between the endosteal layer of the dura externally and the meningeal layer internally. Two sinuses—the straight and inferior sagittal sinuses—are entirely enclosed in the meningeal layers of the dura which passes between the parts of the brain. The dural venous sinuses drain the nervous system and the surrounding bone, and communicate with the external veins through many foramina. There are no valves in this system, so blood can flow in either direction depending on the pressure gradient. The sinuses drain eventually to the internal jugular veins. Most of the sinuses form shallow grooves on the internal surface of the cranial cavity [see Figs. 3.8, 3.9].

The dural venous sinuses also drain the CSF through the arachnoid villi and granulations in the superior sagittal sinus and its lateral lacunae.

Arachnoid villi and granulations

These small, granular bodies lie along the sides of the superior sagittal sinus. They are protrusions of the arachnoid mater through the dura into the superior sagittal sinus and its lateral lacunae [Figs. 8.3, 8.4]. The granulations are normal enlargements of the arachnoid villi which are smaller and finger-shaped. In the elderly, the arachnoid granulations may reach considerable proportions and even erode the inner table of the skull. Small perforations on the surface of the arachnoid villi and granulations allow for the passage of CSF from the subarachnoid space into the superior sagittal sinus. (At the same time, they prevent the reflux of blood into the subarachnoid space.) ➲ Clotting of blood in the superior sagittal sinus blocks the drainage of CSF and causes a rapid rise in intracranial pressure due to the build-up of CSF.

Using the instructions given in Dissection 8.3, cut through the dura and open into the subdural space.

Superior cerebral veins

These extremely thin-walled veins lie in the subarachnoid space immediately superficial to the pia mater. (The meningeal veins lie superficial to the dura.) They run upwards towards the midline and converge on the superior sagittal sinus [see Fig. 26.1]. They have a short course in the subdural space before piercing the dura to enter the sinus [Fig. 8.3].

DISSECTION 8.3 Reflection of the dura

Objective

I. To cut and reflect the dura covering the brain.

Instructions

1. Make two longitudinal incisions through the dura mater along each side of the superior sagittal sinus. From the midpoint of each incision, make another incision down to the cut edge of the skull above the auricle. As these cuts are made, raise the dura to avoid incising the underlying arachnoid, pia, and brain.

2. Turn the four flaps of dura down over the cut edges of the skull, to avoid its sharp edges injuring the brain or your fingers during subsequent dissection.

3. The subdural space is now opened and should be examined.

4. Examine the pia-arachnoid and blood vessels on the upper parts of the cerebral hemispheres now exposed.

Objective

I. To expose the falx cerebri.

Instructions

1. Expose the falx cerebri by dividing the superior cerebral veins on one side, and displacing the upper part of that cerebral hemisphere laterally.

Superior sagittal sinus

The superior sagittal sinus begins anteriorly at the crista galli. At the origin, it communicates with the veins of the frontal sinus and the veins of the nose, through the foramen caecum. The sinus runs posteriorly, forming a median groove on the cranial vault. It becomes continuous with the right transverse sinus at the internal occipital protuberance [Fig. 8.2].

Lateral lacunae

Lateral lacunae are cleft-like lateral extensions of the superior sagittal sinus, between the endosteal and meningeal layers of the dura mater. The largest lacuna is 2–3 cm in diameter and overlies the upper part of the motor area of the brain. Lacunae and arachnoid granulations both increase in size with age and may produce shallow depressions in the skull vault on both sides of the groove for the superior sagittal sinus.

Expose the falx cerebri following the instructions provided in Dissection 8.4.

Falx cerebri

The falx cerebri is a median, sickle-shaped fold of the dura mater, which lies between the two cerebral hemispheres. The superior margin of the falx is attached to the lips of the groove for the superior sagittal sinus on the calvaria. Anteriorly, the falx is narrow and attached to the crista galli. Posteriorly, it increases in depth and becomes continuous with the upper surface of the tentorium cerebelli—an approximately horizontal fold of the dura mater. (The tentorium cerebelli lies between the posterior parts of the cerebral hemispheres and the cerebellum [Figs. 8.2A, 8.5, 8.6, 8.7. 8.8].) From this attachment, the falx descends between the two cerebral hemispheres. The lower border of the falx is free and concave, and overhangs the corpus callosum [p. 356]. The **superior sagittal sinus** lies in the fixed upper margin of the falx, and the **inferior sagittal sinus** lies in its free margin. The **straight sinus** lies at the attachment to the falx cerebri to the tentorium cerebelli [Figs. 8.2A, 8.8].

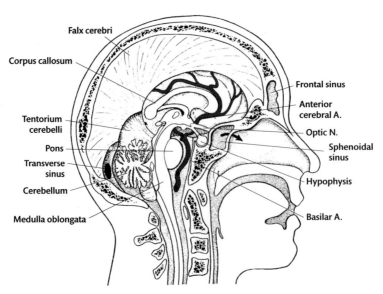

Fig. 8.5 Sagittal section through the head and neck, slightly to the right of the median plane.

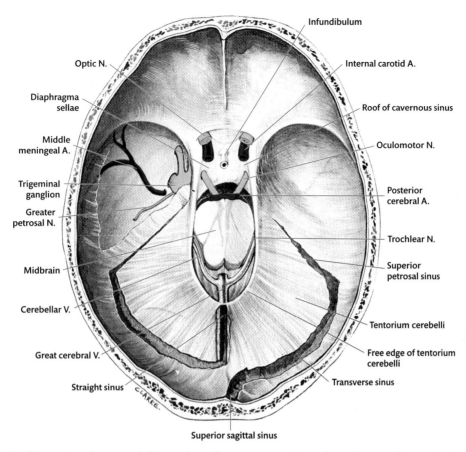

Optic N.

Diaphragma sellae

Middle meningeal A.

Trigeminal ganglion

Greater petrosal N.

Midbrain

Cerebellar V.

Great cerebral V.

Straight sinus

Infundibulum

Internal carotid A.

Roof of cavernous sinus

Oculomotor N.

Posterior cerebral A.

Trochlear N.

Superior petrosal sinus

Tentorium cerebelli

Free edge of tentorium cerebelli

Transverse sinus

CLARKE.

Superior sagittal sinus

Fig. 8.6 Interior of the cranium after removal of the cerebrum. The transverse, straight, and superior petrosal sinuses have been opened, and the dura mater has been removed from the floor of the left middle cranial fossa.

Removal of the brain

Dissection 8.5 provides instructions on how to detach the brain from the base of the skull and remove it.

Structures seen after removal of the cerebrum

With the help of a skull, identify the boundaries of the anterior and middle cranial fossae and the taut, but resilient, tentorium cerebelli [Fig. 8.6].

In the **anterior cranial fossa**, note:

1. The **crista galli** with the falx cerebri attached to it.
2. The **cribriform plate of the ethmoid** which lodges the olfactory bulb. The olfactory nerves pass from the nasal mucosa through the cribriform plate into the olfactory bulb.
3. The **orbital part of the frontal bone** which forms most of the floor of the anterior cranial fos-

sa. It is closely fitted to the irregularities of the orbital surface of the frontal lobe which it separates from the orbit.

4. The **lesser wing of the sphenoid bone**, with the sphenoparietal venous sinus running along its posterior margin towards the **anterior clinoid process**. The free margin of the tentorium is attached to the anterior clinoid process [Figs. 8.2B, 8.6].

In the middle cranial fossa, note:

1. The deep depression for the tip of the temporal lobe of the brain, posterolateral to the orbit.
2. The **middle meningeal vessels** seen through the dural floor of the lateral part of the fossa. Note that there are no branches piercing the dura mater.
3. The **diaphragma sellae** is the raised central area formed by the dura stretched between the four clinoid processes of the sphenoid bone. It is perforated by:
   (i) The **infundibulum** as it passes to the hypophysis.

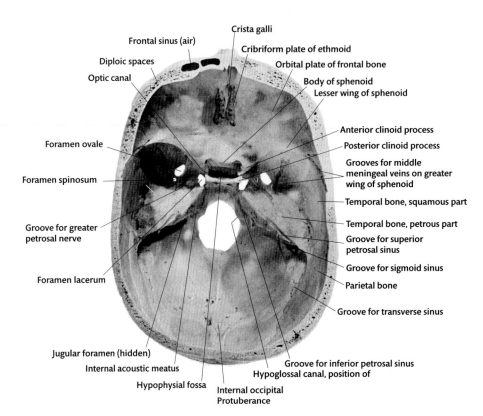

Fig. 8.7 Internal surface of the base of the skull.

Labels (clockwise from top):
Crista galli
Frontal sinus (air)
Cribriform plate of ethmoid
Orbital plate of frontal bone
Body of sphenoid
Lesser wing of sphenoid
Anterior clinoid process
Posterior clinoid process
Grooves for middle meningeal veins on greater wing of sphenoid
Temporal bone, squamous part
Temporal bone, petrous part
Groove for superior petrosal sinus
Groove for sigmoid sinus
Parietal bone
Groove for transverse sinus
Groove for inferior petrosal sinus
Hypoglossal canal, position of
Internal occipital Protuberance
Hypophysial fossa
Internal acoustic meatus
Jugular foramen (hidden)
Foramen lacerum
Groove for greater petrosal nerve
Foramen spinosum
Foramen ovale
Optic canal
Diploic spaces

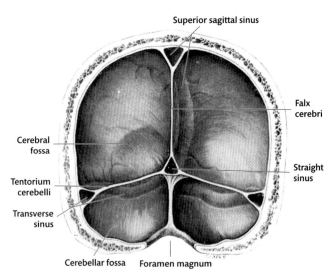

Fig. 8.8 The floor of the cranial cavity after removal of the brain, but with the arteries at the base of the brain *in situ*.

Labels:
Superior sagittal sinus
Falx cerebri
Straight sinus
Cerebral fossa
Tentorium cerebelli
Transverse sinus
Cerebellar fossa
Foramen magnum

(ii) The **oculomotor nerves** as they pierce the dura, medial to the free border of the tentorium.

(iii) The **optic nerves** and **internal carotid arteries** as they pierce the dura, medial to the anterior clinoid processes [Fig. 8.6].

(iv) The **great cerebral vein** at the junction of the free edges of the falx and tentorium [Fig. 8.6].

Tentorium cerebelli

This wide, sloping fold of the dura has a free, curved margin surrounding the midbrain, and

DISSECTION 8.5 Removal of the brain

Objective

I. To remove the brain in one piece.

Instructions

Fig. 8.5 is a sagittal section of the head which shows the relationship of the main parts of the brain to the dural folds and the base of the brain. Identify the cerebrum (largely hidden by the falx cerebri), cerebellum, pons, and medulla on this section prior to starting the dissection.

1. Detach the falx cerebri from the crista galli, and pull the falx up posteriorly from between the hemispheres.

2. Place a block under the shoulders to allow the head to fall back. This makes the frontal lobes fall away from the anterior cranial fossae and exposes the **olfactory bulbs**. Elevate the olfactory bulbs gently from the cribriform plate of the ethmoid, tearing the olfactory nerves which pierce them.

3. The large **optic nerves** then come into view and should be divided close to the optic canal [Fig. 8.6].

4. Step 3 exposes the internal carotid arteries, with the infundibulum passing vertically to the hypophysis between them. Divide all three structures [Fig. 8.6].

5. Allow the brain to fall backwards as each structure is divided, but support it posteriorly so as to avoid damaging it on the skull.

6. Posterior to the infundibulum, identify the dorsum sellae with a posterior clinoid process at each lateral extremity [Fig. 8.6] and the **oculomotor nerves** passing forwards, one on each side of it [Fig. 8.6].

7. Lateral to each oculomotor nerve is the **free edge of the tentorium cerebelli**. Turn the margin of the tentorium laterally, and divide the slender **trochlear nerve** which lies just under its free margin [Fig. 8.2B].

8. Turn the head forcibly to one side, and raise the posterior part of the cerebral hemisphere from the tentorium with your fingers. Divide the **tentorium** along its attachment to the petrous temporal bone [Figs. 8.6, 8.9], taking care not to injure the cerebellum beneath.

9. Then turn the head to the opposite side, and repeat the procedure on the other side.

10. Let the brain fall backwards, so as to draw the brainstem away from the anterior wall of the posterior cranial fossa, and bring the lower cranial nerves into view.

11. Divide the oculomotor nerves and, allowing the brain to fall first to one side and then to the other, identify and divide the trigeminal, abducens, facial, and vestibulocochlear nerves. The last two enter the internal acoustic meatus [Figs. 8.2B, 8.9].

12. Identify and cut the nerves passing to the jugular foramen [Figs. 8.2B, 8.10], but leave the accessory nerve on one side by detaching it from the brain.

13. Look for the hypoglossal nerves, which are deeper and more medial, and cut them also [Fig. 8.10].

14. Press the pons [Fig. 8.5] further posteriorly, and identify the two vertebral arteries ascending to form the basilar artery on its surface.

15. Pass a knife into the vertebral canal in front of the medulla oblongata, and cut the spinal cord and the vertebral arteries.

16. Remove the brain from the cranial cavity, dividing any roots of the accessory nerve still attached to the spinal cord.

17. Removal of the brain in this way, without complete separation of the tentorium from the skull, ruptures the great cerebral vein. Find the cut end of the great cerebral vein where it enters the straight sinus at the junction of the free margins of the falx and tentorium.

a fixed margin attached to the skull at the edge of the posterior cranial fossa. The free margin of the tentorium extends almost horizontally backwards from each anterior clinoid process, forming the **tentorial notch**. At the notch, the posterior cranial fossa continues with the supratentorial compartments of the cranial cavity [Fig. 8.6].

At the attached margin, the two layers of the dural fold diverge to enclose: (1) the wide **transverse sinus** between the internal occipital protuberance and the base of the petrous temporal bone; and (2) the superior petrosal sinus on the superior margin of the petrous temporal bone [Figs. 8.2B, 8.8, 8.9].

At the apex of the petrous temporal bone, the free and attached margins of the tentorium cross

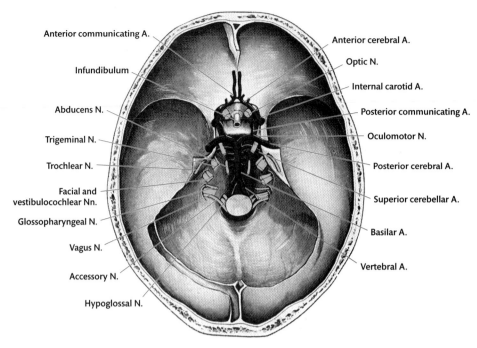

Fig. 8.9 Oblique section through the posterior cranial fossa. The brain and spinal cord have been removed.

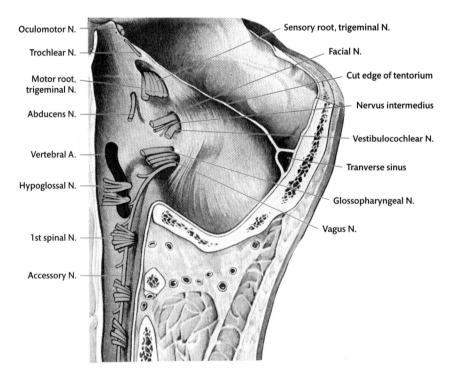

Fig. 8.10 Coronal section through the skull at the level of the foramen magnum. The brain has been removed to show the fossae which lodge the occipital lobes of the hemispheres and the cerebellum.

each other. The free margin passes forwards to the **anterior clinoid process** above the attached margin. The attached margin passes medially to the **posterior clinoid process**. The dura mater which unites these two margins, anteromedial to the crossing, forms the roof of the hypophysial fossa and the lateral wall of the cavernous sinus [Fig. 8.6].

DISSECTION 8.6 Straight, transverse, and sigmoid sinuses

Objective

I. To open and explore the extent of the straight, trans-verse, sigmoid, and superior petrosal sinuses.

Instructions

1. Open the straight sinus by incising the falx cerebri along the left side of its union with the tentorium. Carry this incision forwards along the free edge of the falx to open the small inferior sagittal sinus.

2. Open the transverse sinus by continuing the first incision laterally from the internal occipital protuberance along the fixed margin of the tento-rium cerebelli [Figs. 8.2B, 8.6].

3. Carry the incision down from the lateral end of the transverse sinus along the edge of the sigmoid sinus [Figs. 8.2B, 8.6].

4. Open the superior petrosal sinus by cutting along the fixed margin of the tentorium cerebelli [Figs. 8.2B, 8.6].

5. On the right side, follow the superior sagittal sinus into the transverse sinus, and check for continuity of all the sinuses at the internal occipital protuberance.

The **great cerebral vein** pierces the dura ma-ter and joins the inferior sagittal sinus to form the **straight sinus** [Fig. 8.2A].

Functions of the falx cerebri and tento-rium cerebelli

The falx cerebri and tentorium cerebelli are tough folds of the dura mater which play an important part in stabilizing the brain within the cranial cav-ity. They prevent the brain from moving freely when the head is moved suddenly.

Dissection 8.6 provides instructions on dissection of the straight, transverse, and sigmoid sinuses.

Dural venous sinuses

Inferior sagittal sinus

The narrow inferior sagittal sinus lies in the poste-rior two-thirds of the free margin of the falx cerebri. It drains the falx and part of the medial surface of the hemisphere into the straight sinus [Fig. 8.2A].

Straight sinus

The straight sinus is formed by the union of the great cerebral vein and the inferior sagittal sinus at the point where the free margins of the falx cer-ebri and tentorium cerebelli meet. It runs postero-inferiorly in the line of union of these two folds. At the internal occipital protuberance, it becomes continuous with one of the transverse sinuses, usu-ally the left [Figs. 8.2A, 8.8]. It drains the posterior and central parts of the cerebrum, part of the cer-ebellum, the falx, and the tentorium.

The four sinuses (superior sagittal, straight, and two transverse) may meet in the **confluence of the sinuses** at the internal occipital protuberance.

Transverse sinus

On each side, a transverse sinus runs horizontal-ly in the fixed margin of the tentorium, from the internal occipital protuberance to the base of the petrous temporal bone. It grooves the occipital, par-ietal, and temporal bones. Usually the right trans-verse sinus is a continuation of the superior sagittal sinus, and the left a continuation of the straight sinus. The transverse sinus which receives the su-perior sagittal sinus is larger than the other, but if the sinuses communicate, they may be of equal size. The transverse sinus receives veins from the cerebrum (occipital lobe) and cerebellum, the oc-cipital diploic vein, and the superior petrosal sinus. Anteriorly, it drains into the sigmoid sinus [Figs. 8.2A, 8.2B, 8.8].

Superior petrosal sinus

The narrow superior petrosal sinus drains the pos-terior end of the cavernous sinus [p. 85] to the junction of the transverse and sigmoid sinuses. It lies in that margin of the tentorium cerebelli which is fixed to the petrous temporal bone [Fig. 8.2B].

Paranasal air sinuses

The paranasal air sinuses are air-filled extensions of the nasal cavities. They replace the marrow cavi-ties of the maxilla, ethmoid, frontal, and sphenoid bones, either partly or completely. Each sinus is lined by mucosa which is adherent to the endos-teum lining the bone—a **muco-endosteum**. Cilia on the mucous membrane move the surface mu-cus towards the opening of the sinus into the nasal

Objective

I. To explore the frontal air sinus.

Instructions

1. One or other of frontal sinuses was probably opened when the calvaria was removed. If not, chisel off part of the frontal bone close to the median plane till one of the sinuses is opened.

2. Explore the cavity with a probe, and attempt to find its opening into the nasal cavity.

cavity and keep the sinus empty of secretions. Sinuses tend to enlarge with age. ➲ The openings of the sinuses are relatively narrow and easily obstructed, even by swelling of the vascular endosteum. When blocked, the sinus tends to fill with secretions which readily become infected.

The frontal air sinus is described and dissected in this chapter. The ethmoid air sinuses with the orbit [Chapter 11], and the maxillary and sphenoid air sinuses with the nasal cavity [Chapter 19].

Frontal air sinuses

Dissection 8.7 provides instructions on exploring the frontal air sinus.

The frontal sinuses are paired, asymmetrical cavities in the frontal bone, immediately above the root of the nose and the upper margins of the orbits. They lie between the inner and outer tables of the bone and are separated from each other by a bony septum [see Fig. 3.1B; Figs. 8.5, 8.7]. The sinuses are normally about 2–3 cm in height and width. In addition to expanding into the forehead, they may pass posteriorly between the two tables of the roof of the orbit. The sinuses drain into the nasal cavity through a funnel-shaped passage called the **infundibulum**.

Anterior cranial fossa

Expose the cribriform plate of the ethmoid and the anterior ethmoidal nerve using the instructions given in Dissection 8.8.

Anterior ethmoidal nerve

The anterior ethmoidal nerve is a terminal branch of the nasociliary branch of the ophthalmic nerve.

Objective

I. To expose the cribriform plate of the ethmoid and the anterior ethmoidal nerve.

Instructions

1. Carefully remove the dura mater from the cribriform plate of the ethmoid.

2. Attempt to find the anterior ethmoidal nerve running anteriorly on the lateral margin of the cribriform plate.

It arises in the orbit and enters the cranial cavity with the anterior ethmoidal artery between the frontal and ethmoid bones [Fig. 8.7]. It runs forward on the lateral edge of the cribriform plate, and enters the nose through a small aperture at the side of the crista galli. The nerve and artery supply the mucous membrane of the upper anterior part of the nasal cavity and end as the external nasal artery and nerve.

The small **posterior ethmoidal artery** follows the same course from the orbit, but further posteriorly. Along with the anterior ethmoidal and middle meningeal arteries, it supplies the dura mater of the anterior cranial fossa.

Middle cranial fossa

Using the instructions given in Dissection 8.9, remove the pituitary gland from the hypophysial fossa.

Hypophysis or pituitary gland

The pituitary is an exceedingly important endocrine gland with a wide range of functions, including the control of the other ductless glands and of body growth.

It is a flattened ovoid structure lying in the hypophysial fossa and connected to the inferior surface of the hypothalamus by the **infundibulum** [Fig. 8.11]. The **posterior lobe** of the pituitary is the expanded inferior end of the infundibulum and is developed from the brain. The **anterior lobe** is much larger than the posterior lobe and partly surrounds the posterior lobe and infundibulum.

The pituitary lies posterosuperior to the sphenoidal air sinuses, below the optic chiasma, in front of

DISSECTION 8.9 Pituitary gland

Objective

I. To remove and study the pituitary gland.

Instructions

1. Cut the diaphragma sellae radially, and dislodge the pituitary gland from the hypophysial fossa. Examine its shape with a hand lens, and then make a median section through it.

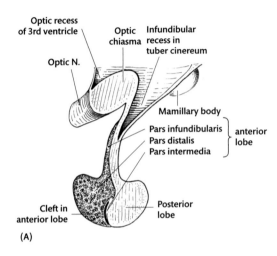

(A)

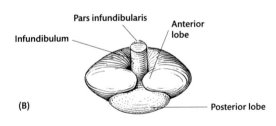

(B)

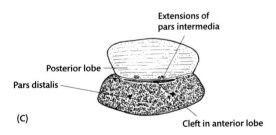

(C)

Fig. 8.11 Diagrammatic views of the hypophysis. (A) In median section; (B) from above and behind; (C) in horizontal section.

the dorsum sellae, and between the two cavernous sinuses. Several venous channels (**intercavernous sinuses**) connect the two cavernous sinuses around the pituitary [Figs. 8.2B, 8.5].

Blood supply of the pituitary

The pituitary is supplied by twigs from the internal carotid and anterior cerebral arteries. The anterior lobe also receives venous blood from the hypothalamus via the **hypothalamo-hypophysial portal system** of veins. The veins of the pituitary drain into the cavernous sinuses.

Cavernous sinus

The paired cavernous sinuses are dural venous sinuses which lie between the endosteal and meningeal layers of the dura on the lateral side of the sphenoid body. They consist of a large number of incompletely fused venous channels surrounding the structures which lie within them, and are important because of the structures which are in and around them.

Position and contents

Each cavernous sinus lies lateral to the pituitary and the sphenoidal air sinus. It extends from the medial end of the superior orbital fissure anteriorly to the apex of the petrous temporal bone posteriorly. Lateral to it is the trigeminal ganglion. The following nerves lie on the lateral wall—the oculomotor, trochlear, ophthalmic, and maxillary divisions of the trigeminal nerve. Within the sinus, but separated from it by the endothelium, lie the internal carotid artery and the abducens nerve [Figs. 8.2B, 8.12].

Tributaries and communications

The cavernous sinus communicates with a number of other veins [Fig. 8.2B]. Anteriorly, it communicates with the ophthalmic veins and the sphenoparietal sinus. Posteriorly, it communicates with the superior and inferior petrosal sinuses. Medially, it is connected to its fellow on the opposite side by intercavernous sinuses in the hypophysial fossa. Superiorly, the superficial middle cerebral vein and one or two small cerebral veins enter it. Inferiorly, it communicates with: (1) the pharyngeal plexus through the carotid canal; and (2) the pterygoid plexus through the foramen ovale and the sphenoidal emissary foramen. The cavernous sinus forms a route of communication between the veins of the face, cheek, brain, and the internal jugular vein.

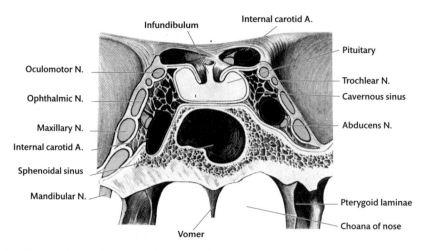

Infundibulum Internal carotid A. Pituitary Trochlear N. Cavernous sinus Abducens N. Oculomotor N. Ophthalmic N. Maxillary N. Internal carotid A. Sphenoidal sinus Mandibular N. Pterygoid laminae Choana of nose Vomer

Fig. 8.12 Coronal section through the sella turcica and cavernous sinuses.

86

➲ The carotid artery may be damaged in injuries to the skull and lead to arterial bleeding within the cavernous sinus. Such a bleed would raise the pressure in the sinus and in the veins entering it. Back pressure in the ophthalmic veins may cause the eyeball to protrude and even to pulsate.

Fig. 8.13 is an axial section through the pituitary gland.

Using the instructions given in Dissection 8.10, expose the structures on the floor of the middle cranial fossa.

Trigeminal nerve

The trigeminal nerve is the fifth cranial nerve. It has three divisions: the ophthalmic, maxillary, and mandibular divisions. It is the principal sensory nerve of the head, supplying: (1) the skin of the face and anterior half of the head; (2) the mucous membrane of the nose, paranasal air sinuses, mouth, and anterior two-thirds of the tongue; (3) the teeth and temporomandibular joint; (4) the contents of the orbit, except the retina; and (5) parts of the dura mater.

DISSECTION 8.10 Middle cranial fossa

Objectives

I. To remove the dura from the cavernous sinus and the rest of the middle cranial fossa. **II.** To identify and trace the structures in the cavernous sinus. **III.** To open the cavum trigeminale and dissect the trigeminal ganglion and its branches. **IV.** To trace the greater and lesser petrosal nerves.

Instructions

1. Turn each half of the tentorium anterolaterally on its attachment to the petrous temporal bone.

2. Find the **trochlear nerve** [Fig. 8.10]. It pierces the inferior surface of the tentorium, close to its free border and near the apex of the petrous temporal bone.

3. Inferior to the trochlear nerve, find the large **trigeminal nerve** [Figs. 8.10, 8.14]. Pass a blunt probe forwards along the nerve. The probe enters the dural sac, the **cavum trigeminale** which surrounds the nerve, and the trigeminal ganglion underneath the

dural floor of the middle cranial fossa. Elevate the probe to raise the dural floor of the middle cranial fossa, and outline the position of the nerve and ganglion [Fig. 8.15].

4. Carefully remove the dura mater from the floor of the middle cranial fossa by cutting through it on the probe in the cavum trigeminale.

5. Strip the dura forwards and laterally to uncover the trigeminal nerve, the ganglion, and the three large branches of the nerve [Fig. 8.15]. The branches arise from the convex anterior border of the ganglion. Remove the dura from the ganglion with care, because the ganglion is a loose mass of cells which is easily destroyed.

6. Trace the **mandibular nerve** inferolaterally to the foramen ovale, close to the entry of the middle meningeal artery.

7. Follow the **maxillary nerve** to the foramen rotundum.

8. Follow the **ophthalmic nerve** into the lateral wall of the cavernous sinus where it divides into three branches which can be traced to the superior orbital fissure [Fig. 8.14].

9. Find the **trochlear** and **oculomotor nerves** in the lateral wall of the cavernous sinus. Pick them up as they pierce the dura, and gently pull on them to identify their more peripheral parts.

10. Preserve the dura where the nerves enter it, but remove it in front of that point so as to follow the nerves to the superior orbital fissure.

11. Remove the remains of the lateral wall of the cavernous sinus from around the nerves, and expose the **internal carotid artery** and the **abducens nerve** within the sinus. Note that the nerve passes

forwards, lateral to the artery. Follow the nerve forwards and backwards.

12. Carefully strip the remainder of the dura from the anterior surface of the petrous temporal bone, and look for the greater and lesser **petrosal nerves**. These slender nerves emerge through slits in the temporal bone and run anteromedially in shallow grooves. The lesser petrosal nerve pierces the skull near the foramen ovale; the greater petrosal nerve is larger and more medial. It disappears under the trigeminal ganglion [Fig. 8.2B].

13. Lift the trigeminal ganglion, and try to identify the **motor root of the trigeminal nerve** on its inferior surface. It runs deep to the ganglion to the foramen ovale.

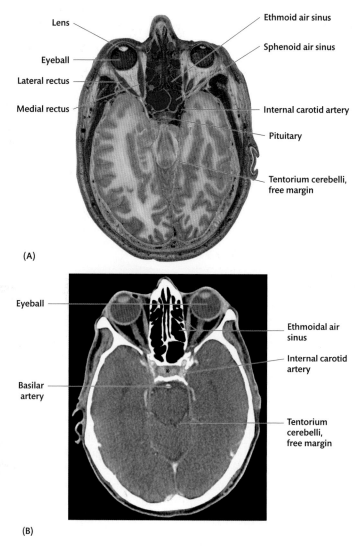

(A)

Lens
Eyeball
Lateral rectus
Medial rectus

Ethmoid air sinus
Sphenoid air sinus
Internal carotid artery
Pituitary
Tentorium cerebelli, free margin

(B)

Eyeball
Basilar artery

Ethmoidal air sinus
Internal carotid artery
Tentorium cerebelli, free margin

Fig. 8.13 (A) Transverse section through the head at the level of the pituitary gland. (B) Axial contrast computerized tomography (CT) through the pituitary (asterisk) and orbit.

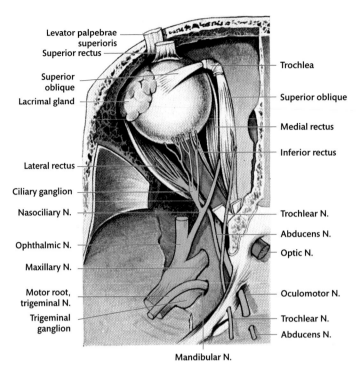

Levator palpebrae superioris
Superior rectus
Superior oblique
Lacrimal gland
Lateral rectus
Ciliary ganglion
Nasociliary N.
Ophthalmic N.
Maxillary N.
Motor root, trigeminal N.
Trigeminal ganglion
Trochlea
Superior oblique
Medial rectus
Inferior rectus
Trochlear N.
Abducens N.
Optic N.
Oculomotor N.
Trochlear N.
Abducens N.
Mandibular N.

Fig. 8.14 Orbit and middle cranial fossa. The trigeminal nerve and ganglion have been turned laterally to expose the motor root.

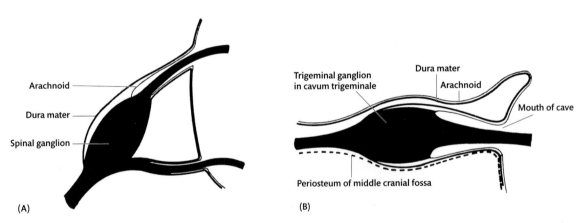

Arachnoid
Dura mater
Spinal ganglion

Trigeminal ganglion in cavum trigeminale
Dura mater
Arachnoid
Mouth of cave
Periosteum of middle cranial fossa

(A)
(B)

Fig. 8.15 Diagram to show the relations of the meninges to: (A) a spinal nerve; and (B) the trigeminal ganglion in the cavum trigeminale.

The **motor fibres** arise in the pons and pass into the mandibular nerve. They supply the four muscles of mastication—the temporalis, masseter, and medial and lateral pterygoids—and the mylohyoid, anterior belly of the digastric, tensor palati, and tensor tympani.

Almost all of the **sensory fibres** in the trigeminal nerve are processes of the cells in the large trigeminal ganglion. The central processes converge to form the **sensory root** of the nerve which enters the pons. The peripheral processes enter the ophthalmic, maxillary, and mandibular nerves. Proprioceptive nerve fibres from the same three nerves pass through the ganglion to cells in the midbrain—a unique arrangement where primary sensory nerve cells have their cell bodies within the central nervous system. (The sensory and motor nuclei of the trigeminal nerve are described in Chapter 28.)

Trigeminal ganglion

The trigeminal ganglion is a semilunar sensory ganglion. It lies in a shallow depression on the anterior surface of the petrous temporal bone (near the apex) and on the adjacent margin of the greater wing of the sphenoid [Fig. 8.14]. Like other sensory ganglia, it lies in a pocket of dura mater—the **cavum trigeminale**. The dura mater forming the cave is tucked forwards from the posterior cranial fossa between the meningeal and endosteal layers on the floor of the middle cranial fossa [Fig. 8.15]. Posteriorly, the narrow neck of the cavum contains the sensory and motor roots of the nerve enclosed in a sleeve of the pia and arachnoid. They groove the upper margin of the petrous temporal bone close to the apex. The distal part of the roots lie above the internal carotid artery in the carotid canal. The superomedial part of the ganglion lies lateral to the cavernous sinus and the artery [Figs. 8.14, 8.15].

Mandibular nerve

The mandibular nerve is the largest of the three branches of the trigeminal nerve. It arises from the inferolateral part of the ganglion, gives a meningeal twig to the floor of the middle cranial fossa, and immediately leaves the skull through the foramen ovale. The small motor root of the mandibular nerve leaves the pons beside the sensory root and passes under the ganglion to the foramen ovale [Fig. 8.14].

Maxillary nerve

The maxillary nerve arises from the anterior surface of the ganglion, inferior to the ophthalmic nerve. It runs forwards between the dura and the lower border of the cavernous sinus, gives off a fine meningeal branch to the middle cranial fossa, and leaves the skull by passing through the foramen rotundum [Fig. 8.7].

Ophthalmic nerve

The ophthalmic nerve is the smallest of the three nerves. It arises from the ganglion, runs forwards in the lateral wall of the cavernous sinus, and divides into three branches—the **nasociliary**, **lacrimal**, and **frontal nerves**—which enter the orbit through the superior orbital fissure [Fig. 8.14]. Near its origin, the ophthalmic nerve communicates with the oculomotor, trochlear, and abducens nerves in the lateral wall of the cavernous sinus.

It also gives off a small **tentorial branch** which curves back into the tentorium cerebelli.

Oculomotor nerve

The oculomotor nerve is the third cranial nerve. It supplies four of the six muscles that move the eyeball, and two of the three muscles within the eyeball [Chapters 11 and 12]. It emerges through the ventral surface of the midbrain, passes anterolaterally between the posterior cerebral and superior cerebellar arteries, and pierces the dura mater in the roof of the cavernous sinus. It then runs forwards in the lateral wall of the cavernous sinus (above the other nerves) and divides into superior and inferior branches which enter the orbit through the superior orbital fissure [Figs. 8.12, 8.14].

Trochlear nerve

This slender fourth cranial nerve supplies one extraocular muscle of the eyeball [Chapter 11]. It emerges from the dorsal surface of the midbrain and curves forwards on the side of the lower midbrain, between the posterior cerebral and superior cerebellar arteries. It pierces the tentorium below the free margin and runs anterosuperiorly in the lateral wall of the cavernous sinus [Fig. 8.12]. It crosses the lateral aspect of the oculomotor nerve to enter the orbit through the superior orbital fissure.

Abducens nerve

The sixth cranial nerve supplies one extraocular muscle of the eyeball [Chapter 11]. It emerges at the lower border of the pons, bends upwards between the pons and the clivus of the skull, and pierces the dura mater 1 cm below the root of the dorsum sellae [Figs. 8.8, 8.9]. Outside the dura, it runs superolaterally to the apex of the petrous temporal bone and crosses the sphenopetrous suture to enter the cavernous sinus. In the sinus, it runs anteriorly, lateral to the internal carotid artery, and leaves the sinus to enter the orbit through the superior orbital fissure [Fig. 8.12].

Intracranial part of the internal carotid artery

Course

The internal carotid artery traverses the carotid canal in the petrous part of the temporal bone. It passes anteromedially in the carotid canal into the upper part of the foramen lacerum [Fig. 8.7] and enters the cavernous sinus by piercing the dural floor. In the cavernous sinus, it turns sharply forwards and runs anteriorly. At the root of the lesser wing of the sphenoid, the artery again turns sharply upwards and backwards and pierces the dura and arachnoid mater on the roof of the cavernous sinus, medial to the anterior clinoid process and behind the optic canal. It then divides into the anterior and middle cerebral arteries on the surface of the brain. The tortuous course of the internal carotid artery produces a sinuous groove on the side of the body of the sphenoid [Fig. 8.16]. The internal carotid artery is surrounded by the internal carotid plexus of sympathetic nerves [see Fig. 9.13].

Branches of the internal carotid artery

The internal carotid artery gives off the following branches at the base of the brain: (1) the **ophthalmic artery** to the orbit; (2) small twigs to the pituitary, trigeminal ganglion, and dura mater in the cavernous sinus; (3) the posterior communicating artery; (4) the anterior choroidal artery; and (5) and (6) the middle and anterior cerebral arteries.

Meningeal vessels of the middle cranial fossa

The meningeal vessels are embedded on the external surface of the dura mater. They protrude from its surface and groove the skull [Fig. 8.1]. They supply the bone and dura mater but do not cross the subdural space to supply the brain or the pia-arachnoid.

The **middle meningeal artery** is a branch of the maxillary artery. It enters the skull through the foramen spinosum and runs anterolaterally on the floor of the middle cranial fossa. It divides into **frontal** and **parietal** branches on the greater wing of the sphenoid. The parietal branch turns posteriorly, and across the lateral wall of the cranial cavity towards the lambda. The larger frontal branch runs towards the lateral end of the lesser wing of the sphenoid [Fig. 8.7]. At the pterion (area where the greater wing of the sphenoid, frontal, parietal, and temporal bones meet), the frontal branch of the middle meningeal artery grooves the skull deeply or even tunnels through the bone, increasing the

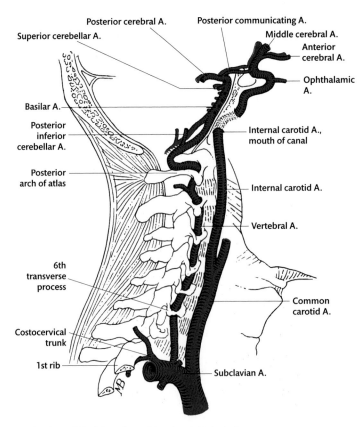

Fig. 8.16 The course and communications of the internal carotid and vertebral arteries.

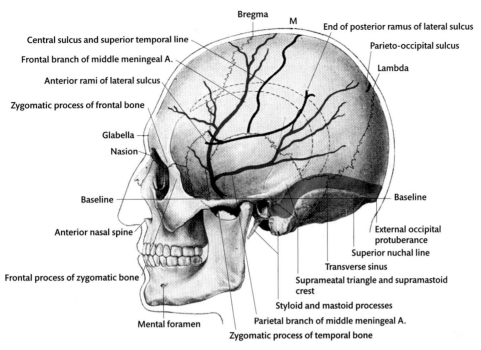

Fig. 8.17 Lateral view of the skull to show the position of certain important intracranial structures. M = midpoint between the nasion and inion.

probability of damage to it in fractures. It then runs obliquely upwards and backwards, parallel to, and slightly behind, the coronal suture and frequently sends a large branch posteriorly on the deep surface of the parietal bone [Fig. 8.17]. The parietal branch is a small, but important, artery because it is a common source of extradural haemorrhage, and lies adjacent to an important area in the brain—the motor cortex.

The middle meningeal vein accompanies the artery through the foramen spinosum to the pterygoid venous plexus.

Accessory meningeal vessels

A small branch of the maxillary or middle meningeal artery—the **accessory meningeal artery**—often traverses the foramen ovale to supply the trigeminal ganglion and adjacent dura. The **ophthalmic** and **lacrimal arteries** from the orbit also send twigs through the superior orbital fissure to the middle cranial fossa.

Petrosal nerves

The greater and lesser petrosal nerves carry preganglionic parasympathetic secretomotor fibres to the lacrimal, nasal, palatine, nasopharyngeal, and parotid glands, and sensory (taste) fibres from the palate.

The **greater petrosal nerve** arises from the genu of the facial nerve in the petrous temporal bone. It runs on the anterior surface of the petrous bone into a narrow groove leading to the foramen lacerum, inferior to the trigeminal ganglion [Fig. 8.7]. Here the nerve is joined by the **deep petrosal nerve** from the sympathetic plexus on the internal carotid artery. It then runs across the foramen lacerum, through the pterygoid canal (a canal in the petrous temporal bone) to the pterygopalatine ganglion. In the canal, it is called the **nerve of the pterygoid canal** [see Fig. 13.8]. (Note: the nerve of the pterygoid canal contains post-ganglionic sympathetic fibres from the internal carotid nerve, and preganglionic parasympathetic fibres from the greater petrosal nerve.) The preganglionic parasympathetic fibres by synapsing in the pterygopalatine ganglion. The sympathetic fibres pass through the ganglion without synapsing in it.

The slender **lesser petrosal nerve** arises from the glossopharyngeal nerve. It emerges on the anterior surface of the petrous temporal bone lateral to the greater petrosal nerve and runs on the bony floor of the middle cranial fossa to leave the skull through

DISSECTION 8.11 Cranial nerves in the posterior cranial fossa

Objective

I. To identify the cut ends of the trigeminal, facial, vestibulocochlear, glossopharyngeal, vagus, spinal accessory, and hypoglossal nerves.

Instructions

1. Using Fig. 8.2B and a dry skull, identify the cranial nerves in the posterior cranial fossa. (1) The **trigeminal nerve** passes into the cavum trigeminale on the superior margin of the petrous temporal bone. (2) The **facial** and **vestibulocochlear nerves** enter the internal acoustic meatus. (3) The **glossopharyngeal**, **vagus**, and **accessory nerves** pass through the jugular foramen. The **spinal part of the accessory nerve** ascends beside the spinal cord, posterior to the ligamentum denticulatum [see Fig. 21.3], to join the vagus. It passes out through the jugular foramen with the glossopharyngeal nerve. The hypoglossal nerve enters the hypoglossal canal, close to the anterolateral margin of the foramen magnum.

the foramen ovale. Its fibres synapse with the cells of the otic ganglion on the medial side of the mandibular nerve [see Fig. 13.8].

Posterior cranial fossa

Using the instructions given in Dissection 8.11, identify the cut ends of the cranial nerves in the posterior cranial fossa.

Structures seen in the posterior cranial fossa

1. The upper end of the spinal cord, which is attached to the margin of the foramen magnum by the first tooth of the ligamentum denticulatum [Fig. 8.2B].
2. The **vertebral artery** which pierces the spinal dura mater near the skull and ascends through the foramen magnum, anterior to the first tooth of the ligamentum denticulatum. It gives a men-

DISSECTION 8.12 Dural venous sinuses in the posterior cranial fossa

Objectives

I. To explore the occipital and sigmoid sinuses.
II. To find and trace the abducens nerve.

Instructions

1. Slit up the falx cerebelli, and look for the **occipital sinus**.
2. Open the **sigmoid sinus** by passing a knife into it at the anterior end of the transverse sinus, and cutting along it to the base of the skull and then forwards to the jugular foramen.
3. Pull gently on the cut end of the abducens nerve, and trace it to the apex of the petrous temporal bone by slitting the dura.

ingeal branch to the posterior cranial fossa before piercing the dura mater, and passes superomedially between the first cervical and hypoglossal nerves [Fig. 8.8].
3. The **first cervical nerve**, in front of the vertebral artery.
4. The **hypoglossal nerve** superior to the first cervical, which pierces the dura at the hypoglossal canal [Fig. 8.8].
5. The spinal part of the **accessory nerve** which ascends through the foramen magnum and turns laterally to join the cranial part of the accessory and vagus nerves. Together, they pierce the dura mater at the jugular foramen, beside the separate aperture for the glossopharyngeal nerve [Fig. 8.8].
6. The **facial nerve**, **nervus intermedius**, and **vestibulocochlear nerve** which enter the internal acoustic meatus [Fig. 8.8].
7. The **falx cerebelli**, a small fold of dura mater on the internal occipital crest. It contains the occipital sinus and fits into the posterior cerebellar notch [Fig. 8.1].

Using the instructions given in Dissection 8.12, open the sigmoid sinus and trace the abducens nerve.

Dura mater of the base of the skull

The dura mater of the base is firmly attached to the bone and is continuous through the foramina, with the periosteum on the external surface of the skull. At the foramen magnum, the meningeal layer of the dura mater becomes continuous with the spinal dura mater.

Venous sinuses of the posterior cranial fossa

Sigmoid sinus

The S-shaped **sigmoid sinus** begins as a continuation of the transverse sinus at the base of the petrous temporal bone [Figs. 8.1, 8.2B]. It curves downwards and grooves the mastoid and petrous parts of the temporal bone. The sinus is medial to the mastoid air cells, posterior to the mastoid antrum and the vertical part of the facial nerve and lateral to the cerebellum.

On the base of the skull, the sigmoid sinus curves forwards on the occipital bone. It joins the inferior petrosal sinus at the jugular foramen to form the internal jugular vein.

It communicates with: (1) the **occipital veins**, through the mastoid emissary vein in the mastoid foramen; (2) the **suboccipital plexus**, by the emissary veins in the condylar canal; and (3) with the beginning of the **transverse sinus**, through the occipital sinus [Fig. 8.2B].

Occipital sinus

When present, this narrow sinus descends in the falx cerebelli from the beginning of the transverse sinus. It communicates through the foramen magnum with the internal vertebral venous plexus [Fig. 8.2B].

Inferior petrosal sinus

The inferior petrosal sinus lies in the groove between the basilar part of the occipital bone and the petrous temporal bone. It drains the posterior end of the cavernous sinus through the jugular foramen to the internal jugular vein [Fig. 8.2B].

Basilar plexus of veins

The basilar plexus of veins lies on the clivus of the skull and unites the inferior petrosal sinuses with the internal vertebral venous plexus through the foramen magnum [Fig. 8.2B].

Diploic veins

These are wide venous spaces of the marrow cavity between the outer and inner tables of the flat bones of the skull. They communicate with the venous sinuses of the dura mater and with the emissary veins.

Emissary veins

Emissary veins are small veins which pass through foramina in the skull and connect the dural venous sinuses with veins outside the skull. They do not have valves, and blood flows through them in both directions. Not all named emissary veins are always present—the parietal, condylar, and sphenoidal emissary veins are frequently absent.

The superior sagittal sinus may be connected to the veins of the frontal air sinus through emissary veins in the foramen caecum, and to the veins of the scalp through the **parietal emissary foramina** in the top of the skull. The **sigmoid sinus** is connected to the occipital or posterior auricular veins through the **mastoid emissary vein** behind the auricle, and to the vertebral veins through the **condylar emissary vein**. The **cavernous sinus** has the greatest number of such communications. It is connected: (1) through the **ophthalmic veins** to the veins of the face; (2) through a plexus of veins along the internal carotid artery to the **pharyngeal veins**; and (3) through the foramen ovale to the **pterygoid venous plexus** in the infratemporal region [Fig. 8.16].

➲ The emissary veins may transmit extracranial infections into the venous sinuses.

Meningeal veins

The meningeal veins are very thin-walled veins which lie between the meningeal arteries and the bone. They end either in the venous sinuses or in veins outside the skull by passing through foramina with the corresponding arteries.

See Clinical Applications 8.1, 8.2, and 8.3 for the practical implications of the anatomy discussed in this chapter.

CLINICAL APPLICATION 8.1 Cavernous sinus thrombosis

A 52-year-old lady with dental caries and a persistent root abscess presented to the emergency department with severe unilateral throbbing headache, double vision, loss of sensation over the upper face, periorbital swelling, and pain on the right side.

Study question 1: what is the likely diagnosis? (Answer: cavernous sinus thrombosis (CST). Other differential diagnosis includes migraine headache and orbital cellulitis.)

Study question 2: what is cavernous sinus thrombosis? (Answer: CST is thrombosis—clot formation—in the cavernous sinus, resulting from spread of infection from the nose, paranasal air sinuses, tonsils, or tooth. It has high morbidity and can have residual visual impairment and cranial nerve deficits.)

Study question 3: what are the veins connected with the cavernous sinus? (Answer: the cavernous sinus receives the superior and inferior ophthalmic veins, the central retinal vein of the retina, the middle meningeal veins, and the pterygoid venous plexus via emissary veins. It also receives

venous blood from the brain through the superficial middle cerebral veins. It drains into the sigmoid sinus via the superior petrosal sinus, and into the internal jugular vein via the inferior petrosal sinus.)

Study question 4: explain the anatomical basis for the symptoms experienced by this patient. (Answer: the headache is a result of meningeal irritation. Swelling and periorbital oedema occur due to venous congestion of the ophthalmic veins. Visual impairment may occur due to papilloedema and retinal haemorrhage secondary to retinal congestion. Other symptoms of CST occur because of the close relationship between the cavernous sinus and the third, fourth, fifth—ophthalmic and maxillary divisions—and sixth cranial nerves in the lateral wall of the cavernous sinus. Pain and loss of sensation over the upper face are the result of stretching/pressure of the ophthalmic and maxillary divisions of the trigeminal nerve. Double vision (diplopia) usually persists due to involvement of the sixth cranial nerve.)

CLINICAL APPLICATION 8.2 Pituitary adenoma

A 28-year-old unmarried woman presented with a history of amenorrhoea (lack of menstruation) and spontaneous secretion of milk from her breasts for the past year. She also reported recent onset of headache and visual disturbances. Testing for visual fields revealed bitemporal hemianopia—loss of temporal field of vision. Computerized tomography (CT) scans showed a large pituitary adenoma [Fig. 8.18].

Study question 1: why does the patient experience visual disturbance? (Answer: a large pituitary adenoma can compress the optic chiasma above and disrupt the nasal fibres from the retina. This causes bitemporal hemianopia.)

Study question 2: what cell type could this tumour be composed of? (Answer: the history suggests a prolactin-secreting tumour called prolactinoma. This causes secretion of breast milk, even in non-lactating women (galactorrhoea). High content of prolactin in the circulating blood can cause suppression of the menstrual cycle (amenorrhoea) and anovular cycles leading to infertility.)

Study question 3: what are the other tumours of the pituitary gland? (Answer: other common hormone-secreting tumours are somatotrophic adenomas—secrete growth hormone; corticotrophic adenomas—secrete adrenocorticotrophin; and

gonadotrophic adenomas—secrete follicle-stimulating hormone (FSH) or luteinizing hormone (LH).)

Study question 4: how are these tumours treated? (Answer: most tumours resolve with medicines. Others can be treated with surgery. The endonasal trans-sphenoidal approach to the pituitary is commonly used.)

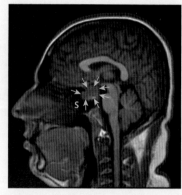

Fig. 8.18 T1-weighted sagittal magnetic resonance imaging (MRI) of a pituitary macroadenoma, sagittal view. Arrows = boundary of macroadenoma; S = sphenoid air sinus.

A 23-year-old man sustained a head injury in a road traffic accident. He was conscious for a short while and then lapsed into a coma. He was suspected of having an intracranial haemorrhage. Intracranial haemorrhages can be classified according to location as: (1) extradural; (2) subdural; (3) subarachnoid; and (4) intracerebral.

Study question 1: use your knowledge of anatomy and Figs. 8.1 and 8.3 to determine which vessels would be the source of bleeding in: (1) extradural; (2) subdural; and (3) subarachnoid haemorrhage. (Answer: (1) extradural haemorrhage = meningeal vessels; (2) subdural haemorrhage = bridging veins as they run from the subarachnoid space to the superior sagittal sinus; and (3) subarachnoid haemorrhage = cerebral vessels.)

With time, blood from ruptured vessels collects within the confines of the space and forms a haematoma. **Epidural haematomas** are formed by high-pressure arterial blood rapidly filling the space between the dura mater and bone. On CT, they are shaped like a biconvex lens and are confined to the area bound by sutures (as the dura is firmly adherent to the bone at the sutures and does not separate easily). If the dura mater is torn, bleeding from extradural vessels can spread into the subdural space.

Subdural haematomas result in slowly developing brain compression and unconsciousness, and are formed by venous blood. They lie between the dura and arachnoid mater. On CTs, they are crescent-shaped and follow the contours of the brain.

Dura mater of the base of the skull

95

CHAPTER 9
Deep dissection of the neck

Introduction

This chapter deals with the description and dissection of the trachea and oesophagus, the thyroid and parathyroid glands, the large vessels of the head and neck, the lower cranial nerves, and the cervical lymph nodes [Fig. 9.1]. These important structures lie deep to the anterior and posterior triangles, and in front of the prevertebral structures described in Chapter 10.

Dissection 9.1 provides instructions on dissection of the trachea, oesophagus, thyroid gland, and related structures.

Thymus

This important lymphoid structure is particularly large in the child. In the adult, it consists chiefly of fat and fibrous tissue. Its two lobes are two slender, elongated, yellowish bodies that lie side by side, anterior to the pericardium and great vessels in the upper part of the thorax [see Figs. 4.20, 4.21, Vol. 2]. The thymus develops as lateral outgrowths of the pharynx and subsequently descends into the thorax. As such, the superior parts of the thymus may be found in the neck, anterior to the trachea, attached to the lower ends of the thyroid gland.

Thyroid gland

The thyroid gland is a highly vascular endocrine gland which partially surrounds the upper part of the trachea. It consists of a pair of **lobes** joined across the midline by a narrow **isthmus** [Fig. 9.2]. It extends from the oblique line on the thyroid cartilage down to the fifth or sixth tracheal ring. It is enclosed in a **sheath** of pre-tracheal fascia which is attached above to the oblique line of the thyroid cartilage and to the arch of the cricoid cartilage. This attachment to the thyroid cartilage means that the thyroid moves with the larynx in swallowing and speaking—a feature which helps to differentiate swellings of the thyroid gland from those of adjacent structures. Deep to the covering formed by the pre-tracheal fascia is the **fibrous capsule** of the gland. Between the pre-tracheal fascia and the fibrous capsule are the arteries and veins. The gland varies greatly in size and is relatively larger in women and children than in men.

Lobes of the thyroid gland

Each of the two conical lobes of the thyroid gland has three surfaces. The convex superficial surface is covered by the sternohyoid, sternothyroid, and omohyoid muscles, and overlapped by the anterior border of the sternocleidomastoid. The inferior aspect of the medial surface is related to the trachea and oesophagus, with the **recurrent laryngeal nerve** between them. Superiorly, the medial surface is related to the cricoid and thyroid cartilages, with the cricothyroid, inferior constrictor muscle, and **external branch of the superior laryngeal nerve** between them. The posterior surface of the thyroid lobe lies on the prevertebral fascia, anterior to the longus colli, and overlaps the medial part of the carotid sheath. The **parathyroid glands** are embedded in the posterior surface [see Fig. 5.2; Figs. 9.3, 9.4, 9.5].

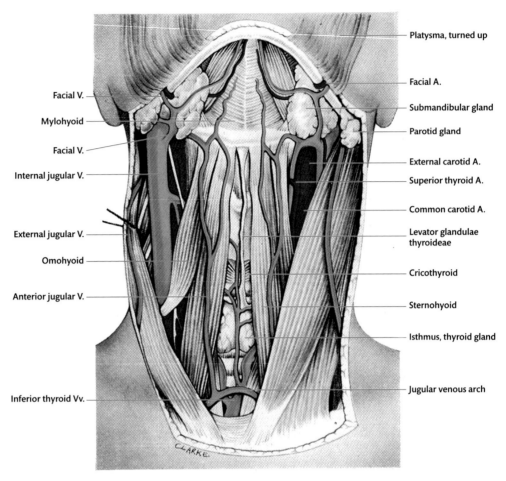

Facial V.

Mylohyoid

Facial V.

Internal jugular V.

External jugular V.

Omohyoid

Anterior jugular V.

Inferior thyroid Vv.

Platysma, turned up

Facial A.

Submandibular gland

Parotid gland

External carotid A.

Superior thyroid A.

Common carotid A.

Levator glandulae thyroideae

Cricothyroid

Sternohyoid

Isthmus, thyroid gland

Jugular venous arch

CLARKE

Fig. 9.1 Dissection of the front of the neck. The right sternocleidomastoid has been retracted.

Isthmus of the thyroid gland

The isthmus of the thyroid gland is of variable width and lies on the second to fourth tracheal rings. It is closer to the lower border of the thyroid lobes and is covered by skin and fasciae of the neck. A slender **pyramidal lobe** frequently extends superiorly from the upper border of the isthmus, usually to the left of the midline. It may be attached to the hyoid bone by a narrow slip of muscle—the **levator glandulae thyroideae**—or by a fibrous strand [Figs. 9.1, 9.2]. This strand is a remnant of the median diverticulum from which the thyroid gland developed. (The diverticulum originates in the foramen caecum of the tongue as a median epithelial downgrowth. It descends in front of the body of the hyoid, hooks up posterior to it, and continues to descend in front of the thyroid and cricoid cartilages. The lower end of the diverticulum expands to form the thyroid

gland. The suprahyoid part of this structure rarely persists.)

Arteries of the thyroid gland

The apex of each lobe receives the **superior thyroid artery** (branch of the external carotid artery) which divides into two or three branches. The base and deep surfaces of each lobe receive branches from the **inferior thyroid arteries** (branches of the thyrocervical trunk of the subclavian artery). A small **thyroidea ima** artery may arise from the brachiocephalic trunk, aortic arch, or left common carotid artery, and ascend on the anterior surface of the trachea to the isthmus. The arteries anastomose freely, especially on the posterior surface of each lobe. (The thyroid arteries are arteries of the gut tube, so they also supply the larynx, laryngeal part of the pharynx, trachea, and oesophagus [Figs. 9.1, 9.5, 9.6].)

DISSECTION 9.1 Thyroid gland, trachea, oesophagus, and related structures

Objectives

I. To expose the thyroid gland and the blood vessels supplying it.   **II.** To identify and trace the trachea, oesophagus, thoracic duct, and recurrent laryngeal nerves.

Instructions

Most of the structures dealt with in this dissection are under cover of the sternocleidomastoid. Others are hidden by the infrahyoid muscles or by the parotid gland and adjacent structures. Try to retain the sternocleidomastoid as far as possible during the dissection, for it is an important landmark in the neck.

1. Identify again the infrahyoid muscles—sternohyoid, sternothyroid, thyrohyoid, and omohyoid.

2. Displace the sternocleidomastoid and the superior belly of the omohyoid laterally. Cut through the sternothyroid near its lower end, and turn it upwards with the nerve which supplies it.

3. Before removing the fat from in front of the trachea, find the inferior thyroid veins in this fat.

Note if any parts of the right and left lobes of the **thymus** extend up into the fat. These are difficult to differentiate from the fat but are darker and ensheathed in the fascia.

4. Remove the fascia from the lobes of the thyroid gland, and expose the arteries and veins supplying it. Lift the lower part of the gland to expose the lateral surfaces of the trachea and oesophagus, with the recurrent laryngeal nerves in the groove between them.

5. On the left side, look for the thoracic duct on the oesophagus. If the thorax has been dissected, the thoracic duct and recurrent laryngeal nerve can often be followed upwards.

6. Pull the upper part of the thyroid gland laterally, and trace the external laryngeal branch of the superior laryngeal nerve to the cricothyroid muscle.

7. Find the lower part of the inferior constrictor muscle arising from a fibrous arch crossing the cricothyroid muscle and hiding its posterior part [see Fig. 6.5].

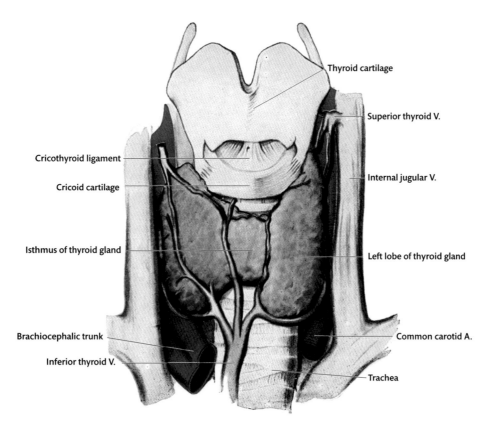

Fig. 9.2 The thyroid gland, anterior surface.

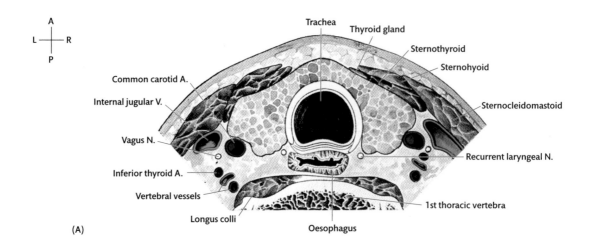

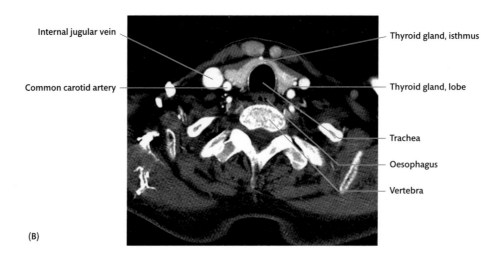

Fig. 9.3 (A) Schematic drawing of a transverse section and (B) axial computerized tomography (CT) through the anterior part of the neck at the level of the first thoracic vertebra.

Veins of the thyroid gland

Three pairs of veins drain the thyroid gland. A **superior thyroid vein** arises near the upper end of each lobe. It either crosses the common carotid artery and drains into the internal jugular vein, or ascends with the superior thyroid artery to drain into the facial vein. A short **middle thyroid vein** arises from the lower part of each lobe and crosses the common carotid artery to drain into the internal jugular vein. The **inferior thyroid vein** descends in front of the trachea from the isthmus and lower parts of the lobes to the corresponding brachiocephalic veins. Occasionally, the inferior thyroid veins unite [Fig. 9.2] and end in one or other of the brachiocephalic veins. They also receive tributaries from the trachea, larynx, and oesophagus.

Lymph vessels of the thyroid gland

The lymph vessels of the thyroid gland drain mostly to nodes on the carotid sheath—the upper and lower deep cervical nodes.

Examine the posterior surface of the thyroid gland, following the instructions given in Dissection 9.2.

Parathyroid glands

These two pairs of small yellowish-brown endocrine glands are embedded in the posterior surface of the capsule of the thyroid gland. They measure approximately $6 \times 3 \times 2$ mm. Their important secretion stimulates the mobilization of calcium from

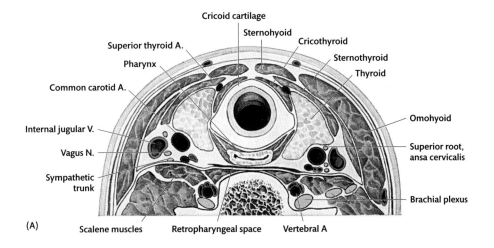

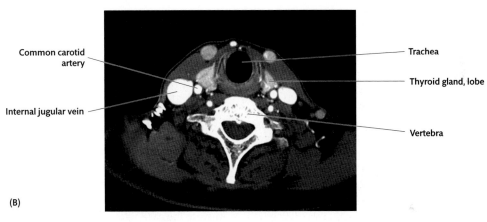

Fig. 9.4 (A) Schematic drawing of a transverse section and (B) axial CT through the anterior part of the neck at the level of the cricoid cartilage.

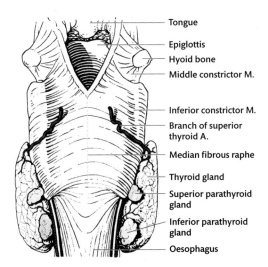

Fig. 9.5 Posterior surface of the thyroid gland to show the para-thyroid glands.

the bones to maintain the normal blood calcium level.

The **superior parathyroid glands** are more constant in position than the inferior and lie at about the middle of the posterior surface of each lobe. Each **inferior parathyroid** is close to the inferior surface of the lobe [Fig. 9.5].

Using the instructions given in Dissection 9.3, study the trachea, oesophagus, and related structures.

Trachea and oesophagus

The trachea and oesophagus begin at the lower border of the cricoid cartilage anterior to the sixth cervical vertebra, and descend into the thorax.

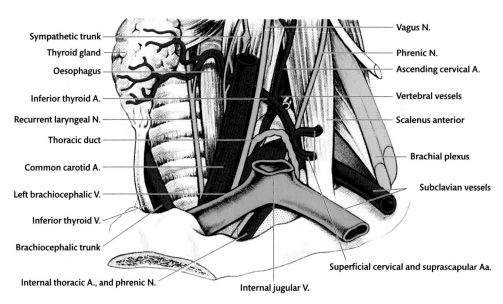

Sympathetic trunk

Thyroid gland

Oesophagus

Inferior thyroid A.

Recurrent laryngeal N.

Thoracic duct

Common carotid A.

Left brachiocephalic V.

Inferior thyroid V.

Brachiocephalic trunk

Internal thoracic A., and phrenic N.

Internal jugular V.

Vagus N.

Phrenic N.

Ascending cervical A.

Vertebral vessels

Scalenus anterior

Brachial plexus

Subclavian vessels

Superficial cervical and suprascapular Aa.

Fig. 9.6 Deep dissection of the root of the neck on the left side. The clavicle, sternocleidomastoid, and infrahyoid muscles have been removed, and the thyroid gland is displaced anteriorly. Pleura, blue stipple.

DISSECTION 9.2 Thyroid and parathyroid glands

Objective

I. To examine the posterior surface of a lobe of the thyroid gland, and identify the blood vessels and parathyroids.

Instructions

1. Cut through the isthmus and the vessels of one lobe, and remove that lobe.

2. Find the anastomotic vessel between the superior and inferior thyroid arteries on the medial part of the posterior surface. Look for the yellowish-brown parathyroid glands immediately lateral to it. The best guide to the parathyroids is the small parathyroid artery which arises from the inferior thyroid artery.

3. Make a cut through the lobe of the thyroid gland, and examine the surface with a hand lens.

DISSECTION 9.3 Trachea and oesophagus

Objective

I. To re-examine the trachea, oesophagus, recurrent laryngeal nerves, and thoracic duct after the thyroid is mobilized.

Instructions

1. Complete the exposure of the trachea and oesophagus.

2. Identify the recurrent laryngeal nerves on either side between the trachea and oesophagus.

3. Identify the thoracic duct on the left of the oesophagus.

Trachea

The trachea is a wide tube, approximately 12 cm long. It is kept constantly patent by the U-shaped cartilaginous bars embedded in its walls. Posteriorly, where the cartilage is deficient, the flat wall of the trachea lies against the oesophagus. Superiorly, the trachea is continuous with the larynx. Laterally are the common carotid arteries and the lobes of the thyroid gland, and on the right side the brachiocephalic trunk. The recurrent laryngeal nerves lie in the groove between the oesophagus and the trachea [Figs. 9.2, 9.3, 9.7].

Oesophagus

The oesophagus is a thick, distensible, muscular tube, approximately 25 cm long. It extends from

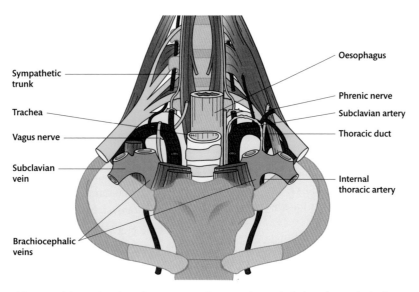

Fig. 9.7 Dissection of the root of the neck to show the structures adjacent to the cervical pleura (green shading).

the pharynx to the stomach [Figs. 9.3, 9.4, 9.5, 9.6, 9.7]. It is surrounded by loose connective tissue which permits distension of the tube. In the neck, the oesophagus lies between the trachea and the prevertebral fascia overlying the prevertebral muscles. On the right, it is in contact with the thyroid gland and the cervical pleura. On the left, it is in contact with the thyroid gland, but the subclavian artery and the thoracic duct separate it from the pleura. The oesophagus inclines to the left as it descends in the neck [Figs. 9.6, 9.7]. Thus, it is more readily accessible to the surgeon on that side.

Dissection 9.4 provides instructions on dissecting the vessels and nerves of the neck.

DISSECTION 9.4 Vessels and nerves of the neck

Objectives

I. To expose the contents of the carotid sheath.
II. To expose the vessels and nerves at the root of the neck.

Instructions

1. Remove the fat, lymph nodes, and the remains of the carotid sheath from the common carotid artery and internal jugular vein.

2. Separate the vessels, and find the vagus nerve between and behind the vein and the artery.

3. Expose the vagus, and find the **right recurrent laryngeal nerve** arising from it as it crosses the subclavian artery. Follow it to the groove between the trachea and oesophagus.

4. On the left side, find the **thoracic duct** entering the junction of the internal jugular and subclavian veins [Fig. 9.6] from above and behind. Trace it backwards and downwards to where it lies behind the left common carotid artery.

5. On both sides, expose the small cervical part of the brachiocephalic vein and its tributaries.

6. On the right side, expose the small part of the brachiocephalic trunk which lies in the neck.

7. Identify the phrenic nerve behind the internal jugular vein and prevertebral fascia. Trace it to the thorax.

8. Displace the internal jugular vein medially to expose the subclavian artery and the cervical pleura. Avoid injury to the thoracic duct and the vertebral veins.

9. Trace the internal thoracic artery, the thyrocervical trunk, and its branches from the first part of the subclavian artery [Fig. 9.6].

10. Pull the scalenus anterior laterally to expose the **costocervical trunk** arising from the subclavian artery at the medial border of the muscle. Trace the trunk over the cervical pleura to the neck of the first rib.

11. Separate the internal jugular vein and the common carotid artery. Carefully dissect deep to the vertebral veins and thoracic duct to find the **vertebral artery** posterior to them.

12. Trace the vertebral artery superiorly in front of the transverse process of the seventh cervical vertebra till it passes into the foramen transversarium of the sixth cervical vertebra.

13. Remove the fat posterior to the vertebral artery to expose the ventral rami of the seventh and eighth cervical nerves, above and below the seventh cervical transverse process respectively [Fig. 9.8].

14. Displace the common carotid artery laterally to expose the **sympathetic trunk** posteromedial to it [Fig. 9.6]. Trace the trunk superiorly and inferiorly.

15. Find the **cervicothoracic ganglion** between the seventh cervical transverse process and the neck of the first rib, posterior to the vertebral artery.

16. Find the small **middle cervical ganglion** anterior to the inferior thyroid artery, close to the sixth cervical transverse process.

17. Find the grey rami communicantes passing from these ganglia to the ventral rami of the spinal nerves.

Brachiocephalic trunk

The brachiocephalic trunk is a large artery which arises from the arch of the aorta and passes superiorly and to the right. For the most part, it lies in the thorax and divides into the right subclavian and right common carotid arteries behind the right sternoclavicular joint.

Subclavian artery

On the left, the subclavian artery arises from the arch of the aorta and ascends on the pleura to enter the neck behind the left sternoclavicular joint. On the right, it arises from the brachiocephalic artery behind the right sternoclavicular joint. On both sides, it arches laterally across the anterior surface of the cervical pleura on to the first rib, posterior to the scalenus anterior [Figs. 9.6, 9.7, 9.8]. It becomes the axillary artery at the outer border of the first rib. The subclavian artery is arbitrarily divided into three parts by the scalenus anterior. The first part is medial to the muscle; the second part is posterior to it, and the third part is lateral. (The third part has been described in Chapter 6.)

First part of the subclavian artery

On the right, the first part runs superolaterally at the medial edge of the scalenus anterior. At its origin, it lies posterior to the sternocleidomastoid, sternohyoid, sternothyroid, and vagus nerve. The **right recurrent laryngeal nerve** arises from the vagus and hooks around the first part of the subclavian artery. In addition, a loop from the sympathetic trunk—the **ansa subclavia**—loops around the subclavian artery at this point. The ansa subclavia are fibres which unite the inferior and middle cervical sympathetic ganglia around the subclavian artery. Near the medial border of the scalenus anterior, the subclavian artery lies posterior to the internal jugular and vertebral veins. It lies anterior to the suprapleural membrane covering the anterior surface of the cervical pleura [Fig. 9.7]. (If the lung has already been removed, investigate the position of the artery from the pleural cavity.)

On the left, the first part of the subclavian artery ascends vertically from the aortic arch, posterior to the vagus, phrenic, and cardiac nerves. It lies behind the left brachiocephalic vein at the sternoclavicular joint. From then onwards, the course of the left subclavian artery is the same as that of the right, except that the thoracic duct and phrenic nerve also descend anterior to it [Fig. 9.6]. The **left recurrent laryngeal nerve** is medial to the artery as it ascends from the aortic arch in the groove between the trachea and oesophagus.

Second part of the subclavian artery

The second part of the subclavian is curved upwards and rises 1.5–2.5 cm above the clavicle. Anteriorly, it has the scalenus anterior and phrenic nerve. Postero-inferiorly, it lies on the suprapleural membrane [Figs. 9.6, 9.7].

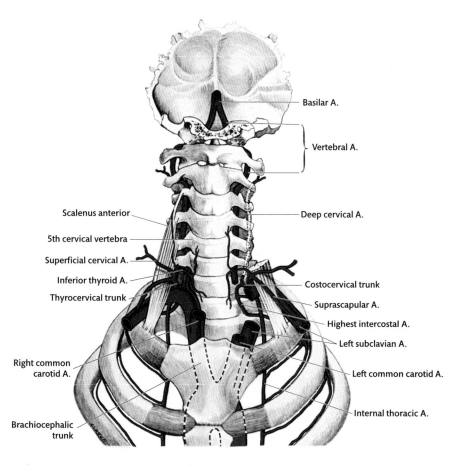

Fig. 9.8 Diagram of the branches of the subclavian arteries. (The deep cervical artery lies deep among the muscles of the back of the neck.)

Branches of the subclavian artery

The first part gives rise to the **vertebral artery**, the **thyrocervical trunk**, and the **internal thoracic artery**. The thyrocervical trunk gives rise to the **inferior thyroid, superficial cervical**, and **suprascapular arteries**. The second part gives rise to the **costocervical trunk**, from which arise the **highest intercostal** and **deep cervical arteries** [Fig. 9.8].

Vertebral artery

The vertebral artery is the first branch of the subclavian artery and mainly supplies the brain. It arises at the level of the sternoclavicular joint, ascends between the longus colli and scalenus anterior muscles, and enters into the foramen transversarium of the sixth cervical vertebra. It is posterior to the common carotid and inferior thyroid arteries and to its own vein, and anterior to the ventral rami of the seventh and eighth cervical nerves and the seventh cervical transverse process. The sympathetic trunk lies along its medial side, and the

cervicothoracic ganglion, which is partly behind the artery, sends branches to form a plexus on it. It is crossed anteriorly by the thoracic duct on the left [see Fig. 8.15; Figs. 9.6, 9.7, 9.8].

Thyrocervical trunk

The short thyrocervical trunk arises from the subclavian artery at the medial margin of the scalenus anterior, posterior to the internal jugular vein. It branches immediately into the inferior thyroid artery, superficial cervical and suprascapular branches.

The **inferior thyroid artery** ascends along the medial border of the scalenus anterior. Just below the transverse process of the sixth cervical vertebra, it turns medially in front of the vertebral artery and posterior to the vagus, sympathetic trunk, and common carotid artery, to reach the middle of the posterior surface of the thyroid gland. Then it descends to the lower pole of the gland and branches close to the recurrent laryngeal nerve. It supplies the thyroid and parathyroid glands, and anastomoses with the superior thyroid artery [Figs. 9.6, 9.8].

The **ascending cervical branch** of the inferior thyroid artery passes upwards on the cervical transverse processes. It supplies the prevertebral muscles and sends branches to the spinal cord [Fig. 9.8].

The **inferior laryngeal artery** also arises from the inferior thyroid artery and accompanies the recurrent laryngeal nerve to the larynx. Other branches from the thyrocervical trunk pass to the trachea, oesophagus, pharynx, and infrahyoid muscles.

Internal thoracic artery

The internal thoracic artery arises from the inferior surface of the subclavian artery near the medial border of the scalenus anterior. It passes inferomedially to the back of the first costal cartilage. In the neck, it lies anterior to the pleura behind the medial part of the clavicle [Fig. 9.7].

Costocervical trunk

The **costocervical trunk** arises from the posterior surface of the second part of the subclavian artery [Fig. 9.8]. It arches posteriorly over the pleura and divides at the neck of the first rib into the deep cervical and superior intercostal arteries.

The **deep cervical artery** passes into the back of the neck above the neck of the first rib. Together with the descending branch of the occipital artery, it is the main source of blood supply to the muscles of the back of the neck.

The **superior intercostal artery** descends anterior to the neck of the first rib and gives posterior intercostal arteries to the first and second intercostal spaces. If the lung has been removed, examine these from the interior of the thorax [Fig. 9.8].

Fig. 9.10 is a schematic section through the neck at the level of C. 5, showing the areas supplied by branches of the external carotid and subclavian arteries.

Subclavian vein

The subclavian vein is a continuation of the axillary vein at the outer border of the first rib. It unites with the internal jugular vein behind the sternoclavicular joint to form the brachiocephalic vein. It receives the external jugular vein. None of the veins corresponding to the branches of the subclavian artery drain into the subclavian vein. The vertebral vein descends posterior to the internal jugular vein from the foramen transversarium of the sixth cervical vertebra and drains into the brachiocephalic vein. The **internal thoracic vein** joins the brachiocephalic vein near the superior aperture of the thorax. The deep cervical vein joins the vertebral vein [Figs. 9.6, 9.7].

Brachiocephalic veins

The brachiocephalic veins collect blood from the head and neck, upper limbs, walls of the thorax, and the anterior abdominal wall (internal thoracic veins). They are formed behind the medial end of the clavicle by the union of the corresponding internal jugular and subclavian veins [Figs. 9.7, 9.9]. They descend into the thorax and end by uniting with each other to form the superior vena cava. They have no valves.

In the neck, the right brachiocephalic vein lies on the cervical pleura with the phrenic nerve and internal thoracic artery intervening. It is lateral to the brachiocephalic trunk (with the vagus behind and between them) and posterior to the medial end of the clavicle. It enters the thorax behind the right first costal cartilage. On the left, the vein is first posterior to the clavicle and anterior to the pleura and internal thoracic artery. It then descends posterior to the sternoclavicular joint, anterior to the phrenic and vagus nerves, and the arteries arising from the aortic arch [Figs. 9.7, 9.10].

Tributaries in the neck

Both brachiocephalic veins receive the vertebral, highest intercostal, and frequently the inferior thyroid veins, and one or two lymph trunks. The thoracic duct and left superior intercostal vein enter the left vein.

Thoracic duct

The thoracic duct is a large lymph vessel which drains lymph into the venous system. It drains lymph from: (1) all the regions below the diaphragm, except for the upper part of the right lobe of the liver and the upper half of the anterior abdominal wall; (2) the posterior thoracic wall on both sides; and (3) the left half of the body above the diaphragm. The lymph in the duct has a milky appearance due to the fat from the small intestine.

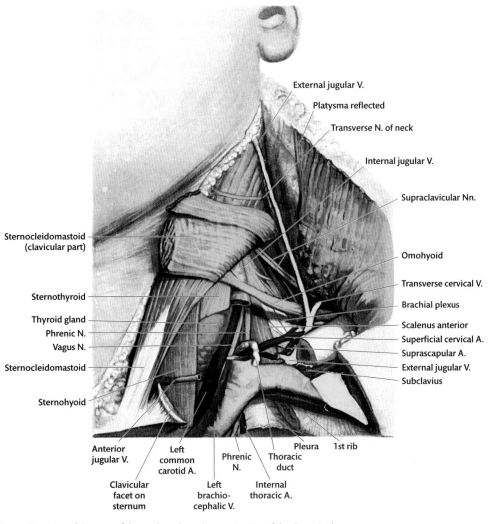

External jugular V.

Platysma reflected

Transverse N. of neck

Internal jugular V.

Supraclavicular Nn.

Sternocleidomastoid (clavicular part)

Omohyoid

Transverse cervical V.

Sternothyroid

Brachial plexus

Thyroid gland

Scalenus anterior

Phrenic N.

Superficial cervical A.

Vagus N.

Suprascapular A.

Sternocleidomastoid

External jugular V.

Subclavius

Sternohyoid

Anterior jugular V.

Left common carotid A.

Phrenic N.

Thoracic duct

Pleura   1st rib

Clavicular facet on sternum

Left brachio-cephalic V.

Internal thoracic A.

Fig. 9.9 Deep dissection of the root of the neck to show the termination of the thoracic duct.

The thoracic duct is slender, thin-walled, and frequently mistaken for a vein. It ascends from the thorax along the left margin of the oesophagus. At the level of the seventh cervical vertebra, it arches anterolaterally between the carotid sheath and the cervical pleura, and turns inferiorly to enter the left brachiocephalic vein in the angle between the internal jugular and subclavian veins [Figs. 9.7, 9.9]. Its opening into the vein is guarded by a valve.

There are three other lymph trunks in the root of the neck on each side: (1) the **subclavian lymph trunk** which drains the upper limb; (2) the **jugular lymph trunk** which drains the head and neck; and (3) the **bronchomediastinal lymph trunk** which drains the lung, mediastinum, and part of the anterior walls of the thorax and abdomen through the **internal thoracic lymph vessels**. None of these vessels is visible by dissection. The mode of termination of these lymph trunks is variable. The bronchomediastinal trunks usually enter the corresponding brachiocephalic veins. On the left side, all three lymph trunks may end in the thoracic duct. Commonly, the subclavian lymph trunk ends in the subclavian vein. On the right side, the jugular and subclavian lymph trunks may end separately in the corresponding veins but frequently unite to form a **right lymph duct** which drains into the venous system at the junction of the right internal jugular and subclavian veins. The mode of termination of the three lymph trunks alters the territory drained by the thoracic duct.

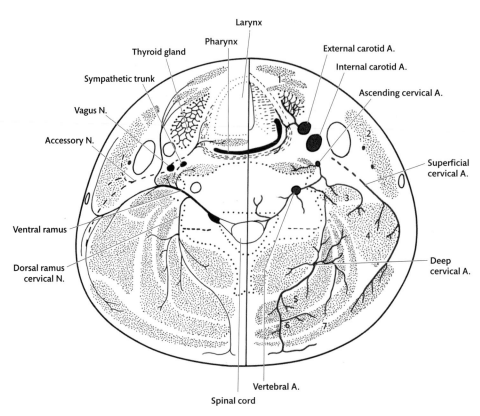

Larynx
Pharynx
Thyroid gland
Sympathetic trunk
Vagus N.
Accessory N.
Ventral ramus
Dorsal ramus
cervical N.
External carotid A.
Internal carotid A.
Ascending cervical A.
Superficial
cervical A.
Deep
cervical A.
Vertebral A.
Spinal cord

Fig. 9.10 Diagrammatic transverse section through the neck to show the distribution of nerves (left) and arteries (right). The diagram is constructed from a number of adjacent levels. The part of the accessory nerve shown by an interrupted line is at a still higher level. 1. Infrahyoid muscles. 2. Sternocleidomastoid. 3. Scalenus medius. 4. Levator scapulae. 5. Semispinalis capitis. 6. Splenius capitis. 7. Trapezius.

Cervical pleura

On each side, the parietal pleura forms the dome of the pleura and bulges upwards into the root of the neck [Fig. 9.7]. Superiorly, it reaches up to the level of the neck of the first rib, which is 2.5–5.0 cm above the sternal end of the first rib. A thickening of the fascia—the **suprapleural membrane**—stretches from the transverse process of the seventh cervical vertebra to the inner margin of the first rib and covers the cervical pleura. This membrane may contain some muscle fibres—the **scalenus minimus**.

The upper two ribs, the first intercostal space, and the sympathetic trunk lie posterior to the cervical pleura. The great vessels of the upper limb and head and neck lie anterior to it. The vertebral artery curves superiorly over the dome of the pleura to reach the vertebral column [Fig. 9.7].

The vertebral bodies, oesophagus, and trachea, and on the left side the thoracic duct and the recurrent laryngeal nerve, lie medial to the cervical pleura. The scalenus anterior, subclavian artery, and the lower trunk of the brachial plexus lie lateral to it. Because the subclavian artery lies on the anterior surface of the cervical pleura, its ascending and descending branches—the vertebral artery, inferior thyroid artery, and internal thoracic artery—also lie on the anterior surface. The costocervical trunk and its superior intercostal branch arch over the dome of the pleura from the anterior to the posterior surface.

Vertical neurovascular bundles of the neck

A neurovascular bundle lies on each side of the trachea and oesophagus. In the lower part of the neck, the bundle consists of the **internal jugular vein** laterally, the **common carotid artery** medially, and the **vagus nerve** behind and between them. Above the level of the thyroid cartilage, the neurovascular bundle consists of the **internal carotid artery**, internal jugular vein, **glossopharyngeal**,

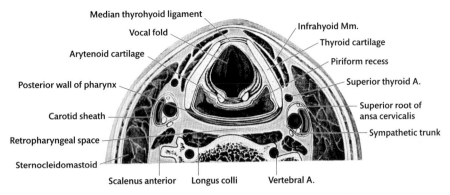

Median thyrohyoid ligament

Vocal fold

Arytenoid cartilage

Posterior wall of pharynx

Carotid sheath

Retropharyngeal space

Sternocleidomastoid

Scalenus anterior   Longus colli   Vertebral A.

Infrahyoid Mm.

Thyroid cartilage

Piriform recess

Superior thyroid A.

Superior root of ansa cervicalis

Sympathetic trunk

Fig. 9.11 Transverse section through the anterior part of the neck at the level of the upper part of the thyroid cartilage.

vagus, **spinal accessory**, and **hypoglossal nerves**. The bundle is enclosed in a fascial sheath— the **carotid sheath** [see Fig. 5.2; Fig. 9.11]—which extends from the root of the neck to the base of the skull. It lies on the sympathetic trunk, prevertebral fascia, prevertebral muscles, and cervical transverse processes. Parts of this neurovascular bundle have been seen and described in the carotid triangle in Chapter 6.

Dissection 9.5 provides instructions on dissection of the neurovascular structures of the neck.

Before beginning the dissection, identify the carotid canal, jugular foramen, hypoglossal canal, and foramen magnum on the base of a dried skull, and note the openings of these foramina on its internal aspect [see Fig. 8.7]. The **carotid canal** lies furthest anteriorly and transmits the internal carotid artery. Immediately posterior to it is the **jugular foramen** which transmits the sigmoid and inferior petrosal sinuses and the glossopharyngeal, vagus, and accessory nerves between the two veins. The hypoglossal nerve traverses the **hypoglossal**

DISSECTION 9.5 Neurovascular structures of the neck

Objectives

I. To remove the right half of the skull and related structures, so as to gain approach to the cavities of the nose, mouth, pharynx, and larynx from the medial side.   **II.** To expose the superior parts of the internal carotid artery, the internal jugular vein, and the lower four cranial nerves in the upper part of the carotid sheath.

Instructions

1. On the right side, free the greater occipital nerve from the scalp, and turn it inferiorly. Cut through the great auricular, lesser occipital, and transverse nerve of the neck on the sternocleidomastoid. Leave sufficient nerve on both sides of the cuts to allow the ends to be identified subsequently.

2. In the suboccipital triangle, separate the superior oblique and rectus capitis posterior major and the minor muscles from their bony attachments, and remove them. This exposes the posterior atlanto-occipital membrane [see Fig. 22.4]. Cut across this membrane close to the skull, but

avoid damage to the vertebral arteries on the posterior arch of the atlas.

3. Detach the longissimus muscle from the skull [see Fig. 7.4].

4. Cut across the sternocleidomastoid 2–3 cm above the clavicle, and turn it superiorly. Clean the deep surface of the sternocleidomastoid as far as the skull, and identify the accessory nerve entering it. Cut the nerve in the posterior triangle, so that the superior part of the nerve remains with the sternocleidomastoid.

5. Pass a finger behind the carotid sheath and pharynx, and separate them from the prevertebral fascia and the sympathetic trunk as far superiorly as the superior cervical ganglion. Note how easily the loose fascia behind the pharynx is torn. (In the living, this loose areolar tissue permits the pharynx to slide on the vertebral column.)

6. Saw through the mandible in the midline, and continue this cut through the tongue and epiglottis with a knife. Cut through the hyoid bone in the

midline, and extend the incision inferiorly through the larynx, pharynx, and trachea to the inferior border of the isthmus of the thyroid gland.

7. Cut transversely through the right half of the trachea, oesophagus, and neurovascular bundle. (Do not cut the sympathetic trunk, phrenic nerve, and scalenus anterior.)

8. Separate the upper parts of the transected structures from those behind them.

9. Make a mid-sagittal saw cut through the anterior part of the skull up to the foramen magnum. Do not damage the atlas vertebra.

10. Within the skull, detach the dura mater and membrana tectoria [see Fig. 22.4] from the anterior margin of the foramen magnum, and turn it inferiorly to expose the alar ligaments and the longitudinal fibres of the cruciate ligament [see Fig. 22.1].

11. Cut across the right alar ligament, and flex the right half of the head on the vertebral column. Divide the tight posterior part of the capsule of the atlanto-occipital joint. Now lever the occipital condyle out of its articulation, cutting any remaining parts of the capsule of the joint as they are exposed.

12. Free the vertebral artery and the first cervical nerve from the posterior arch of the atlas, and cut across the artery where it emerges from the transverse process of the atlas. Cut through the rectus capitis lateralis, rectus capitis anterior, longus capitis [see Fig. 10.1], and anterior atlanto-occipital membrane [see Fig. 22.4].

13. Complete the median division of the soft palate and of the posterior pharyngeal wall with a knife. Gently lift away the right half of the skull and attached structures. (Leave the ganglion and sympathetic trunk on the vertebral column.)

On the right side:

14. Find the internal laryngeal nerve piercing the thyrohyoid membrane. Trace it superiorly to the superior laryngeal nerve, medial to the external and internal carotid arteries. Trace the superior laryngeal nerve to the vagus. Above its origin from the vagus, find the pharyngeal branch of the vagus, and trace it between the carotid arteries to the pharynx [see Fig. 6.5; Fig. 9.12].

15. Find the glossopharyngeal, accessory, and hypoglossal nerves in the upper part of the neurovascular bundle, and trace them distally. The nerves separate inferiorly [Figs. 9.12, 9.13]. The accessory (spinal part) runs postero-inferiorly, either superficial or deep to the internal jugular vein. The glossopharyngeal nerve passes antero-inferiorly with the stylopharyngeus muscle, lateral to the internal carotid artery. The hypoglossal nerve curves anteriorly, superficial to the internal and external carotid arteries. The vagus descends vertically between the artery and vein in the carotid sheath.

16. When following the glossopharyngeal nerve, identify the stylopharyngeus muscle on which it runs to the pharynx. Trace the muscle to its origin from the styloid process.

17. The **stylopharyngeus** enters the pharynx between the superior and middle constrictor muscles of the pharynx. The upper margin of the **middle constrictor** can be defined and followed forwards to the hyoid bone [see Fig. 6.5].

18. Trace a branch from the glossopharyngeal and vagus nerves down between the two carotid arteries to the carotid sinus [Fig. 9.12]. This branch is the **carotid sinus nerve** and may be followed to the carotid body in the bifurcation of the common carotid artery.

19. Find the branches of the sympathetic ganglion (grey rami communicantes) passing posteriorly to the upper four cervical ventral rami.

20. Trace the occipital artery from the occiput to its origin.

21. Expose the posterior belly of the digastric from behind, and find the hypoglossal nerve hooking round the origin of the occipital artery, superficial to both carotid arteries [Fig. 9.14].

On the left side:

22. Cut through the posterior belly of the digastric, close to its origin. Turn it antero-inferiorly to expose the stylopharyngeus [see Fig. 6.5], but avoid damage to the glossopharyngeal nerve which curves round the lateral aspect of the muscle.

23. Lift the neurovascular bundle from the sympathetic trunk, and trace the trunk upwards to the **superior cervical ganglion**. Attempt to find the branches of the ganglion to the internal carotid artery, the external carotid artery, and the cranial nerves in the bundle.

canal, immediately above the occipital condyle, and joins the other nerves between the internal carotid artery and internal jugular vein close to the skull.

Common carotid artery

The right common carotid artery arises from the brachiocephalic trunk behind the right sternoclavicular joint. The left common carotid artery arises from the arch of the aorta and ascends into the neck, posterior to the left sternoclavicular joint. From behind the sternoclavicular joint, each artery ascends to the upper border of the thyroid cartilage at the level of the disc between the third and fourth cervical vertebrae [Figs. 9.2, 9.3, 9.4, 9.6, 9.12].

Here it ends by dividing into the internal and external carotid arteries.

In the neck, the common carotid artery ascends anterior to the subclavian and vertebral arteries to lie on the prevertebral fascia on the sixth cervical transverse process—the **carotid tubercle**. (The anterior tubercle of the sixth cervical vertebra is longer than the others and is called the carotid tubercle. The carotid artery can be forcibly compressed on this bony prominence.)

The common carotid arteries lie in the carotid sheath. The lower part of both common carotid arteries is overlapped anteriorly by the sternocleidomastoid, the infrahyoid muscles, and the thyroid gland. They lie lateral to the thyroid cartilage, thyroid gland, pharynx, larynx, trachea, and oesophagus [see Fig. 5.2; Fig. 9.1].

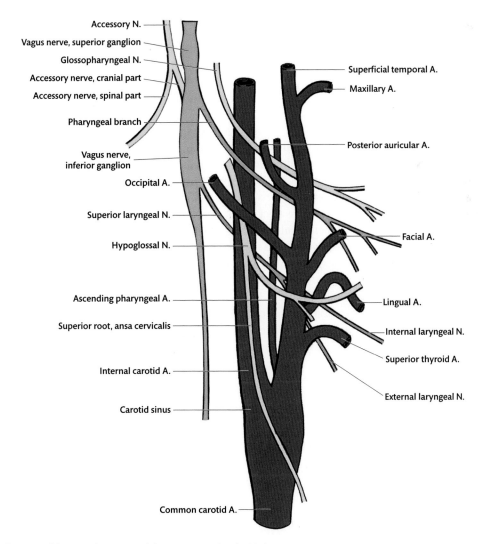

Fig. 9.12 Diagram of the carotid arteries and the nerves associated with them.

The **carotid sinus** is a slight dilatation of the upper part of the common carotid and the adjacent part of the internal carotid artery. At the sinus, the wall of the arteries is more elastic than elsewhere and is heavily innervated. The carotid sinus is a pressure receptor. Distension of the sinus wall stimulates the nerve endings and leads to a reflex slowing of the heart and a fall in blood pressure.

The **carotid body** is a small gland-like structure situated in the carotid bifurcation. It consists of clusters of epithelial-like cells arranged around capillaries. The carotid body responds to changes in blood gas tension and brings about reflex changes in respiration. The carotid body may be seen by twisting the arteries round and dissecting between them.

Both the carotid sinus and the carotid body are innervated principally by the **glossopharyngeal nerve** through the **carotid sinus nerve**, but they are also supplied by the vagus and sympathetics.

External carotid artery

The external carotid artery begins as a branch of the common carotid artery in the carotid triangle (Chapter 6). It ascends on the lateral aspect of the pharynx, anteromedial and parallel to the internal carotid artery. The transverse nerve of the neck, cervical branches of the facial nerve, facial and lingual veins, and hypoglossal nerve lie superficial to it. Branches of the superior laryngeal nerve are deep to it [see Figs. 6.4, 6.6; Fig. 9.12]. Above the carotid triangle, the external carotid artery is covered by the angle of the mandible, posterior belly of the digastric, and the stylohyoid. Superior to the stylohyoid, the external carotid artery and its facial branch turn laterally, away from the internal carotid artery, and enter the deep surface of the parotid gland. Before it enters the parotid gland, the styloid process of the temporal bone, stylopharyngeus muscle, glossopharyngeal nerve, styloglossus muscle, and the pharyngeal branch of the vagus lie between the internal and external carotid arteries [Fig. 9.15]. In the parotid gland, the external carotid artery ascends to the back of the neck of the mandible and divides into the **superficial temporal** and **maxillary arteries**. In the gland, it lies deep to the facial nerve and retromandibular vein.

The external carotid artery is surrounded by the **external carotid plexus** of sympathetic nerve fibres. These nerve fibres arise in the cells of the superior cervical ganglion of the sympathetic trunk. Like the internal carotid nerve on the corresponding artery, this plexus is one of the main routes of distribution of sympathetic nerves to the head. (Similar plexuses on the vertebral and subclavian arteries and sympathetic fibres from the cervical sympathetic ganglia in the spinal and cranial nerves complete the sympathetic distribution to the head and neck.)

Branches of the external carotid artery

Superior thyroid artery

The **superior thyroid artery** arises from the anterior surface of the external carotid, close to its origin. It runs antero-inferiorly in the carotid triangle, deep to the infrahyoid muscles. The initial segment of the artery has been seen in the carotid triangle. It divides into anterior and posterior branches at the apex of the lobe of the thyroid gland. It gives rise to: (1) small muscular branches; (2) the small **infrahyoid artery** which runs along the lower border of the hyoid bone; (3) the larger **superior laryngeal artery** which pierces the thyrohyoid membrane with the internal laryngeal nerve; (4) the small **sternocleidomastoid branch** which runs postero-inferiorly across the carotid sheath; and (5) the **cricothyroid branch** which arises deep to the sternothyroid muscle and runs anteriorly across the cricothyroid muscle to anastomose with its fellow on the cricothyroid membrane [see Fig. 6.7].

Occipital artery

The occipital artery arises from the posterior surface of the external carotid artery, opposite the origin of the facial branch [Figs. 9.12, 9.14]. It runs along the lower border of the posterior belly of the digastric, deep to the sternocleidomastoid, to reach and groove the base of the skull, medial to the mastoid notch. Its further course and branches are described in Chapter 4. In the neck, it lies superficial to the internal carotid artery, hypoglossal nerve (which hooks anteriorly round its origin), internal jugular vein, and accessory nerve [Fig. 9.15]. It gives off several muscular branches, one of which accompanies the accessory nerve to the sternocleidomastoid, and a meningeal branch which enters the skull through the jugular foramen.

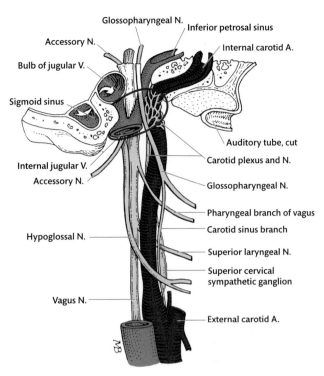

Fig. 9.13 Diagram of structures in and below the right jugular foramen. Circle = jugular foramen.

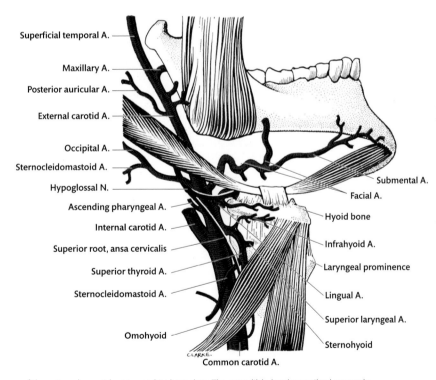

Fig. 9.14 Diagram of the external carotid artery and its branches. The mandible has been tilted upwards.

Posterior auricular artery

The posterior auricular artery is a small branch which lies along the upper border of the posterior belly of the digastric [Fig. 9.14]. It passes superficial to the mastoid process with the posterior auricular nerve. It supplies the adjacent muscles and the parotid gland, and sends a **stylomastoid branch** superiorly into the stylomastoid foramen to supply

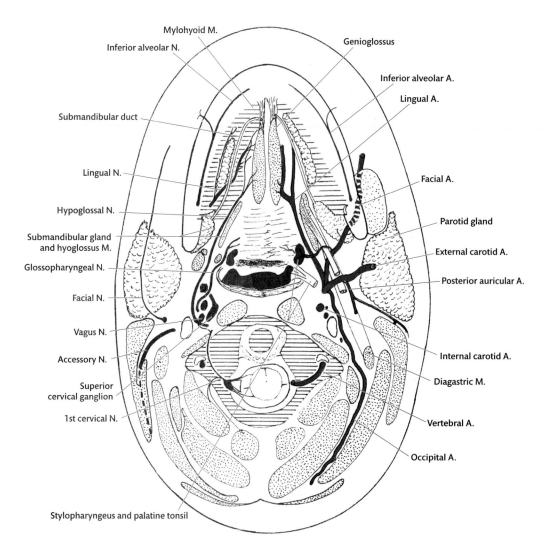

Mylohyoid M.

Inferior alveolar N.

Genioglossus

Inferior alveolar A.

Lingual A.

Submandibular duct

Lingual N.

Facial A.

Hypoglossal N.

Parotid gland

Submandibular gland
and hyoglossus M.

External carotid A.

Glossopharyngeal N.

Posterior auricular A.

Facial N.

Vagus N.

Internal carotid A.

Accessory N.

Diagastric M.

Superior
cervical ganglion

1st cervical N.

Vertebral A.

Occipital A.

Stylopharyngeus and palatine tonsil

Fig. 9.15 A diagrammatic section through the first cervical vertebra and the floor of the mouth to show the course of nerves (left) and arteries (right). The diagram is constructed from a number of adjacent levels. The muscle immediately superior to the facial artery is the styloglossus; that inferior to it is the stylohyoid.

the **facial nerve** and other structures within the temporal bone.

Ascending pharyngeal artery

The ascending pharyngeal artery is the first and smallest branch of the external carotid artery. It ascends on the pharynx, medial to the carotid arteries [Fig. 9.12].

Internal carotid artery

The cervical part of the internal carotid artery lies on the longus capitis and the sympathetic trunk [see Fig. 5.2]. The vagus lies postero-lateral to it in the neck, with the glossopharyngeal, accessory, and hypoglossal nerves also posterior at the base

of the skull. The artery lies between the internal jugular vein and the pharynx.

More inferiorly, the artery lies deep to the sterno-cleidomastoid, lingual and facial veins, hypoglossal nerve, and the occipital artery [Fig. 9.13]. The superior root of the ansa cervicalis is anterior, and the external carotid is anteromedial to it. The internal carotid artery ascends deep to the posterior belly of the digastric, the styloid process, and the muscles attached to it. These structures separate it from the parotid gland. It then passes anterior to the internal jugular vein and enters the carotid canal. It is accompanied by the **internal carotid nerve** from the superior cervical ganglion of the sympathetic trunk.

Of the common, internal, and external carotid arteries on each side, only the external carotid artery gives branches to structures in the neck (mainly to the parts of the respiratory and digestive systems). The remainder of the neck—principally muscles and bone—is supplied by the subclavian arteries [Fig. 9.10]. The internal carotid arteries supply a considerable part of the brain, the orbital contents, the forehead, the anterior part of the scalp, and parts of the external nose and walls of the nasal cavities. The remainder of the structures in the head is supplied by the external carotid arteries.

Internal jugular vein

The internal jugular vein is usually the largest vein in the neck. It begins at the jugular foramen by the union of the sigmoid and inferior petrosal sinuses [Fig. 9.13]. It descends vertically on the lateral side of the internal and common carotid arteries, enclosed with them and the vagus nerve in the carotid sheath [Fig. 9.11]. It ends behind the medial part of the clavicle by uniting with the subclavian vein to form the brachiocephalic vein [see Fig. 6.7; Fig. 9.9]. In the lower part of the neck, the left internal jugular vein overlaps the left common carotid artery, while on the right, the right internal jugular vein remains lateral to the common carotid artery.

The upper end of the internal jugular vein is dilated to form the **superior bulb**. At the lower end of the vein, there is a smaller dilatation—the **inferior bulb**—with a valve just above it [see Fig. 6.13].

The right internal jugular vein is usually larger than the left because it usually drains the superior sagittal sinus. At the base of the skull, the internal jugular vein lies postero-lateral to the internal carotid artery, with the last four cranial nerves between them. Along its course, the longus capitis, sympathetic trunk, roots of the cervical plexus, scalenus anterior, and phrenic nerve lie posterior to the vein. The internal carotid artery, common carotid artery, glossopharyngeal nerve, pharyngeal branch of the vagus, hypoglossal nerve, and superior root of the ansa cervicalis lie medial to it. The spinal part of the accessory nerve may run anterior to the upper part of the vein, and the inferior root of the ansa cervicalis may be lateral or medial to its lower part [Fig. 9.13].

Tributaries of the internal jugular vein

1. The **pharyngeal plexus** drains into the upper part by two or more veins.

2. The **facial**, **lingual**, and **superior thyroid veins** enter the internal jugular vein in the carotid triangle.

3. The **middle thyroid vein** and sometimes the **jugular lymph trunk** enter it at the root of the neck.

Nerves of the neck

The structures in the neck are derived from one of two embryological sources, each with its own source of nerve supply. The vertebral column and its associated muscles, the muscles of the tongue, and the infrahyoid muscles are derived from the occipital and upper cervical somites (somatic in origin). They are supplied by the hypoglossal and upper cervical spinal nerves.

The walls of the respiratory and digestive systems—nasal cavities, oral cavity, pharynx, larynx, trachea, oesophagus, and their associated glands—are derived from the pharyngeal or branchial arches (visceral in origin). They are supplied by cranial nerves of **branchiomeric origin**—the **trigeminal** (V), **facial** (VII), **glossopharyngeal** (IX), **vagus** (X), and **accessory** (XI) nerves. (The territory supplied by the branchiomeric nerves extends from the oral and nasal orifices to the upper part of the gut tube in the abdomen.) **Muscles of facial expression** (VII) and the **sternocleidomastoid** and **trapezius muscles** (XI) are also innervated by cranial nerves of branchiomeric origin, as they originate from the wall of the gut tube. Table 9.1 gives the distribution of the branchiomeric cranial nerves supplying the head and neck.

The glossopharyngeal, vagus, and spinal accessory nerves enter the neurovascular bundle through the jugular foramen. They descend between the internal carotid artery and internal jugular vein, and either leave the bundle (IX and spinal part of XI) or send branches from it (X and cranial part of XI). The hypoglossal nerve also enters the bundle but leaves it shortly to supply the muscles of the tongue.

Glossopharyngeal nerve

The glossopharyngeal (ninth) cranial nerve arises from the side of the upper medulla oblongata and passes through the jugular foramen in its own dural

Table 9.1 Distribution of branchiomeric nerves in the neck

Nerve	Area supplied in head and neck		
	Sensory	Striated muscle	Parasympathetic
Trigeminal (V)	Skin and mucous membrane of oronasal region, face, forehead, scalp, dura mater	Muscles of mastication, anterior belly of digastric, mylohyoid, tensor tympani, tensor palati	–
Facial (VII)	Anterior two-thirds of tongue and palate—taste	Muscles of facial expression, posterior belly of digastric, stylohyoid, stapedius	Submandibular, sublingual, nasal, lacrimal, palatine, oral glands
Glossopharyngeal (IX)	Posterior one-third of tongue, epiglottis, palate—taste and general sensation, middle ear, auditory tube, mastoid antrum, carotid sinus, carotid body	Stylopharyngeus	Parotid and glands in posterior one-third of tongue
Vagus (X)	Pharynx, larynx, oesophagus, trachea, dura mater, external acoustic meatus	Muscles of pharynx, larynx, and soft palate except tensor palati	Glands and smooth muscle of pharynx, larynx, trachea, oesophagus (also many thoracic and abdominal viscera)
Accessory, cranial part (XI)	Larynx, pharynx, oesophagus, trachea	Muscles of pharynx and larynx	–
Accessory, spinal part (XI)	–	Sternocleidomastoid and trapezius	–

sheath, between the sigmoid and inferior petrosal sinuses. At the base of the skull, it has two small sensory ganglia—the **superior** and **inferior ganglia**. It descends between the internal jugular vein and the internal carotid artery, curves around the lateral surface of the stylopharyngeus, between the internal and external carotid arteries, and passes with that muscle into the pharynx [see Fig. 6.5; Figs. 9.12, 9.13]. In the wall of the pharynx, it lies external to the mucous membrane of the lower part of the **tonsillar fossa** and runs forwards into the tongue, deep to the hyoglossus. It receives taste and general sensation from the posterior third of the tongue, vallate papillae [see Fig. 18.1], palatine tonsil, part of the soft palate and adjacent pharynx, and the anterior surface of the epiglottis.

Branches of the glossopharyngeal nerve

1. The slender **tympanic branch** of the glossopharyngeal nerve enters a minute canal on the ridge of the bone between the jugular foramen and the carotid canal. It ascends to the middle ear and forms the **tympanic plexus** on the medial wall of the middle ear cavity, with minute **carotico-tympanic nerves** from the sympathetic plexus on the internal carotid artery [see Fig. 13.8]. The tympanic plexus supplies the mucous membrane of the middle ear, auditory tube, mastoid antrum, and mastoid air cells and sends preganglionic parasympathetic (secretomotor) nerves through the **lesser petrosal nerve** to the otic ganglion. (The otic ganglion innervates the parotid gland.)

2. The **nerve to the stylopharyngeus** supplies the stylopharyngeus and passes through it to the pharyngeal mucous membrane.

3. The **pharyngeal branches** supply the pharyngeal mucous membrane and run with the pharyngeal branch of the vagus to the pharyngeal plexus.

4. One branch from the glossopharyngeal nerve joins a branch of the vagus to form the **carotid sinus nerve** to the carotid sinus and body.

Vagus nerve course

The vagus arises by a row of rootlets from the side of the medulla oblongata [see Fig. 24.2], immediately inferior to the glossopharyngeal nerve. It leaves the skull with the accessory nerve through the middle compartment of the jugular foramen. Like the glossopharyngeal nerve, it has two **sensory ganglia**, superior and inferior, at the base of the skull. The vagus descends vertically in the carotid sheath, posteromedial to the internal jugular vein and postero-lateral to the internal and common carotid arteries [Figs. 9.12, 9.13].

At the root of the neck, each vagus crosses the anterior surface of the corresponding subclavian artery. The right vagus then descends, posterior to the brachiocephalic vein, to the right side of the trachea in the thorax. The left vagus descends between the subclavian and common carotid arteries, posterior to the left brachiocephalic vein [Figs. 9.7, 9.9].

Branches of the vagus nerve

1. The vagus communicates with the other nerves in the jugular foramen.
2. It is joined by the cranial part of the accessory and gives branches to the larynx.
3. A small **meningeal branch** passes back through the jugular foramen to the dura mater of the posterior cranial fossa.
4. The slender **auricular branch** runs through a minute canal in the lateral wall of the jugular fossa to the tympanomastoid fissure. It pierces the cartilage of the external acoustic meatus and supplies the skin lining of the lower half of the meatus and the tympanic membrane. ➲ Irritation of the skin in this region may give rise to an intractable cough or cause other vagal reflexes.
5. The **pharyngeal branch** of the vagus arises immediately below the skull. It runs antero-inferiorly between the internal and external carotid arteries, to form a large part of the **pharyngeal plexus** in the fascia covering the middle constrictor muscle of the pharynx. The plexus also receives branches from the glossopharyngeal nerve and superior cervical sympathetic ganglion. It supplies the pharyngeal wall [Figs. 9.12, 9.13].
6. The **superior laryngeal nerve** is larger than the pharyngeal branch and arises inferior to it. It descends deep to both carotid arteries and divides into two branches: the **internal** and **external** laryngeal nerves [Figs. 9.12, 9.13]. The internal laryngeal nerve descends on the lateral wall of the pharynx and pierces the thyrohyoid membrane. It descends deep to the mucous lining of the piriform recess of the pharynx and supplies the mucous membrane of the pharynx and the upper part of the larynx. The thin **external branch** descends on the side of the pharynx, deep to the carotid and superior thyroid arteries, sternothyroid muscle, and thyroid gland. It supplies the cricothyroid muscle [see Fig. 6.5] (the only intrinsic laryngeal muscle not supplied by the recurrent laryngeal nerve) and the inferior constrictor muscle [see Fig. 6.5].
7. Two slender **cardiac branches** arise from each vagus, one in the upper and the other in the lower part of the neck. They descend with the vagus into the thorax and join the superficial and deep cardiac plexuses.
8. The right **recurrent laryngeal nerve** arises as the vagus crosses the first part of the subclavian artery (the left as it crosses the arch of the aorta). Each nerve hooks below the corresponding artery and ascends in the groove between the oesophagus and trachea. The nerve passes deep to the lobe of the thyroid gland and enters the larynx, deep to the inferior border of the inferior constrictor muscle [Figs. 9.6, 9.7]. Within the larynx, it communicates with the internal branch of the superior laryngeal nerve and supplies the mucous membrane below the level of the vocal folds and all the intrinsic muscles, except the cricothyroid. The recurrent laryngeal nerve also gives off cardiac branches near its origin and supplies the trachea, the oesophagus, and the inferior part of the pharynx.

Accessory nerve

The eleventh cranial nerve—the spinal accessory—is mainly motor. The **cranial roots** emerge from the side of the medulla oblongata as a vertical row in series with those of the vagus. The **spinal roots** arise from the upper five cervical segments of the spinal cord and ascend through the foramen magnum. The spinal roots join the cranial rootlets within the skull [see Fig. 8.8].

The accessory nerve leaves the skull through the jugular foramen in the same dural sheath as the vagus. At the jugular foramen, the cranial part continues with the vagus and enters its laryngeal branches. The spinal part turns postero-inferiorly, crosses the tip of the transverse process of the atlas and the upper part of the carotid triangle to enter and supply the sternocleidomastoid [Fig. 9.12]. The nerve then runs through the sternocleidomastoid and emerges in the posterior triangle from its posterior border. It continues postero-inferiorly in the investing layer of the deep fascia of the posterior triangle, and enters the deep surface of the trapezius and supplies it [see Fig. 5.4]. It receives sensory branches from the second to fourth cervical ventral rami.

Hypoglossal nerve

The **hypoglossal nerve** arises as a row of rootlets from the anterior surface of the medulla oblongata [see Fig. 24.2]. The rootlets unite to form the hypoglossal nerve which leaves the skull through the hypoglossal canal. At the base of the skull, the hypoglossal nerve lies medial to the structures in the carotid sheath. The nerve then enters the neurovascular bundle, adheres briefly to the lateral surface of the vagus, and receives a branch from the first cervical ventral ramus [Figs. 9.12, 9.13, 9.14]. It descends with the vagus, deep to the posterior belly of the digastric, curves anteriorly on the root of the occipital artery, and enters the anterior triangle, lateral to the external carotid artery.

Branches of the hypoglossal nerve

1. A **meningeal branch**, composed of nerve fibres of the first cervical nerve, runs back through the hypoglossal canal to supply the dura mater near the foramen magnum.
2. A descending branch—the **superior root of the ansa cervicalis** (C. 1).
3. Nerves to **thyrohyoid** and **geniohyoid** (C. 1).

4. Branches to all the intrinsic and extrinsic **muscles of the tongue**, except the palatoglossus [Figs. 9.15, 9.16].

Cervical sympathethic trunk

The dissection of the cervical sympathetic ganglion is described in Dissection 9.6.

Start by reviewing the general features of the sympathetic trunk [Vol. 2, p. 7]. In the neck, the sympathetic trunk consists of **preganglionic sympathetic fibres** which ascend from the upper thoracic segments to the cervical ganglia. The trunk runs almost vertically, anterior to the longus colli and longus capitis muscles on the roots of the transverse processes, posterior to the common and internal carotid arteries. Inferiorly, it is medial to the vertebral artery and is crossed by the inferior thyroid artery posteriorly. (The thoracic duct lies anteriorly on the left.)

Superiorly, the trunk ends in the superior cervical ganglion. Nerve fibres from the ganglion extend into the skull as the **internal carotid nerve** on the internal carotid artery [Fig. 9.13]. Inferiorly, the sympathetic trunk enters the thorax by passing in front of the neck of the first rib.

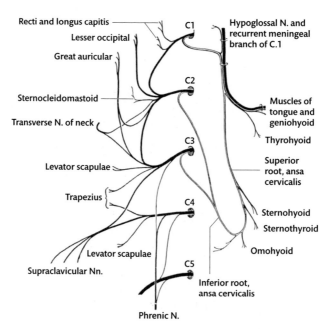

Fig. 9.16 A diagram of the cervical plexus and ansa cervicalis. C. 1 to C. 5, ventral rami of the upper five cervical nerves. Note that the nerves to the geniohyoid and thyrohyoid muscles and the superior root of the ansa are derived from the first cervical ventral ramus, although they appear to arise from the hypoglossal nerve.

Sympathetic ganglia and rami communicantes

There are three cervical ganglia—superior, middle, and inferior cervical ganglia. The inferior cervical ganglion is often fused with the first thoracic ganglion to form the **cervicothoracic ganglion**. **Preganglionic sympathetic fibres** from the upper thoracic segments enter the ganglion and synapse in it. **Post-ganglionic sympathetic** fibres from the ganglia pass in the **grey rami communicantes** to the ventral rami of the cervical nerves. The post-ganglionic sympathetic fibres are distributed to the head, neck, and upper limbs through: (1) the grey rami communicantes; (2) communications with the cranial nerves; and (3) plexuses around the branches of the major arteries.

Superior cervical ganglion

The superior cervical ganglion is the largest (2.5 cm long) ganglion of the trunk. It lies between the internal carotid artery and the longus capitis, at the level of the second and third cervical vertebrae.

It gives a number of branches: (1) communicating branches to the ninth, tenth, and twelfth cranial nerves; (2) the **grey rami communicantes** to the upper four cervical ventral rami; (3) the **internal carotid nerve** which runs on the internal carotid artery; (4) the **laryngopharyngeal branches** to the pharyngeal plexus; (5) the **external carotid nerves** which form the external carotid plexus on the external carotid artery and its branches; and (6) the **superior cervical cardiac nerve** to the

cardiac plexus. On the left, this nerve ends in the superficial cardiac plexus. On the right, it passes anterior or posterior to the subclavian artery and descends behind the brachiocephalic trunk to end in the deep cardiac plexus.

Middle cervical ganglion

This small ganglion lies on the inferior thyroid artery at the level of the cricoid cartilage. It gives rise to: (1) the **grey rami communicantes** to the fifth and sixth cervical nerves; (2) **thyroid branches** which form a plexus on the inferior thyroid artery and communicate with the recurrent and external laryngeal nerves; (3) the **middle cervical cardiac nerves** to the deep cardiac plexus; and (4) the **ansa subclavia**, a slender branch which loops round the subclavian artery and sends nerve fibres to the phrenic nerve.

Inferior cervical or cervicothoracic ganglion

The cervicothoracic ganglion represents the fused inferior cervical and first thoracic ganglia. It lies across the neck of the first rib. It receives a **white ramus** from the first thoracic ventral ramus and sends a grey ramus to the first, and sometimes to the second thoracic ventral ramus. When the inferior cervical ganglion is not fused with the first thoracic ganglion, it is small and lies behind the common carotid and vertebral arteries, anterior to the eighth cervical ventral ramus. The inferior cervical ganglion has the following branches, which arise from the cervicothoracic ganglion when they are fused: (1) the **grey rami communicantes** to the seventh and eighth cervical ventral rami; (2) fine filaments from the ansa subclavia to form the **subclavian plexus** on the subclavian artery; (3) larger filaments to form the **vertebral plexus** on the vertebral artery; and (4) the **inferior cervical cardiac nerves** which pass with the middle cervical nerve to the deep cardiac plexus.

All the sympathetic ganglia send post-ganglionic nerve fibres to structures in the head, neck, and upper limbs. They receive preganglionic fibres through the white rami communicantes of the upper thoracic ventral rami which ascend in the trunk and reach its ganglia. ➲ Destruction of the sympathetic trunk at the root of the neck, as a result of surgery (cervical sympathectomy) or of some pathological condition, isolates these sympathetic ganglion cells from the central nervous system and eliminates

119

Objective

I. To identify and trace the ventral rami of the cervical spinal nerves.

Instructions

1. Expose the prevertebral muscles and the cervical plexus on the right side.

2. Follow the ventral rami of the cervical nerves and their branches, noting the communications between the upper five.

3. Define the attachments of the scalene muscles [see Fig. 10.1], and trace the lower cervical and first thoracic ventral rami as far medially as possible, detaching the scalenus anterior if necessary.

the reflex responses to sympathetic stimuli. Thus, sweating from heat or fear, vasoconstriction from cold or fright, and dilation of the pupils as a result of darkness or terror are lost on the side of the injury. In addition, there is loss of cutaneous vasodilation in response to heat, and drooping of the upper eyelid (**ptosis**) due to paralysis of the smooth muscle in the upper eyelid.

Using the instructions given in Dissection 9.7, trace the ventral rami of the cervical spinal nerves.

Cervical plexus

The cervical plexus is formed by communications between the ventral rami of the upper four cervical nerves. These nerves emerge from the vertebral canal, superior to the corresponding vertebrae. The **ventral rami of the first cervical nerve** emerge between the rectus capitis anterior and rectus capitis lateralis. The **ventral rami of the second to fourth cervical nerves** emerge anterior to the scalenus medius. They communicate serially with each other. The communication between the fourth and fifth ventral rami unite the cervical and brachial plexuses. When C. 4 makes a large contribution to the brachial plexus, the brachial plexus is said to be **prefixed**. The cervical plexus lies posterior to the internal jugular vein and the prevertebral fascia [Fig. 9.16].

Branches of the cervical plexus

(a) **Communicating branches**: (1) the superior cervical ganglion gives a grey **ramus communicans** to the first four cervical ventral rami; (2) a branch from the first cervical ventral ramus descends to join the **hypoglossal nerve**. This branch usually supplies the geniohyoid and thyrohyoid, and forms the **superior root of the ansa cervicalis**; (3) sensory branches from the second, third, and fourth cervical ventral rami join the **accessory nerve** and supply the sternocleidomastoid (C. 2, 3) and trapezius (C. 3, 4).

(b) **Cutaneous branches**: lesser occipital, great auricular, transverse cervical, and supraclavicular nerves [Chapter 5].

(c) **Muscular branches** to the diaphragm (**phrenic nerve**—C. 3, 4, 5), infrahyoid muscles, prevertebral muscles, scalene, intertransverse, and levator scapulae [Fig. 9.16].

Phrenic nerve (C. 3, 4, 5)

The phrenic nerve arises mainly from the fourth cervical ventral ramus, with a contribution from C. 3 and C. 5 [Fig. 9.16]. At its origin, it is at the lateral border of the scalenus anterior and posterolateral to the internal jugular vein. On both sides, the nerve descends with the internal jugular vein obliquely across the scalenus anterior, to reach the medial border of the scalenus anterior, just inferior to the subclavian artery [Figs. 9.6, 9.7, 9.9]. The right phrenic nerve enters the thorax, posterolateral to the right brachiocephalic vein and the superior vena cava. The left phrenic nerve enters the thorax between the common carotid artery and the pleura.

The root from the fifth cervical ventral ramus may not join the phrenic nerve on the surface of the scalenus anterior but may descend into the thorax before joining it, or reach it through a communication from the nerve to the subclavius.

Scalene muscles

The three scalene muscles—**scalenus anterior, scalenus medius**, and **scalenus posterior**—form a thick muscular mass behind the prevertebral fascia. They extend inferolaterally from the cervical transverse processes to the first two ribs. **Nerve**

supply: twigs from the ventral rami of the lower five or six cervical ventral rami. **Actions**: they elevate the first two ribs on inspiration and produce lateral flexion of the cervical vertebrae when acting unilaterally [Fig. 9.7].

Scalenus anterior

The scalenus anterior takes origin from the anterior tubercles of the transverse processes of the third to sixth cervical vertebrae. It descends between the subclavian artery and vein, to be inserted into the scalene tubercle on the first rib [Figs. 9.7, 9.17].

It is separated from the scalenus medius posteriorly by the roots of the brachial plexus and the subclavian artery. Anteriorly, it is crossed obliquely by the internal jugular vein and the phrenic nerve. More superficially, it is crossed by the inferior belly of the omohyoid and the superficial cervical and suprascapular arteries. The scalenus anterior lies lateral to the thyrocervical trunk [Fig. 9.8], suprapleural membrane, pleura, and has the vertebral artery in contact with it superiorly [Figs. 9.6, 9.7, 9.8].

Scalenus medius

The scalenus medius is larger than the scalenus anterior. It takes origin from the posterior tubercles of all the cervical transverse processes and is inserted into a rough area on the superior surface of the first rib, posterior to the groove for the subclavian artery [Fig. 9.17]. It lies deep to the prevertebral fascia in the posterior triangle of the neck, immediately posterior to the ventral rami of the spinal nerves and the third part of the subclavian artery. It lies anterior to the levator scapulae muscle. The scalenus medius is pierced by the **dorsal scapular nerve** and by the upper two roots of the **long thoracic nerve** [see Figs. 5.4, 5.6]. Inferiorly, it is in contact with the cervical pleura.

Scalenus posterior

This small muscle is a part of the scalenus medius which is inserted into the external surface of the second rib [Fig. 9.17].

Cervical fascia

The three layers of the deep fascia—the **investing layer**, **pre-tracheal layer**, and **prevertebral layer**—enclose the muscles and other moving structures, and are adherent to them and to the surrounding structures by loose areolar tissue. The presence of the cervical fascia permits movement between and within the layers. The layers also form planes which tend to direct the spread of infection in the neck. The layers of the cervical fascia are difficult to dissect.

Investing fascia

The investing layer of the deep fascia encircles the neck and splits to enclose the sternocleidomastoid and trapezius muscles. It forms the roof of the posterior triangle. It is attached to the body and greater horn of the hyoid bone. Above the hyoid, it splits into two layers to enclose the submandibular gland. The thin, deeper layer passes deep to the gland and gets attached to the mylohyoid line of the mandible [see Figs. 5.2, 6.3]. The thick, superficial layer passes to the inferior border of the body and ramus of the mandible. Posterior to the submandibular gland, the superficial layer is partially disrupted by the parotid gland. Its deepest part extends inwards to the styloid process and forms the **stylomandibular ligament**.

Inferiorly, the investing fascia splits to enclose the suprasternal space above the manubrium sternum [see Fig. 6.3] and is attached to the sternum, clavicle, acromion, and spine of the scapula. The fascia of the infrahyoid muscles is in contact with the deep surface of the investing layer. It also forms a sling around the intermediate tendon of the omohyoid and binds it down to the clavicle.

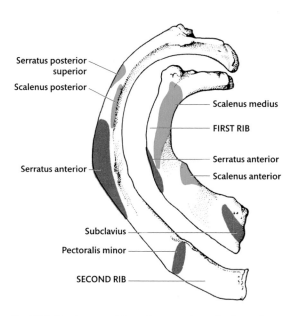

Fig. 9.17 Attachments of the scalene muscles to the first and second ribs.

Pre-tracheal fascia

The pre-tracheal fascia covers the front and sides of the trachea and splits to enclose the **thyroid gland**. It is attached to the oblique line on the thyroid cartilage and to the arch of the cricoid cartilage superiorly. These attachments cause the thyroid gland to rise and fall with the larynx in swallowing. Inferiorly, the pre-tracheal fascia surrounds the inferior thyroid veins and fuses with the pericardium [see Fig. 6.3].

Carotid sheath

The carotid sheath is a tubular condensation of the fascia which extends from the base of the skull to the root of the neck. It encloses the common and internal carotid arteries, the internal jugular vein, the vagus nerve, and the ansa cervicalis. It is wedged between the investing, pre-tracheal, and prevertebral fasciae [see Fig. 5.2].

Prevertebral fascia

The prevertebral layer encloses the vertebral column and its muscles. Anteriorly, it extends from the base of the skull to the level of the third thoracic vertebra where it fuses with the anterior longitudinal ligament [see Fig. 6.3]. Laterally, it covers the scalene muscles, the levator scapulae, and the splenius capitis, and forms the fascial floor of the posterior triangle. It descends on the scalene muscles to the outer border of the first rib. An extension of the prevertebral fascia—the **axillary sheath**—is carried outwards from the outer border of the first rib around the brachial plexus and the subclavian artery as they emerge through the cervico-axillary canal between the scalene muscles [see Fig. 5.7]. Medial to the scalenus anterior, the prevertebral fascia is continuous with the **suprapleural membrane**. The prevertebral fascia is separated from the pharynx and oesophagus by loose areolar tissue—**retropharyngeal space**. This space allows the pharynx and oesophagus to be distended with food and to slide on the prevertebral fascia during swallowing and speaking.

The **alar fascia** lies anterior to the prevertebral fascia on the anterior surface of the vertebrae, behind the pharynx and oesophagus. Laterally, it is attached to the transverse process of the cervical vertebra. It extends from the base of the skull to the seventh cervical vertebra.

Buccopharyngeal fascia

The buccopharyngeal fascia is a delicate, distensible fascial layer covering the constrictor muscles of the pharynx and buccinator. It extends from the base of the skull to the oesophagus.

Lymph nodes and lymph vessels of the head and neck

Some of the lymph nodes along the carotid sheath and in the root of the neck may have been seen already, but the nodes and vessels cannot be demonstrated satisfactorily by routine dissection. The following account gives a brief description of the lymphatic system in the head and neck [Fig. 9.18].

The lymph nodes of the head and neck are numerous and may be divided into superficial and deep groups. The **superficial groups** are situated around the junction of the head with the neck. They drain all the superficial structures and some deep tissue of the head. Most of the efferent lymph vessels from the superficial nodes pass to the deep group. The **deep group** consists of a chain of lymph nodes—the **deep cervical lymph nodes**—arranged along the internal jugular vein, from the level of the digastric to the root of the neck. They are arbitrarily divided into the upper deep cervical and lower deep cervical nodes by the omohyoid. A few scattered, superficial nodes are found along the external and anterior jugular veins. These drain to the deep cervical nodes.

Superficial lymph nodes of the head

Occipital lymph nodes

The few, small occipital lymph nodes lie on the upper end of the trapezius and on the fascia at the apex of the posterior triangle. They drain the occipital part of the scalp and the upper part of the back of the neck to the upper deep cervical lymph nodes.

Retro-auricular lymph nodes

The retro-auricular nodes lie on the superior part of the sternocleidomastoid, posterior to the auricle. They drain the posterior side of the head and the posterior surface of the auricle, to the deep nodes under the sternocleidomastoid.

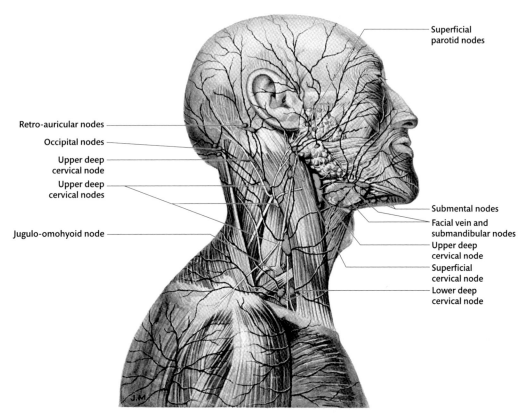

Superficial
parotid nodes

Retro-auricular nodes

Occipital nodes

Upper deep
cervical node

Upper deep
cervical nodes

Jugulo-omohyoid node

Submental nodes

Facial vein and
submandibular nodes

Upper deep
cervical node

Superficial
cervical node

Lower deep
cervical node

Fig. 9.18 Lymph nodes of the head and neck, shown with the sternocleidomastoid in position.

Parotid lymph nodes

Several small lymph nodes are scattered through the parotid gland. The superficial nodes drain the area between a vertical line through the auricle and an oblique line joining the medial angle of the eye to the angle of the mandible. This area includes most of the auricle and the external acoustic meatus. Deeper nodes in this region drain the temporal and infratemporal fossae, the middle ear, the auditory tube, and the upper molar teeth and gums. Efferent vessels from these nodes drain either to nodes on the external jugular vein or to the upper deep cervical lymph nodes.

Submandibular lymph nodes

The submandibular lymph nodes lie along the submandibular gland, mainly under cover of the mandible. They receive superficial lymph vessels from the area below the line joining the medial angle of the eye and the angle of the mandible. They also receive lymph from the submandibular and sublingual salivary glands, the side of the tongue and posterior part of the floor of the mouth, most of the teeth and gums, part of the palate, and the anterior parts of the walls of the nasal cavity. They drain to the deep cervical nodes under the sternocleidomastoid. Some small nodes lie along the course of the facial vein. One of these—the mandibular node—lies at the anterior border of the masseter and drains the cheek and lateral parts of the lips to the submandibular nodes.

Submental lymph nodes

The submental nodes lie on the fascia covering the mylohyoid, between the anterior bellies of the digastric muscles [see Fig. 6.1]. They receive lymph from a wedge-shaped area, including the lower incisor teeth, gums, and the anterior part of the floor of the mouth. They drain to the deep cervical lymph nodes. Though small, some of these nodes may be palpable, even in healthy individuals.

Retropharyngeal lymph nodes

A few nodes lie in the fascia of the posterior wall of the upper pharynx, at the level of the mastoid process. They receive lymph from the oropharynx, nasopharynx, palate, nose, paranasal sinuses, auditory tube, and middle ear. These nodes drain postero-inferiorly to the nodes in the posterior triangle.

Superficial cervical lymph nodes

1. Three or four **superficial cervical nodes** lie along the external jugular vein. They drain the parotid nodes and the adjoining skin to the deep nodes in the carotid triangle or at the root of the neck.
2. A few small nodes lie on the anterior jugular vein and drain the skin and muscles along the vein to the lower deep cervical nodes.
3. Small anterior cervical lymph nodes lie on the front and sides of the trachea. They are continuous with the tracheobronchial nodes in the thorax. They drain lymph from the larynx, trachea, and thyroid gland to the lower deep cervical lymph nodes.

Deep cervical lymph nodes

The deep cervical lymph nodes form a broad strip of nodes extending from the digastric muscles to the root of the neck. Most of them lie under cover of the sternocleidomastoid. The deep cervical nodes receive lymph from all the other groups. Two of the nodes are particularly large—the **jugulodigastric nodes** which drain the palatine tonsil and tongue, and the **jugulo-omohyoid nodes**. Both are named after their relation to the corresponding muscles.

Some of the deep nodes extend into the posterior triangle: (1) along the accessory nerve (draining the retropharyngeal nodes); and (2) on the superficial cervical artery across the upper part of the brachial plexus. The final efferent pathway for all the lymph of the head and neck is the **jugular lymph trunk** at the root of the neck. This trunk enters the thoracic duct on the left side and the internal jugular vein on the right.

See Clinical Applications 9.1, 9.2, and 9.3 for the practical implications of the anatomy discussed in this chapter.

Table 9.2 provides an overview of the movements of the hyoid bone.

CLINICAL APPLICATION 9.1 Tracheostomy

A 53-year-old male was rescued from a burning building by the fire rescue team. He suffered burn injuries to his face, trunk, and upper limbs. He was breathless, partially conscious, and in severe pain. Examination revealed severe laryngeal oedema and possible inhalational injury to the lungs due to inhaled smoke. At the hospital, his condition deteriorated, and a tracheostomy was done.

Study question 1: what is laryngeal oedema? (Answer: laryngeal oedema is inflammation and damage to the mucosa of the larynx.)

Study question 2: what is tracheostomy? (Answer: tracheostomy is an emergency procedure done to create a passage into the trachea in someone with an impending airway obstruction. A surgical incision is made in the anterior neck into the cervical trachea. A cuffed tube is introduced into the incision and connected to a ventilator machine.)

Study question 3: what are the important anatomical structures that one must be careful to avoid while doing a tracheostomy? (Answer: important structures in close relation to the cervical trachea include the thyroid gland and its isthmus lying in front of the trachea, carotid vessels and the internal jugular vein on either side, and the recurrent laryngeal nerve in the tracheo-oesophageal groove.)

Study question 4: what are the common indications for a tracheostomy? (Answer: common indications include upper airway obstruction by a foreign body or cancerous growth, laryngeal oedema following burns and anaphylaxis, bilateral paralysis of the vocal cord, and severe fractures of the midface and mandible making orotracheal or nasotracheal intubation impossible.)

CLINICAL APPLICATION 9.2 Thyromegaly

A 35-year old woman presented with a history of weight gain, intolerance to cold, tiredness, excessive sleepiness, lethargy, and constipation. On examination, she has a swelling in front of the neck that moves up on deglutition.

Study question 1: what is the likely diagnosis? (Answer: thyroid swelling, based on the evidence that the swelling moved on deglutition; and hypothyroidism, based on the history.)

Study question 2: what is an enlargement of the thyroid gland called? (Answer: an enlargement of the thyroid is called thyromegaly or goitre. It may be associated with excess or decreased secretion of T3 and T4 hormones, leading to hypothyroidism or hyperthyroidism. Features of hyperthyroidism include weight loss, tachycardia, palpitations, anxiety, tremor, easy muscle fatigue, increased bowel movements, and heat intolerance.)

Study question 3: why does the thyroid gland move up on deglutition? (Answer: the thyroid gland is enveloped by the pre-tracheal fascia that is attached in the midline to the hyoid bone, and laterally to the oblique line of the thyroid cartilage. Further, a thickened band of fascia called the ligament of Berry anchors the medial surface of the thyroid gland to the cricoid cartilage. Elevation of the hyoid bone and thyroid and cricoid cartilage during deglutition causes elevation of the thyroid gland.)

Study question 4: what anatomical structures should the surgeon be careful of during thyroidectomy? (Answer: (1) the external laryngeal branch of the superior laryngeal nerve; (2) the recurrent laryngeal nerve; and (3) accidental removal of the parathyroid glands which can lead to hypoparathyroidism.) See Clinical Application 9.3 for neurological complications of thyroid surgery.

CLINICAL APPLICATION 9.3 Neurological complications of thyroid surgery

The superior and inferior laryngeal nerves are cervical branches of the vagus nerve that are pertinent to thyroid surgery because of their intimate relation to the thyroid gland. The external branch of the superior laryngeal nerve runs with the superior thyroid vessels to the superior pole of the thyroid gland. Injury to the nerve causes paralysis of the cricothyroid muscle and an inability to produce high-pitched sounds. Identifying the nerve during surgery helps avoid accidental transection and excessive stretching. When the nerve is not identified, the superior thyroid artery branches should be ligated close to the thyroid gland.

The recurrent laryngeal nerve runs in the tracheo-oesophageal groove towards the larynx, close to the posterior aspect of the thyroid and the inferior thyroid artery. Injury to this nerve causes paralysis of the vocal cord and sensory loss below the level of the glottis. The patient could experience mild to severe hoarseness of the voice, acute airway obstruction, and difficulty in swallowing [see Fig. 9.6].

Table 9.2 Movements of the hyoid bone

Movement	Muscles	Nerve supply
Elevation	Digastric	Trigeminal and facial
	Stylohyoid	Facial
	Mylohyoid	Trigeminal
Depression	Sternohyoid	Ansa cervicalis
	Omohyoid	Ansa cervicalis
	Thyrohyoid and sternothyroid	C. 1 and ansa cervicalis
Protraction	Geniohyoid	C. 1 ventral ramus
Retraction	Middle constrictor of pharynx	Pharyngeal plexus
	Stylohyoid	Facial

CHAPTER 10
The prevertebral region

Introduction

This chapter describes the muscles and vessels which lie in front of the cervical vertebrae. These muscles are enclosed in the prevertebral fascia [see Fig. 5.2].

Muscles

The prevertebral muscles are most easily seen on the right in the dissected specimen, though the longus capitis, rectus capitis lateralis, and rectus capitis anterior have been cut across. The cut ends of these can be seen on the base of the skull, or the entire muscles can be exposed on the left by displacing the left half of the pharynx. The muscles are covered anteriorly by the prevertebral fascia and are supplied by the ventral rami of the cervical nerves. As a group, they flex the neck, and the head on the neck.

Longus colli

This is the longest and most medial of the muscles. A detailed account of the bony attachments is beyond the scope of this book. The student should know that it extends from the anterior tubercle of the atlas to the third thoracic vertebra. It is attached to the bodies of the intervening vertebrae and to the transverse processes of the third to sixth cervical vertebrae [Figs. 10.1, 10.2].

Longus capitis

The longus capitis is anterolateral to the longus colli. It takes origin from the anterior tubercles of the third to sixth cervical transverse processes and is inserted into the base of the skull in front of the rectus capitis anterior [see Fig. 7.2; Fig. 10.1].

Rectus capitis anterior

The rectus capitis anterior extends from the anterior surface of the lateral mass of the atlas to the base of the skull, immediately anterior to the occipital condyle [see Fig. 7.2; Fig. 10.1].

Rectus capitis lateralis

The rectus capitis lateralis extends from the superior surface of the transverse process of the atlas to the jugular process of the occipital bone. It is immediately posterior to the jugular foramen and is separated from the rectus capitis anterior by the ventral ramus of the **first cervical nerve** which supplies both muscles [see Fig. 7.2; Fig. 10.1]. **Action**: the two rectus muscles act with the muscles of the suboccipital triangle to stabilize the skull on the vertebral column.

Using the instructions given in Dissection 10.1, find and trace the initial segments of the vertebral artery.

Vertebral artery

The vertebral artery is an important branch of the first part of the subclavian artery. The two vertebral arteries join to form the basilar artery within the cranial cavity. Together, they supply the upper part of the spinal cord, medulla oblongata, pons, cerebellum, midbrain, and the posterior part of the cerebrum.

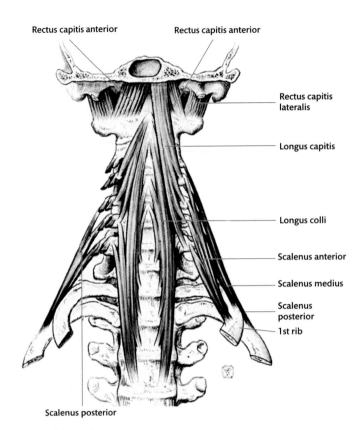

Rectus capitis anterior   Rectus capitis anterior

Rectus capitis lateralis

Longus capitis

Longus colli

Scalenus anterior

Scalenus medius

Scalenus posterior

1st rib

Scalenus posterior

Fig. 10.1 The prevertebral muscles of the neck.

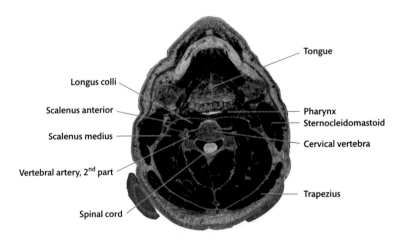

Tongue

Longus colli

Scalenus anterior

Pharynx
Sternocleidomastoid

Scalenus medius

Cervical vertebra

Vertebral artery, 2nd part

Trapezius

Spinal cord

Fig. 10.2 Transverse section at the level of the oropharynx. The position of the prevertebral fascia is shown by the dotted blue line.
Image courtesy of the Visible Human Project of the US National Library of Medicine.

First part of the vertebral artery

The vertebral artery begins as a branch of the first part of the subclavian artery and ascends behind the common carotid artery to the sixth cervical transverse process [Fig. 10.3].

Second part of the vertebral artery

The second part of the vertebral artery ascends through the foramen transversaria of the upper six cervical vertebrae, accompanied by the **vertebral veins** and a **sympathetic nerve plexus** derived

DISSECTION 10.1 Vertebral artery

Objective

I. To trace the first and second parts of the vertebral artery.

Instructions

1. Re-define the attachments of the scalene muscles on both sides.

2. Remove the scalenus anterior to expose the anterior and posterior **intertransverse muscles** which

unite the corresponding tubercles of adjacent cervical transverse processes. They are separated from each other by the ventral rami of the cervical nerves. The dorsal rami pass posteriorly, medial to the posterior intertransverse muscles.

3. The vertebral artery may now be exposed in the intertransverse spaces by removing the anterior intertransverse muscles.

from the cervicothoracic ganglion. Between the transverse processes, it is anterior to the ventral rami of the cervical nerves. The artery runs vertically upwards through the foramen transversaria of the sixth to second cervical vertebrae. In the foramen transversarium of the axis, the artery turns laterally under the superior articular facet, bends upwards, and enters the foramen transversarium of the atlas, which is placed further laterally than the others [see Fig. 9.8; Fig. 10.3].

Third part of the vertebral artery

The third part of the artery emerges on the superior surface of the atlas between the rectus capitis lateralis and the superior articular process of the atlas. It curves horizontally over the lateral and posterior surfaces of the superior articular process with the ventral ramus of the first cervical nerve. It grooves the superior articular process and the root of the posterior arch of the atlas. It leaves this region by

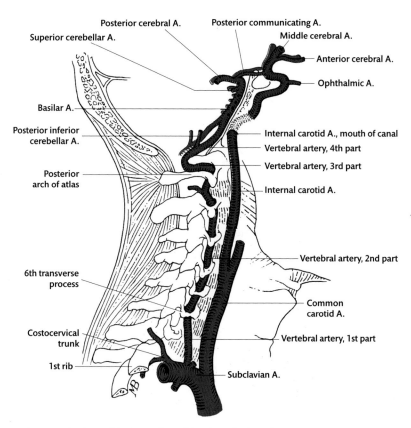

Fig. 10.3 The course and communications of the internal carotid and vertebral arteries.

passing medially in front of the posterior atlanto-occipital membrane [see Figs. 7.4, 7.6; Fig. 10.3].

Fourth part of the vertebral artery

The fourth part of the vertebral artery lies in the vertebral canal and cranial cavity. In the vertebral canal, the artery turns superiorly, pierces the dura mater and arachnoid, and enters the cranial cavity through the foramen magnum, anterior to the uppermost tooth of the ligamentum denticulatum. It then runs anterosuperiorly on the medulla oblongata between the rootlets of the first cervical and hypoglossal nerves. At the lower border of the pons, it unites with the vertebral artery of the opposite side to form the basilar artery [see Fig. 8.8; Fig. 10.3].

Branches of vertebral artery

There are no branches from the first part of the artery. The second and third parts of the artery give rise to **spinal** and **muscular** branches which anastomose with branches of the occipital and deep cervical arteries. The fourth part gives off a meningeal branch, and a series of branches to the medulla oblongata and spinal cord.

Vertebral vein

A plexus of veins is formed around the beginning of the third part of the vertebral artery by the union of veins from the internal vertebral venous plexus and the suboccipital triangle. This plexus runs with the second part of the artery through the foramen transversaria. It anastomoses with the **internal vertebral venous plexus** and the **deep cervical veins**. It ends as one or two vertebral veins, which descend with the artery from the sixth cervical transverse process, and enters the posterior surface of the brachiocephalic vein near its origin. One or two veins pass through the foramen transversarium of the seventh cervical vertebra.

See Clinical Application 10.1 for the practical implications of the anatomy discussed in this chapter.

Table 10.1 provides an overview of the movements of the neck and of the head on the neck.

CLINICAL APPLICATION 10.1 Prevertebral, retropharyngeal, and danger spaces in the neck

The fascia of the neck limits the fascial spaces (or potential spaces) to form closed compartments. Infections tend to remain and spread within these compartments. A thin prevertebral tissue space exists between the vertebral column and the prevertebral fascia. It extends from the skull to the coccyx and encloses the prevertebral muscles. Between the prevertebral and alar fasciae is a space known as the danger space. It is a closed space, and infections can reach it only through penetrating injury. It extends downwards into the posterior mediastinum. (It forms a ready path through which infection can spread to the thorax.) The retropharyngeal space lies between the alar fascia and the pharynx. (The alar fascia lies anterior to the prevertebral fascia on the anterior surface of the vertebra and behind the pharynx and oesophagus [Chapter 9].)

Table 10.1 Movements of the neck and of the head on the neck

Movement	Muscles	Nerve supply
Flexion	Sternocleidomastoid	Accessory
	Longus colli (both muscles acting)	Cervical ventral rami
	Longus capitis	Cervical ventral rami
	Rectus capitis anterior*	C. 1 ventral ramus
Extension	Splenius cervicis and capitis	Cervical dorsal rami
	Erector spinae	Cervical dorsal rami
	Rectus capitis posterior major and minor*	C. 1 dorsal ramus
	Obliquus capitis superior*	C. 1 dorsal ramus
	Trapezius	Accessory
Lateral flexion and rotation	Sternocleidomastoid†	Accessory
	Scalenes	Cervical ventral rami
	Longus colli	Cervical ventral rami
	Rectus capitis lateralis*	C. 1 ventral ramus
	Levator scapulae (shoulder fixed)	Cervical ventral rami
	Splenius†	Cervical dorsal rami
	Longissimus	Cervical dorsal rami
	Obliquus capitis superior† and inferior	C. 1 dorsal ramus

* These muscles act mainly as ligaments of adjustable length and tension.† In rotation (one muscle acting), turns the face towards the opposite side.† In rotation, turns the face to the same side.

CHAPTER 11
The orbit

Introduction

The orbit contains the eyeball, optic nerve, extraocular muscles which move the eye, associated vessels and nerves, orbital fat, and fascia. It also contains the lacrimal gland and the levator palpebrae superioris, the muscle which raises the upper eyelid. The eyeball is described in Chapter 12.

Bony orbit

The bony orbit is pyramidal in shape. The base lies anteriorly at the orbital margin; the apex is directed posteriorly. The **roof** of the orbit is formed mainly by the **orbital plate of the frontal bone** and completed posteriorly by the **lesser wing of the sphenoid** [see Fig. 3.9]. The **medial wall** is formed mainly by the **orbital plate of the ethmoid, body of the sphenoid, lacrimal** and **frontal processes of the maxilla** [Fig. 11.1]. The **floor** of the orbit is formed by the **maxilla** and the **zygomatic bone** laterally [Fig. 11.2]. The **lateral wall** is formed mainly by the **greater wing of the sphenoid** and the **frontal process of the zygomatic bone** [see Fig. 3.9].

Fig. 11.3 shows the relationship of the orbit (2) to the anterior cranial fossa above, the ethmoid air cells medially, and the maxillary air sinus inferiorly.

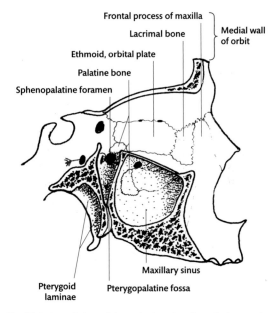

Frontal process of maxilla

Lacrimal bone

Medial wall of orbit

Ethmoid, orbital plate

Palatine bone

Sphenopalatine foramen

Maxillary sinus

Pterygoid laminae

Pterygopalatine fossa

Fig. 11.1 Lateral view of the sagittal section through the anterior part of the skull to show the pterygopalatine fossa and the construction of the medial wall of the orbit. Arrow in foramen rotundum.

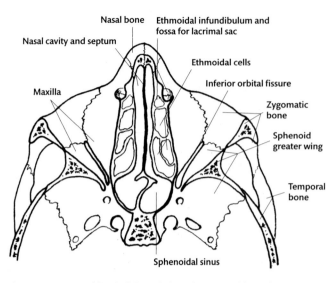

Nasal bone

Ethmoidal infundibulum and fossa for lacrimal sac

Nasal cavity and septum

Ethmoidal cells

Inferior orbital fissure

Maxilla

Zygomatic bone

Sphenoid greater wing

Temporal bone

Sphenoidal sinus

Fig. 11.2 Horizontal section of the anterior part of the skull through the orbits, viewed from above.

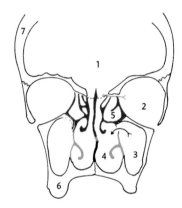

Fig. 11.3 Drawing of a coronal section through the skull to show the relative positions of the orbit, maxillary sinus, nasal cavity, and ethmoidal air cells. Blue arrow shows the route of the anterior ethmoidal vessels and nerve; black arrow is in the opening of the maxillary sinus. Blue = inferior concha and septal cartilage; red = ethmoid bone; solid black = vomer. 1. Anterior cranial fossa. 2. Orbit. 3. Maxillary sinus. 4. Nasal cavity. 5. Ethmoidal air cell. 6. Alveolar process of the maxilla. 7. Frontal bone. [See also Fig. 3.1B.]

Using the instructions given in Dissection 11.1, remove the roof of the orbit, and explore the frontal and ethmoidal air sinuses.

Ethmoidal sinuses

The ethmoidal air cells or sinuses are multiple, thin-walled cavities, which occupy the part of the ethmoid between the orbit and the upper part of the nasal cavity [see Fig. 8.13A; Figs. 11.2, 11.3]. They are in three groups: the anterior, middle, and

DISSECTION 11.1 Roof of the orbit

Objectives

I. To remove the roof of the orbit.   **II.** To explore the frontal and ethmoidal air sinuses.

Instructions

1. Strip the periosteum from the floor of the anterior cranial fossa, except over the cribriform plate of the ethmoid. With a gentle tap of the hammer on a chisel, crack the orbital roof and remove the broken pieces of bone from the underlying orbital periosteum. Extend the opening with bone forceps, keeping outside the orbital periosteum, until all but the anterior margin of the orbital roof is removed.

2. Occasionally, the **frontal air sinus** extends into the roof of the orbit; in this case, two layers of bone and the contained sinus must be removed.

3. The **orbital part of the frontal bone** forms most of the roof of the orbit and extends medially over the ethmoidal air cells.

4. Chip away the frontal bone overlying the ethmoidal air cells. Avoid injury to the vessels and nerves beneath, and expose the mucoperiosteal lining of the **ethmoidal sinuses**. Open some of them.

5. Remove the remains of the lesser wing of the sphenoid, but leave the margin of the optic canal intact. The superior orbital fissure is now opened, and the nerves which have been followed from the wall of the cavernous sinus can be traced into the orbit.

posterior ethmoidal sinuses. The anterior and middle ethmoidal sinuses open into the middle meatus of the nose [see Fig. 19.3], and the posterior ethmoidal sinuses open into the superior meatus [see Fig. 19.6]. Explore them with a blunt probe, and attempt to find their openings into the nasal cavity.

Orbital periosteum

The orbital periosteum lines the bony orbit and encloses the contents of the orbit, except the zygomatic nerve and the infra-orbital nerve and vessels. It forms a funnel-shaped sheath which is loosely attached to the bony walls of the orbit. Posteriorly, it is continuous with the middle cranial fossa through the optic canal and the superior orbital fissure.

Using the instructions given in Dissection 11.2, dissect the muscles and nerves seen immediately deep to the orbital periosteum on the roof of the orbit.

Frontal nerve

The **frontal nerve** is a direct continuation of the ophthalmic nerve. It enters the orbit through the superior orbital fissure and runs forwards, under the orbital periosteum, on the levator palpebrae superioris. It ends by dividing into the supra-orbital and supratrochlear nerves [Fig. 11.4].

Supratrochlear nerve

The supratrochlear nerve is the small medial branch of the frontal nerve. It runs towards the pulley of the superior oblique muscle, pierces the palpebral fascia above it, and leaves the orbit to run upwards into the forehead to supply the scalp [Chapter 4]. In the orbit, it communicates with the infratrochlear nerve.

Supra-orbital nerve

The supra-orbital branch runs forwards, in line with the parent stem. It passes through the supra-orbital

---

DISSECTION 11.2 Orbit

Objectives

I. To identify the levator palpebrae superioris, superior rectus, and superior oblique muscles. **II.** To identify and trace the frontal, trochlear, and lacrimal nerves and the corresponding arteries.

Instructions

1. Cut through the orbital periosteum transversely, close to the anterior margin of the orbit, and then anteroposteriorly along the midline of the orbit.

2. Take care not to injure the nerves which pass through the superior orbital fissure. Find the trochlear nerve, and trace it forwards and medially to the superior oblique muscle in the upper medial part of the orbit. The **trochlear nerve** lies immediately beneath the periosteum and is easily damaged when the periosteum is cut.

3. In the midline of the orbit, find the frontal nerve lying on the levator palpebrae superioris. Trace it forwards to its division into the supra-orbital and supratrochlear nerves, each of which runs with the corresponding artery [Fig. 11.4].

4. Follow the supratrochlear nerve to the medial angle of the orbit where it passes above the pulley (trochlea) of the superior oblique muscle.

5. Identify the levator palpebrae superioris and superior oblique muscles.

6. Expose the superior oblique muscle, and follow its tendon to the pulley at the superomedial angle of the orbit [Fig. 11.5]. The tendon passes through the pulley and then turns posterolaterally to its insertion. It disappears from view beneath the levator palpebrae superioris and the superior rectus.

7. Raise the levator palpebrae superioris, and identify the superior rectus muscle beneath it. Find the branch of the oculomotor nerve which pierces that muscle to enter the levator.

8. Find the lacrimal nerve and artery which lie in the fat along the superolateral part of the orbit. Trace them to the lacrimal gland [Fig. 11.4].

9. Define the extent of the lacrimal gland.

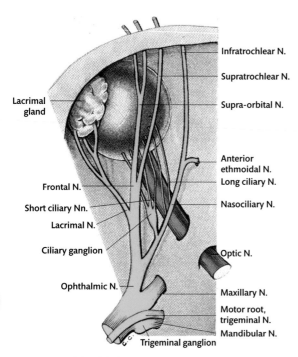

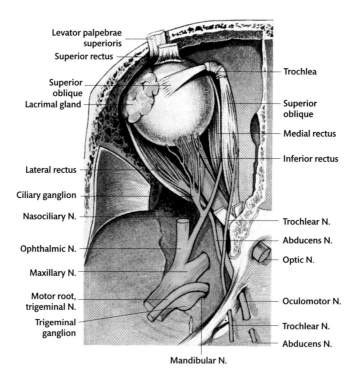

Infratrochlear N.

Supratrochlear N.

Supra-orbital N.

Lacrimal gland

Anterior ethmoidal N.
Long ciliary N.

Frontal N.

Nasociliary N.

Short ciliary Nn.

Lacrimal N.

Ciliary ganglion

Optic N.

Ophthalmic N.

Maxillary N.

Motor root, trigeminal N.

Mandibular N.

Trigeminal ganglion

Fig. 11.4 The left ophthalmic nerve. The trigeminal nerve and ganglion have been turned laterally.

notch or foramen and turns upwards into the fore-head to supply the scalp [Chapter 4].

Lacrimal nerve

The lacrimal nerve is the smallest branch of the ophthalmic nerve. It passes through the lateral part of the superior orbital fissure [Fig. 11.6] and runs forwards and laterally above the lateral rectus muscle. At the anterior part of the orbit, it receives post-ganglionic parasympathetic fibres from the **zygomatic nerve**. It gives branches to the lacrimal gland, and the **palpebral branch** to the skin of the upper eyelid [see Fig 14.5].

Trochlear nerve

The trochlear nerve is the fourth cranial nerve. It supplies only the superior oblique muscle. It enters the orbit through the superior orbital fissure and

Levator palpebrae superioris

Superior rectus

Trochlea

Superior oblique

Lacrimal gland

Superior oblique

Medial rectus

Inferior rectus

Lateral rectus

Ciliary ganglion

Nasociliary N.

Trochlear N.

Ophthalmic N.

Abducens N.

Optic N.

Maxillary N.

Motor root, trigeminal N.

Oculomotor N.

Trigeminal ganglion

Trochlear N.

Abducens N.

Mandibular N.

Fig. 11.5 Dissection of the orbit and middle cranial fossa. The cut ends of the levator palpebrae superioris and superior rectus have been turned anteriorly. The trigeminal nerve and ganglion have been turned laterally.

passes forwards and medially just under the roof of the orbit, to the superior oblique [Fig. 11.5]. (The remaining nerves of the orbit are seen later.)

Lacrimal gland

The lacrimal gland is a lobulated gland situated at the superolateral angle of the orbit. It lies in a depression on the medial side of the zygomatic process of the frontal bone, mostly hidden by the orbital margin [Fig. 11.4]. The concave medial surface of the gland rests on the levator palpebrae superioris and the lateral rectus. These muscles separate it from the eyeball. The small **palpebral part of the lacrimal gland** projects down into the upper lid between the palpebral fascia and the conjunctiva. Nine to ten thin ducts from the gland open on the deep surface of the upper eyelid near the superior conjunctival fornix [see Fig. 4.15]. Parasympathetic secretomotor nerve fibres to the gland arise in the **pterygopalatine ganglion** and reach the gland through a branch of the zygomatic nerve.

Levator palpebrae superioris

The levator palpebrae superioris lies superior to the superior rectus [Fig. 11.6]. It takes origin from the roof of the orbit, immediately anterior to the optic canal. It passes forwards above the rectus superior. Anteriorly, it widens into a broad membranous tendon which is inserted into the skin of the upper eyelid, the anterior surface of the superior tarsus, and the superior conjunctival fornix [see Fig. 4.13]. A layer of **involuntary** (smooth) **muscle** arises from the aponeurosis and is attached to the superior tarsus.

Nerve supply: the skeletal muscle is supplied by the oculomotor nerve, superior division. The smooth muscle is supplied by the cervical sympathetics through the carotid plexus. Denervation of the muscle by injury to the cervical sympathetics or the oculomotor nerve leads to drooping of the eyelid (**ptosis**) [Fig. 4.13]. **Action**: it opens the eye by raising the upper eyelid and the superior conjunctival fornix.

Using the instructions given in Dissection 12.3, define the fascial sheath of the eyeball.

DISSECTION 11.3 Fascial sheath of the eyeball

Objective

I. To try and define the fascial sheath of the eyeball.

Instructions

1. Divide the frontal nerve and the levator palpebrae superioris, and turn them out of the way. If possible, inflate the eyeball through a small cut in the sclera (the white part of the eye).

2. Cut through the superior rectus, and reflect it.

3. Note the amount of loose tissue, posterior to the eyeball. This is the fascial sheath of the eyeball. Insert a blunt seeker between it and the eyeball, and gauge the extent of the sheath.

Extraocular muscles of the eyeball

Six muscles move the eyeball—the medial, lateral, superior and inferior recti, and superior and inferior obliques. The superior rectus and superior oblique have been exposed already and will be described here. The other muscles will be seen after the vessels and nerves are dissected.

Superior rectus

The superior rectus takes origin from the upper margin of the common tendinous ring which surrounds the orbital end of the optic canal and the medial part of the superior orbital fissure [Fig. 11.6]. It passes anterolaterally above the optic nerve and is inserted into the sclera, about 6 mm behind the sclerocorneal junction [Fig. 11.7].

Nerve supply: superior division of the oculomotor nerve. **Action**: elevation of the eye when the eye is turned laterally.

Superior oblique

The superior oblique takes origin from the roof of the orbit, immediately anteromedial to the optic canal, and passes anteriorly along the upper part of the

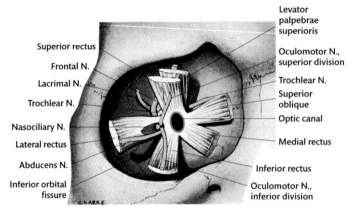

Fig. 11.6 Diagram showing the origin of the ocular muscles and the routes of entry of nerves into the right orbit. Green = common tendinous ring.

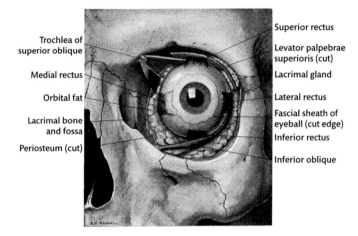

Fig. 11.7 Dissection of the left orbit to show the insertions of the muscles of the eyeball.

medial wall of the orbit. Anteriorly, it forms a thin tendon which enters the trochlea. The **trochlea** is a small fibrocartilaginous ring attached by fibrous tissue to the trochlear fossa on the frontal bone. It is lined with a synovial sheath which allows the tendon to slide freely in it. At the trochlea, the tendon of the superior oblique turns posterolaterally and passes backwards between the superior rectus above and the eyeball below [Figs. 11.5, 11.7]. Lateral to the superior rectus, the tendon flattens out and is inserted into the sclera, midway between the attachment of the optic nerve and the cornea. **Nerve supply**: the trochlear nerve. **Action**: it turns the cornea downwards when it is already turned medially, a position in which the inferior rectus is ineffective as a depressor of the cornea.

Using the instructions given in Dissection 11.4, dissect the optic nerve and ciliary ganglion.

Optic nerve

The optic nerve is a sensory nerve, made up mainly of fibres which originate in the retina (the light-sensitive layer of the eye). It enters the orbit through the optic canal. It is surrounded by sheaths of the dura mater, arachnoid, and pia mater, which enclose extensions of the subdural and subarachnoid spaces between them. The nerve runs anterolaterally and slightly downwards to pierce the sclera, a short distance medial to the centre of the posterior surface. The nasociliary nerve, ophthalmic artery, and superior ophthalmic vein cross above. The ciliary nerves and vessels surround it near the eyeball [Figs. 11.5, 11.8]. The nerve is slightly longer than the distance it has to run, so as to allow for the movements of the eyeball.

DISSECTION 11.4 Optic nerve and ciliary ganglion

Objectives

I. To identify and trace the optic nerve. **II.** To identify the ciliary ganglion, and the long and short ciliary nerves. **III.** To identify and trace the nasociliary nerve.

Instructions

1. Remove the fat beneath the superior rectus, and expose the optic nerve.

2. Look for the structures which cross the optic nerve posteriorly. They are the nasociliary nerve, the ophthalmic artery, and the superior ophthalmic vein. Trace these structures and their branches forwards [Fig. 11.8].

3. Two thread-like branches from the nasociliary nerve—the long ciliary nerves—run along the optic nerve to the eyeball [Fig. 11.4]. Find them.

4. Numerous short ciliary nerves run forwards in the fat around the optic nerve. Find them [Fig. 11.4].

5. Follow the short ciliary nerve posteriorly to the ciliary ganglion, a small collection of nerve cells between the optic nerve and the lateral rectus.

6. With care, find the branches to the ciliary ganglion from the nasociliary and inferior divisions of the oculomotor nerve.

7. Remove the fat lateral to the ganglion, and expose the abducens nerve on the medial side of the lateral rectus muscle [Fig. 11.5].

8. Expose the optic nerve in its sheaths.

Nasociliary nerve

The nasociliary nerve arises from the ophthalmic nerve in the anterior part of the cavernous sinus [Fig. 11.4]. It passes through the superior orbital fissure within the common tendinous ring [Fig. 11.6] and runs anteromedially above the optic nerve to the medial wall of the orbit. It continues forwards between the superior oblique and medial rectus muscles, and ends by dividing into the infratrochlear and anterior ethmoidal nerves.

Branches: it gives off: (1) the **communicating branch to the ciliary ganglion** which runs along the lateral side of the optic nerve to reach the ganglion; (2) two **long ciliary nerves** which run along the medial side of the optic nerve and pierce the sclera in this position—the long ciliary nerves are sensory to all of the eyeball, except the retina, and also carry post-ganglionic sympathetic nerves from the internal carotid plexus to the dilator pupillae; (3) the **posterior ethmoidal nerve** which arises from the nasociliary nerve at the medial wall of the orbit—it runs through the posterior ethmoidal foramen and supplies the mucous membrane of the ethmoid and sphenoid air sinuses; (4) the **infratrochlear nerve** which is the smaller terminal branch of the nasociliary nerve—it runs forwards and leaves the orbit below the trochlea; it appears on the face, above the medial angle of the eye, and supplies the skin of the eyelids and the upper half of the external nose [see Fig. 4.7; Fig. 11.4]; and (5) the **anterior ethmoidal nerve** which leaves the orbit through the anterior ethmoidal foramen, crosses above the ethmoidal sinuses [Fig. 11.8], and appears at the lateral margin of the cribriform plate of the ethmoid [Fig. 11.3]. It turns forwards under the dura mater and descends into the wall of the nasal cavity through a slit-like aperture at the side of the crista galli. It gives **internal nasal branches** to the adjacent mucous membrane of the lateral and septal walls, runs on the deep surface of the nasal bone, and emerges between the nasal bone and the lateral nasal cartilage [see Fig. 4.7] as the **external nasal** nerve. It supplies the skin of the lower half of the nose.

Parasympathetic ganglia

The four small parasympathetic ganglia—ciliary, pterygopalatine, otic, and submandibular ganglion—are associated with the branches of the trigeminal nerve. They belong to the parasympathetic part of the autonomic nervous system. Although only the ciliary ganglion lies in the orbit, the general features to these ganglia are mentioned here.

The parasympathetic ganglia lie closer to the structures they supply than the cervical sympathetic ganglia which send sympathetic nerves to the same structures. The ganglia receive **preganglionic fibres** from either the oculomotor, facial, or glossopharyngeal nerves and give rise to **post-ganglionic nerve fibres**. Post-ganglionic fibres are distributed mainly through the branches of the trigeminal nerve to

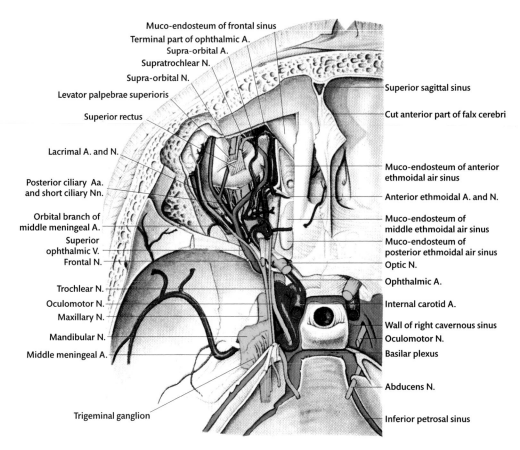

Muco-endosteum of frontal sinus
Terminal part of ophthalmic A.
Supra-orbital A.
Supratrochlear N.
Supra-orbital N.
Levator palpebrae superioris
Superior rectus

Lacrimal A. and N.

Posterior ciliary Aa.
and short ciliary Nn.

Orbital branch of
middle meningeal A.
Superior
ophthalmic V.
Frontal N.

Trochlear N.
Oculomotor N.
Maxillary N.

Mandibular N.

Middle meningeal A.

Trigeminal ganglion

Superior sagittal sinus

Cut anterior part of falx cerebri

Muco-endosteum of anterior
ethmoidal air sinus

Anterior ethmoidal A. and N.

Muco-endosteum of
middle ethmoidal air sinus
Muco-endosteum of
posterior ethmoidal air sinus
Optic N.

Ophthalmic A.

Internal carotid A.

Wall of right cavernous sinus
Oculomotor N.

Basilar plexus

Abducens N.

Inferior petrosal sinus

Fig. 11.8 Dissection of the orbit and middle cranial fossa.

glands of the orbit, nose, nasopharynx, and mouth (see Table 9.1), and to the sphincter of the pupil and ciliary muscle of the eyeball.

Post-ganglionic sympathetic and sensory fibres of the trigeminal nerve frequently run through these ganglia but have no functional connection with them. The post-ganglionic sympathetic nerves reach the ganglia through plexuses on the arteries which supply them.

Ciliary ganglion

The ciliary ganglion consists of a small collection of parasympathetic nerve cells, about the size of a large pinhead. It lies in the fatty tissue between the optic nerve and the lateral rectus muscle.

The ganglion cells receive preganglionic parasympathetic fibres from the oculomotor nerve, and send post-ganglionic parasympathetic fibres through the short ciliary nerves.

Connections of the ciliary ganglion

Different types of nerve fibres—parasympathetic, sympathetic, and sensory fibres—are associated with the ganglion. (1) Preganglionic parasympathetic nerves enter the ganglion, synapse in it, and give rise to post-ganglionic parasympathetic nerves. (2) Post-ganglionic sympathetic nerves pass through the ganglion without synapsing in it. (3) Sensory fibres from the eyeball pass through the ganglion without synapsing in it.

The following nerves are connected to the ciliary ganglion. (1) Long, thin branches from the nasociliary nerve enter the ciliary ganglion. They carry (i) **sensory** fibres from the eyeball; and (ii) post-ganglionic **sympathetic** fibres to the dilator pupillae muscle and blood vessels in the outer coats of the eyeball. (The sympathetic fibres enter the ophthalmic nerve from the internal carotid plexus.) Both the sensory and sympathetic fibres pass through the ganglion without synapsing in it. They reach the eyeball in the short ciliary nerves.

(2) A short, thick branch from the nerve to the inferior oblique muscle (oculomotor nerve) enters the ganglion from below. It carries preganglionic **parasympathetic** fibres which synapse with the cells of the ganglion. (3) Approximately six **short ciliary nerves** arise and pass beside the optic nerve. They divide into 12–20 nerves which pierce the sclera around the entrance of the optic nerve. They carry the post-ganglionic fibres to the eyeball and innervate the **sphincter pupillae** and **ciliary muscle**. (Further details of the intraocular muscles of the eyeball are described in Chapter 12.)

Ophthalmic artery

The ophthalmic artery arises from the internal carotid artery as it pierces the arachnoid mater [Figs. 11.8, 11.9].

Course

It enters the orbit through the optic canal, in the subarachnoid space around the optic nerve, and pierces the arachnoid and dura mater. In its course the ophthalmic artery moves from its position below the optic nerve, to the lateral side and then above it to reach the medial wall of the orbit [Fig. 11.9]. On the medial wall, the artery runs forwards below the superior oblique muscle, and ends by dividing into the supratrochlear and dorsal nasal arteries near the front of the orbit.

Branches of the ophthalmic artery

The branches of the ophthalmic artery are numerous and difficult to display but correspond to the nerves in the orbit [Fig. 11.9]. They supply the contents of the orbit through **muscular branches**, the **central artery of the retina** and the **posterior ciliary** and **lacrimal arteries**. Branches of the ophthalmic artery also extend beyond the orbit to the eyelids—**palpebral arteries**; forehead and scalp—**supra-orbital and supratrochlear arteries**; ethmoidal air cells and walls of the upper nasal cavity—**anterior** and **posterior ethmoidal arteries**; and skin of the nose—**dorsal** and **external nasal arteries**. The most important branch is the central artery of the retina. It enters the optic nerve in the orbit and runs in it to the retina. ➲ It is the only artery to the retina, and its occlusion results in blindness of that eye.

The lacrimal artery communicates with the middle meningeal artery through the superior orbital fissure [Fig. 11.8].

Ophthalmic veins

The orbit is drained by the superior and inferior ophthalmic veins. The **superior** ophthalmic vein begins

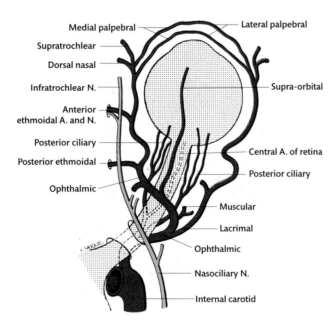

Fig. 11.9 The ophthalmic artery and its branches.

Labels: Medial palpebral, Lateral palpebral, Supratrochlear, Dorsal nasal, Infratrochlear N., Supra-orbital, Anterior ethmoidal A. and N., Posterior ciliary, Central A. of retina, Posterior ethmoidal, Posterior ciliary, Ophthalmic, Muscular, Lacrimal, Ophthalmic, Nasociliary N., Internal carotid in the anterior part of the orbit, close to the ophthalmic artery, and runs with the ophthalmic artery in the orbit. It communicates with the supra-orbital and supratrochlear tributaries of the facial vein.

The **inferior** ophthalmic vein is smaller and lies below the optic nerve. Both superior and inferior ophthalmic veins receive numerous tributaries in the orbit, pass through the superior orbital fissure, and drain into the cavernous sinus, either separately or by a common trunk.

Extraocular muscles of the eyeball (*continued*)

Origin of the extraocular muscles

Using the instructions given in Dissection 11.5, expose the origin of the extraocular muscles.

The four recti arise from a **common tendinous ring** which surrounds the orbital end of the optic canal and the medial part of the superior orbital fissure. The superior, inferior, and medial recti arise from the ring above, below, and medial to the optic canal, respectively. The lateral rectus arises by two heads from the lateral part of the ring and the adjoining margins of the orbital fissure. The two divisions of the oculomotor nerve, nasociliary nerve, abducens nerve, and the ophthalmic veins pass between the two heads of the lateral rectus muscle [Fig. 11.6].

The superior oblique arises from the body of the sphenoid between the superior and medial recti. The inferior oblique is entirely separate from the others. It takes origin from a small area of the floor of the orbit, just lateral to the opening of the nasolacrimal canal. It passes laterally and backwards below the inferior rectus [Figs. 11.7, 11.10].

Insertions of the extraocular muscles

The recti are inserted into the sclera about 6 mm behind the corneoscleral junction. The oblique muscles are inserted into the sclera much further back. The superior oblique is inserted in the upper lateral quadrant of the eyeball behind the equator, and the inferior oblique in the lower lateral quadrant also behind the equator [Fig. 11.7].

Actions of the extraocular muscles

The **medial** and **lateral recti** have the simple function of moving the eye around a vertical axis.

DISSECTION 11.5 Origin of the extraocular muscles

Objectives

I. To expose the origin of the muscles that arise from the common tendinous ring and the superior oblique.   **II.** To display the inferior oblique muscle.

Instructions

1. Divide the optic nerve close to the canal, and turn it forwards with the eyeball. Expose the origin of the recti and the superior oblique.

2. Replace the eyeball. Make an incision through the lower eyelid. Raise the eyeball slightly, and dissect away the fat and loose connective tissue to expose the inferior oblique muscle.

3. Expose the recti muscles, and trace the nerves into the inferior oblique, and inferior and medial recti from the inferior division of the oculomotor nerve.

4. Once again, trace the nerves forwards from the cavernous sinus into the orbit, and note the relative positions in the superior orbital fissure [Fig. 11.6].

The medial rectus turns the cornea medially (adduction of the eye) and the lateral rectus turns it laterally (abduction of the eye).

Elevation and depression of the cornea are brought about by different sets of muscles, depending on whether the eye is abducted or adducted. The **superior** and **inferior recti** produce simple elevation and depression of the cornea only when the eye is abducted. In this position, the **visual axis** corresponds with the axis of these muscles [Fig. 11.11A]. As the cornea is turned medially, the superior and inferior recti become progressively less effective in elevating and depressing the cornea, but tend to turn it further medially [Figs. 11.11B, 11.11C]. When the eye is turned medially, the visual axis moves nearer to the axis of the **oblique muscles**. In the medially turned eye, the inferior oblique produces elevation, and the superior oblique produces depression. Apart from the four primary movements of adduction, abduction, elevation, and depression of the eyeball, the eyeball is also rotated around an anteroposterior axis. Movement of the 12 o'clock position of the cornea inwards or nasally is called **intorsion**. It is

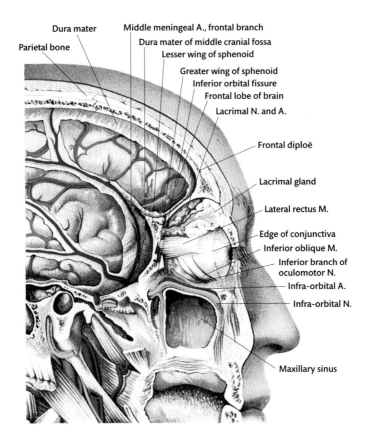

Dura mater
Parietal bone
Middle meningeal A., frontal branch
Dura mater of middle cranial fossa
Lesser wing of sphenoid
Greater wing of sphenoid
Inferior orbital fissure
Frontal lobe of brain
Lacrimal N. and A.
Frontal diploë
Lacrimal gland
Lateral rectus M.
Edge of conjunctiva
Inferior oblique M.
Inferior branch of oculomotor N.
Infra-orbital A.
Infra-orbital N.
Maxillary sinus

Fig. 11.10 Dissection of the orbit and maxillary sinus from the lateral side.

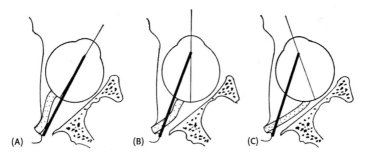

(A)   (B)   (C)

Fig. 11.11 Three diagrams to show the changing relationship and actions of the superior and inferior rectus muscles (thick line) as the cornea is turned from lateral to medial. (A) When the cornea is turned laterally, the two muscles elevate and depress the cornea, respectively. (B) and (C) As the cornea is turned further medially, they become progressively less effective in this action but turn the cornea further medially. It is in this position that the oblique muscles become effective elevators (inferior oblique) and depressors (superior oblique) of the cornea.

brought about by the superior rectus and superior oblique. Movement of the 12 o'clock position of the cornea outwards is called **extorsion**. It is brought about by the inferior rectus and inferior oblique.

The eye muscles may be used in any combination to produce intermediate movements, and delicate control of eye movements is essential for normal vision. See Clinical Application 11.1 for conjugate movements of the eye.

Oculomotor nerve

The oculomotor (third cranial nerve) divides into two—superior and inferior divisions. Both divisions enter the orbit between the two heads of the lateral rectus muscle [Fig. 11.6]. The superior division passes to the superior rectus and, through it, to the levator palpebrae superioris. The larger inferior division supplies the medial rectus, inferior rectus, and inferior oblique, and gives the parasympathetic root to the ciliary ganglion.

Abducens nerve

The abducens (sixth cranial nerve) enters the orbit between the two heads of the lateral rectus and continues forwards, closely applied to the medial surface of that muscle and supplies it [Figs. 11.5, 11.6]. It supplies only the lateral rectus.

Fascial sheath of the eyeball

The fascial sheath of the eyeball is a membranous socket for the eyeball. It is deficient in front over the cornea. It is separated from the eyeball by soft, semi-fluid areolar tissue which allows the eyeball to slide freely in the sheath. The free anterior margin of the sheath fuses with the ocular conjunctiva close to

the margin of the cornea. Posteriorly, the sheath is adherent to the dural sheath of the optic nerve. The sheath is loosely attached to orbital fat [Fig. 11.12].

Each of the extrinsic muscles of the eyeball pierces the fascial sheath at the equator of the eyeball and receives a covering sleeve from it. The sleeve over the recti extend posteriorly and merge with the epimysium. Note the position of the sheath over the medial and lateral recti in Fig. 11.12. Each of these sleeves is attached by fibrous tissue to the bony wall of the orbit and acts as a pulley which prevents the muscle from compressing the eyeball when it contracts. The sheath of the superior oblique passes to the trochlea and fuses with it. The sheath of the inferior oblique reaches the floor of the orbit.

Ligaments in the orbit

(1) The **suspensory ligament** is a hammock-shaped sling stretched below the eyeball in the anterior part of the orbit. It extends between the

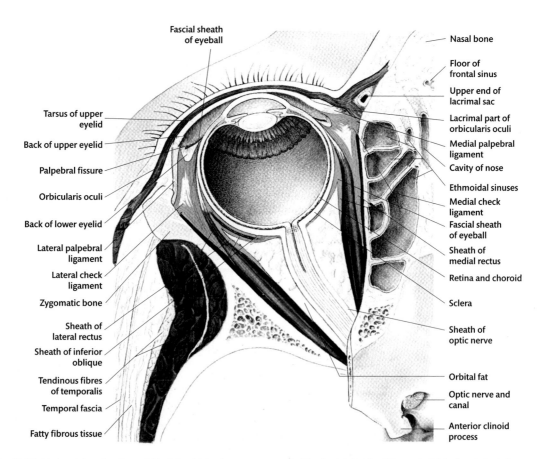

Fig. 11.12 Horizontal section through the left orbit to show arrangement of the fascial sheath of the eyeball (blue) and check ligaments. [See also Fig. 8.13A.]

lacrimal and zygomatic bones. It is broadest beneath the eyeball where it is attached to the fascial sheath and helps to support the eyeball and steady the fascial sheath. (2) The **check ligaments** are strong bands which pass from the sheaths around the lateral and medial rectus muscles to the zygomatic and lacrimal bones respectively, close to the attachments of the suspensory ligament [Fig. 11.12]. These ligaments limit the movement of the lateral and medial recti. Similar checks are present on the superior and inferior rectus muscles.

The zygomatic and infra-orbital nerves, though contents of the orbit, lie outside the orbital periosteum. They are most conveniently dissected later with the maxillary sinus.

See Clinical Applications 11.1 and 11.2 for the practical implications of the anatomy discussed in this chapter.

CLINICAL APPLICATION 11.1 Conjugate eye movements

Movements of the eye and pupil occur constantly to bring the image of the object of visual interest to focus on the retina (fovea). **Conjugate eye movement** is the motor coordination of the eyes which allows both eyes to fix on a single object. **Yoked muscles** are contralaterally paired extraocular muscles which work together to direct the gaze in a particular direction. The movement of the two eyes should be matched accurately to avoid **diplopia**—double vision. Table 11.1 shows the yoked muscles for each direction of gaze. It must be remembered that when one set of muscles contract to act, the antagonists of those muscles will relax to allow movement.

Table 11.1 Yoked muscles

Direction of gaze	Muscle acting in left eye	Muscle acting in right eye
To the left	Lateral rectus	Medial rectus
To the right	Medial rectus	Lateral rectus
To the left and up	Superior rectus	Inferior oblique
To the right and up	Inferior oblique	Superior rectus
To the left and down	Inferior rectus	Superior oblique
To the right and down	Superior oblique	Inferior rectus

CLINICAL APPLICATION 11.2 Paralysis of extraocular muscles

Paralysis of extraocular muscles can occur due to injury of the nerve supplying it, or to the brainstem in the region from where the nerves arise. Injury can be due to trauma, compression by a tumour, or ischaemia. Typically, the individual would present with diplopia (double vision) and a squint. In order to determine which muscle is paralysed, each muscle is isolated by function and tested. For instance, to test the function of the superior oblique muscle, the subject is asked to adduct the eye and look down. In the adducted position, the axis of the eyeball is in line with the oblique muscles, and the inferior rectus will not act as a depressor. Any downward gaze a patient is able to achieve is solely by the action of the superior oblique.

Study question 1: how would you test the remaining extraocular muscles of the eyeball? (Answer: to test the lateral rectus: ask the patient to look laterally. Medial rectus: ask the patient to look medially. Superior rectus: ask the patient to abduct and then elevate the eyeball. Inferior rectus: ask the patient to abduct and then depress the eyeball. Inferior oblique: ask the patient to adduct and then elevate the eyeball.)

Paralysis of the levator palpebrae superioris causes ptosis (drooping of the eyelid).

Study question 2: describe the features of oculomotor paralysis. (Answer: the paralysed eye would be turned down and out, due to unopposed action of the lateral rectus and superior oblique. The patient would also have ptosis due to paralysis of the levator palpebrae superioris, and a dilated pupil due to paralysis of the sphincter pupillae [Chapter 12].)

CHAPTER 12
The eyeball

The eyeball lies in the anterior part of the orbit, enclosed in a fascial sheath which separates it from the orbital muscles and fat. It is about 2.5 cm in diameter but is not perfectly spherical. The anterior clear part—the cornea—has a smaller radius of curvature than the rest of the globe and protrudes from the anterior surface of the eyeball.

For a satisfactory dissection of the eyeball, use one which has been hardened for a few days in formaldehyde. You will need four of these to do all the dissections described here.

General structure of the eyeball

The eyeball consists of three concentric coats or layers, which enclose a cavity.

The coats are: (1) an external fibrous coat made up of the cornea and sclera. The posterior five-sixths of this layer is the white, opaque **sclera**. The anterior one-sixth is the more highly curved, transparent **cornea**; (2) a middle coat which is vascular and muscular; it consists of the **iris** anteriorly, the **choroid** posteriorly, and the thickest part—the **ciliary body**—in between the iris and choroid; and (3) the internal coat—the **retina**; it contains the light-sensitive elements (rods and cones) and gives rise to the nerve fibres of the optic nerve.

The lens is suspended in the eyeball by the suspensory ligament. Together, the lens and suspensory ligament divide the cavity of the eyeball into an aqueous chamber in front, and a vitreous chamber behind. The aqueous chamber is further divided into an **anterior chamber** (between the cornea and the iris) and a **posterior chamber** (between the iris and the lens). The anterior and posterior chambers are continuous with each other through the aperture in the middle of the iris—the **pupil** [Fig. 12.1].

Using the instructions given in Dissection 12.1, clean the surface of the eyeball and section it.

The light rays which enter the eye travel through the following **refracting media**: (1) the cornea; (2) the aqueous humour, a watery medium which fills the **anterior** and **posterior chambers**; (3) the lens; and (4) the vitreous body, which occupies the **vitreous chamber**. Because the greatest change in refractive index is between the air and the cornea, its curved surface plays a very important part in the optical system. ➲ Pathological changes in the shape of the cornea markedly interfere with the ability of the eye to bring an image to focus on the retina.

Fibrous coat

Sclera

The sclera is a dense, collagenous coat, which covers the posterior five-sixths of the eyeball [Figs. 12.1, 12.2]. It is loosely attached to the choroid by delicate, pigmented areolar tissue, but firmly adherent to the ciliary body. The sclera is continuous anteriorly with the cornea [Fig. 12.1].

The point where the optic nerve pierces the sclera is approximately 3 mm to the nasal side of the posterior pole. The bundles of optic nerve fibres, with the blood vessels to the retina among them, pass through a number of holes in the sclera. The optic nerve is covered by all three meninges of the brain, and three meninges fuse with the sclera at the junction of the optic nerve with the sclera. The

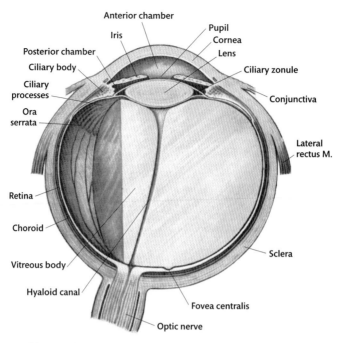

Fig. 12.1 Diagrammatic section of the eyeball.

DISSECTION 12.1 Sectioning of the eyeball

Objectives

I. To clean the surface of the eyeball.   **II.** To section the eyeball for study of the interior.

Instructions

1. Remove the loose tissue from the surface of the eyeball.

2. Pick up the conjunctiva and fascial sheath close to the corneal margin, and cut through these layers around the margin of the cornea. Proceed to strip these soft parts from the surface of the white part of the eye (the sclera), working steadily backwards towards the entry of the optic nerve.

3. Identify the venae vorticosae which pierce the sclera a little posterior to the equator, in the coronal plane [Fig. 12.2].

4. Identify the posterior ciliary arteries and ciliary nerves, as they enter the sclera around the attachment of the optic nerve [Fig. 12.2].

5. To obtain a general idea of the parts of the eyeball, make sections through hardened specimens in different planes: (1) through the equator; (2) a horizontal section. Remove the vitreous body from one-half cut horizontally, and retain it in the other [Fig. 12.1].

6. Place the sections in formaldehyde solution for reference during dissection.

subdural and subarachnoid spaces also end at this point [see Fig. 11.12].

The sclera is also pierced by numerous blood vessels and nerves, which supply the fibrous and vascular coats. They are: (1) the long and short **posterior ciliary arteries** and **ciliary nerves** which pierce the sclera around the optic nerve; (2) 4–5 veins—the **venae vorticosae**—which emerge a short distance posterior to the equator and are spaced equally around the eyeball; and (4) the

anterior ciliary arteries which pierce the sclera near the corneal margin [Fig. 12.2].

Cornea

The cornea is the transparent one-sixth of the fibrous coat of the eyeball. The anterior surface of the cornea is covered with a layer of epithelium which is firmly bound to it and is continuous with the conjunctiva at the margin of the cornea. On the posterior surface of the cornea is the **posterior**

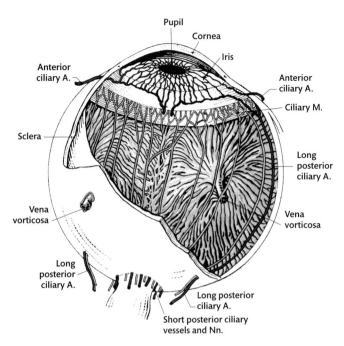

Fig. 12.2 Dissection of the eyeball. Part of the sclera has been removed to show the vascular coat and the arrangement of ciliary nerves and vessels.

limiting lamina, an elastic glassy layer. The iris lies behind the cornea and is separated from it by the aqueous humour [Fig. 12.1].

Middle (vascular) coat choroid

The middle or vascular coat of the eye consists of the iris, the ciliary body, and the choroid.

Iris

The iris is the coloured part of the eye. It lies posterior to the cornea and anterior to the lens. It is separated from the cornea by the anterior chamber and is bathed by the aqueous humour on both surfaces. At its circumference, the iris is continuous with the ciliary body behind and is connected to the cornea by the pectinate ligament of the iris [Fig. 12.1].

The iris varies greatly in colour in light-skinned races. It is circular in outline and surrounds a central circular aperture—the **pupil**. Its anterior surface shows faint radial striations, and its posterior surface is deeply pigmented [Fig. 4.3].

The diameter of the pupil is constantly changing to control the amount of light reaching the retina. Changes in the size of the pupil are brought about by the action of two sets of involuntary muscles in the iris. It is constricted by the circular fibres of the **sphincter pupillae** (which lie in the pupillary margin of the iris), and dilated by fibres which run radially towards the periphery of the iris—the **dilator pupillae**. **Nerve supply**: the sphincter pupillae is supplied by post-ganglionic parasympathetic fibres from the ciliary ganglion which reach it through the short ciliary nerves. The dilator pupillae is supplied by post-ganglionic sympathetic fibres from the carotid plexus, which reach it through the nasociliary and long ciliary nerves [Fig. 11.4].

Pectinate ligament of the iris

At the junction of the cornea and iris is a small, circular venous channel—the **sinus venosus sclerae**. At the margin of the cornea, the posterior limiting lamina of the cornea breaks up into bundles of fibres. Some of these fibres pass posteriorly into the choroid and sclera. Others arch medially into the iris, crossing the angle between the cornea and the iris in the form of a number of separate bundles, known as the **pectinate ligament of the iris** [Fig. 12.3]. Between the bundles are the minute **spaces of the iridocorneal angle**. These spaces form a communication between the

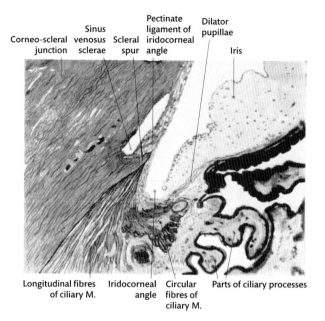

Fig. 12.3 The iridocorneal angle.

anterior chamber of the eyeball and the sinus venosus sclerae, through which the aqueous humour can drain into the venous system. ➲ Blockage of this system is associated with a serious condition called glaucoma, in which the intraocular tension is greatly increased.

Ciliary body

The ciliary body (between the iris anteriorly and the choroid posteriorly) is divisible into: (1) an external part—the **ciliary muscle**; and (2) an internal part—the **ciliary processes** [Figs. 12.1, 12.3, 12.4].

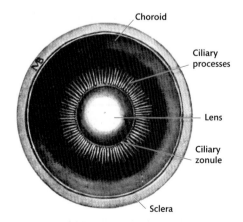

Fig. 12.4 Anterior half of the interior of the eyeball viewed from behind after removal of the vitreous.

Ciliary muscle

The ciliary muscle is composed of involuntary muscle fibres arranged in two groups—radiating and circular [Fig. 12.3].

The **radiating fibres** arise from the deep surface of the sclera, close to the cornea, and radiate posteriorly into the ciliary processes. The **circular fibres** are arranged in two or three bundles that lie on the deep surface of the radiating fibres, and form a muscular ring close to the peripheral margin of the iris. **Nerve supply**: parasympathetic fibres from the ciliary ganglion through the short ciliary nerves. **Action**: accommodation of the eye to focus on near objects. Contraction of the ciliary muscles relaxes the suspensory ligament of the lens [p. 153] and increases the curvature of the lens to enable the eye to focus on near objects.

Using the instructions given in Dissection 12.2, dissect the iris and the ciliary processes.

Ciliary processes

Ciliary processes are radial folds which extend from the anterior margin of the choroid inwards towards the margin of the lens. They end behind the peripheral margin of the iris. They are approximately 70 in number and extend across the posterior surface of the ciliary body. The posterior surface of the processes is applied to the vitreous membrane—the outer condensed part of the vitreous body—and to

DISSECTION 12.2 Iris and ciliary processes

Objective

I. To study the iris and ciliary processes.

Instructions

1. To expose the ciliary processes, make a coronal section through an eyeball anterior to the equator [Fig. 12.4]. Remove the vitreous body from the anterior segment. Then wash out the pigment from the anterior part of the middle coat to expose the ciliary processes more fully.

2. Alternatively, remove the cornea by cutting around the corneoscleral junction, and examine the exposed iris.

3. Make a number of radial cuts into the anterior part of the sclera, and fold each segment of the sclera outwards, stripping it from the ciliary body.

4. Remove the iris.

DISSECTION 12.3 Choroid

Objective

I. To remove the sclera and expose the choroid.

Instructions

1. Start with an undissected eye. Using a sharp knife, make an incision through the sclera at the equator, stopping as soon as the black choroid appears. Introduce one blade of blunt-ended scissors through the cut, and extend the incision through the sclera around the equator. Take care to separate the choroid from its deep surface as you proceed.

2. Raise the anterior and posterior parts of the divided sclera from the choroid, and by careful blunt dissection, turn these parts anteriorly and posteriorly, stripping them from the choroid. Some resistance will be encountered with the anterior part close to the cornea, due to the attachment of the ciliary muscle to the deep surface of the sclera. As this attachment is broken down by continued blunt dissection, the aqueous humour will escape.

3. Remove the posterior part of the sclera by dividing the optic nerve fibres where they enter the deep surface.

4. The eyeball, denuded of its fibrous coat, should be placed in water for further investigation.

5. Gently brush the eyeball under water with a brush. This removes the pigment and exposes the curved tributaries of the venae vorticosae, which appear as white lines [Fig. 12.2].

149

the peripheral part of the ciliary zonule [p. 153] [Fig. 12.4].

Choroid

The choroid is the largest part of the middle coat. It lies between the sclera and the retina. It is thickest posteriorly where it is pierced by the optic nerve and becomes thinner as it approaches the ciliary body. The choroid is connected to the sclera by delicate, pigmented areolar tissue, and also by the blood vessels and nerves which pass between them. The deep surface of the choroid is adherent to the outermost layer of the retina.

The choroid consists mainly of blood vessels which are arranged in two layers: (1) a deep, close-meshed capillary net; and (2) a more superficial venous layer from which the venae vorticosae arise. The short posterior ciliary arteries run between these layers.

Using the instructions given in Dissection 12.3, remove the sclera from one eyeball.

Ciliary nerves

Twelve or more fine **short ciliary nerves** arise from the ciliary ganglion and pierce the sclera around the optic nerve. On the inner aspect of the sclera, they run anteriorly and break up into fine plexiform branches to the ciliary muscle, iris, and cornea [Fig. 12.2]. The short ciliary nerves contain: (1) **post-ganglionic parasympathetic fibres** from the ciliary ganglion to the ciliary muscle and the sphincter pupillae; (2) **post-ganglionic sympathetic fibres** from the internal carotid plexus to the vessels of the eyeball; and (3) **sensory fibres** from the nasociliary nerve. (The sympathetic and sensory fibres have no connection with the cells of the ciliary ganglion.)

The **long ciliary branches** of the nasociliary nerve transmit sensory and sympathetic nerve fibres to the eyeball. They pierce the sclera close to the optic nerve. The sympathetic fibres come from the internal carotid plexus, and some of them supply the dilator pupillae.

Ciliary arteries

The **short posterior ciliary arteries** are branches of the ophthalmic artery. They pierce the sclera close to the optic nerve and end in the choroid [Figs. 12.2, 12.5].

The **long posterior ciliary arteries** are two branches of the ophthalmic artery which pierce the sclera some distance from the optic nerve. They run anteriorly, between the sclera and choroid, on opposite sides of the eyeball. In the region of the ciliary body, they branch and anastomose with the anterior ciliary arteries to form the **greater arterial circle** at the periphery of the iris [Fig. 12.5]. This circle supplies the iris, the ciliary muscle, and the ciliary processes.

The **anterior ciliary arteries** are minute twigs which arise from the arteries to the recti muscles. They pierce the sclera close to the cornea and take part in the formation of the greater arterial circle. The **lesser arterial circle** is a small anastomotic ring in the iris at the margin of the pupil [Fig. 12.5].

Venae vorticosae

Four to five large veins arise from the venous plexus in the choroid and pierce the sclera immediately posterior to the equator. These are the venae vorticosae. They drain into the ophthalmic veins [Fig. 12.2].

Using the instructions given in Dissection 12.4, identify the layers of the retina.

DISSECTION 12.4 Retina

Objective

I. To study the layers of the retina.

Instructions

1. Remove the vitreous body from the posterior segment of the specimen used to show the ciliary processes.

2. Study the white nervous layer of the retina which has been exposed.

3. Gently lift the inner nervous layer of the retina, and appreciate the outer pigmented layer.

Retina

The retina consists of two layers: (1) an outer **pigment layer** which is adherent to the choroid; and (2) a thicker inner **nervous layer**. A potential space (the remnant of the optic cavity in the embryo) exists between the pigment layer of the retina and the nervous layer. The nervous layer is attached to the vitreous and pigment layer only where the optic nerve pierces the sclera. It is readily detached from the pigment layer, even during life. ➡ Such a detachment of the retina makes it

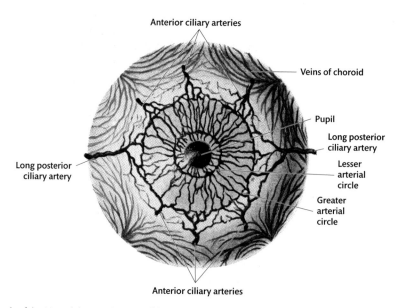

Fig. 12.5 Blood vessels of the iris and the anterior part of the choroid viewed from the front.

impossible to focus an image on the nervous layer and may interfere with nutrition to the retina.

The pigment layer absorbs the light which has passed through the nervous layer and prevents it from being reflected back as scattered rays, which would interfere with the sharpness of the image. (In many nocturnal animals, the choroid forms a reflecting layer known as the tapetum. The presence of the tapetum ensures the passage of low intensities of light twice through the retina, to increase its sensitivity.)

The nervous layer is the light-sensitive part of the retina. It ends anteriorly, at a wavy margin—the **ora serrata**—close to the posterior margin of the ciliary body [Fig. 12.1]. The two layers—the pigment and nervous layers—are continued, anterior to the ora serrata, as a very thin layer on the posterior aspect of the ciliary processes and the posterior surface of the iris. This continuation of the retina on the ciliary processes and iris is known as the **pars ciliaris retinae** and the **pars iridica retinae**, respectively.

The nervous layer of the retina consists of multiple layers of cells. The outermost are the light-sensitive **rods** and **cones**. The innermost are the **ganglion** cells that give rise to the fibres in the optic nerve [Fig. 12.6]. The nerve fibres originating in the ganglion cell run over the inner surface of the retina and converge on the optic nerve.

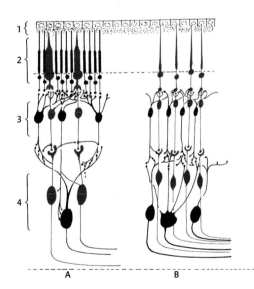

Fig. 12.6 Arrangement of cells in the peripheral (A) and central (B) parts of the retina. Only the rods, cones, bipolar, and ganglion cells are shown. The cones and specific cone connections are shown in red. In (B), the tightly packed cones have been separated for diagrammatic purposes. 1. Pigment layer of the retina. 2. Rods and cones. 3. Bipolar cells. 4. Ganglion cells.

At the commencement of the optic nerve, the retina has a circular elevation, with a slight central depression on it. This is the **optic disc** [Fig. 12.7]. The optic disc is situated approximately 3 mm to the nasal side of the anteroposterior axis of the eyeball and is the site where the nerve fibres turn posteriorly into the optic nerve. At the optic disc, there are no sensory retinal elements and it accounts for the blind spot in the visual field. The central artery of the retina enters the retina at the optic disc.

In the centre of the visual axis is a small yellowish spot on the retina—the **macula lutea**. It has a slight depression at the centre—the **fovea centralis** [Fig. 12.7]. The fovea is the site of maximum visual acuity. At the fovea, the inner layers of the nervous layer of the retina are swept aside to expose the cones. This allows light to fall directly on these elements (without passing through the other layers), and so improves the quality of the image on the cones. [Fig. 12.6B]. The nerve fibres and blood vessels which pass to and from the optic disc do not cross the macula but go around it, so as not to obstruct the light rays.

Central retinal arteries and veins

The central retinal arteries and veins are the only source of blood supply to the inner layers of the retina. (The outer retinal layers receive some nutrition from the choroidal vessels by diffusion.) The central artery is a branch of the ophthalmic artery [see Fig. 11.9]. It pierces the sheaths of the optic nerve and enters the optic nerve in the orbit. It reaches the retina through the optic nerve and appears in the eyeball at the optic disc. In the optic nerve, it runs with the corresponding central vein. At the optic disc, the central artery of the retina divides into superior and inferior branches, each of which divides into a large temporal, and a smaller nasal arteriole [Fig. 12.7]. These branches run on the internal surface of the retina to the ora serrata. They do not anastomose with each other or with any of the other arteries of the eyeball.

The **retinal veins** converge on the optic disc and enter the optic nerve as two small trunks which soon unite to form the **central vein of the retina**. The central vein of the retina drains into the superior ophthalmic vein, after piercing the meningeal sheaths of the optic nerve.

Using the instructions given in Dissection 12.5, examine the ciliary zonule and the lens.

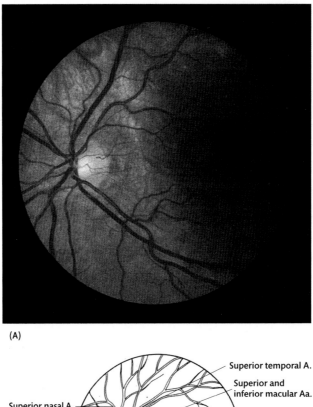

(A)

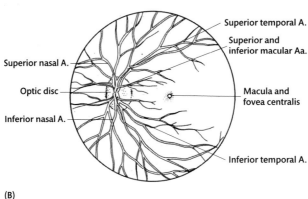

Superior temporal A.

Superior and inferior macular Aa.

Superior nasal A.

Optic disc

Inferior nasal A.

Macula and fovea centralis

Inferior temporal A.

(B)

Fig. 12.7 (A) Retinal blood vessels, as seen through the ophthalmoscope. (B) Diagrammatic representation of (A).

DISSECTION 12.5 Ciliary zonule and lens

Objective

I. To examine the ciliary zonule, capsule of the lens, and lens.

Instructions

1. In the anterior segment of a freshly dissected eye, examine the vitreous membrane, the capsule of the lens, and the ciliary zonule.

2. Remove the lens (which is now hardened), and examine it.

Vitreous body

The vitreous body is a soft, transparent, jelly-like substance which fills the posterior four-fifths of the eyeball. It lies in contact with the retina, the ciliary processes, the ciliary zonule, and the lens. The lens forms a deep depression—the **hyaloid fossa**—on the anterior surface of the vitreous body [Fig. 12.1].

The outer surface of the vitreous body is condensed to form a transparent envelope—the **vitreous membrane**. A minute canal—the **hyaloid canal**—runs through the vitreous body from the optic disc to the posterior surface of the lens [Fig. 12.1]. It represents the remains of a branch of the central artery of the retina—the **hyaloid artery**—which supplied the developing lens in the fetus but which subsequently disappeared. This hyaloid canal cannot be seen in an ordinary dissection but may be visualized in the living with a slit-lamp. The minute remnant of the hyaloid artery attaches the vitreous body to the optic disc, though elsewhere the vitreous body is entirely free from the retina.

Ciliary zonule and suspensory ligament of the lens

The ciliary zonule is a thickened part of the vitreous membrane which is in contact with the posterior surface of the ciliary process [Figs. 12.1, 12.4, 12.8]. At the inner margin of the ciliary processes, it splits into two layers. The posterior layer is extremely thin and lines the hyaloid fossa. The anterior layer is thicker and forms the **suspensory ligament of the lens**. It is attached principally to the anterior surface of the capsule of the lens a short distance from its margin, to the margin of the lens, and the posterior surface close to the margin. [Figs. 12.1, 12.8]. The multiple attachments of the suspensory ligament to the lens result in the formation of a multilocular, fluid-filled space around the margin of the lens—the zonular space.

The suspensory ligament holds the lens firmly in the hyaloid fossa. When the eye is at rest, the suspensory ligament maintains a certain degree of tension on the lens. The lens is drawn out radially and flattens, so as to maintain a long focal length. When the eye focuses on near objects, the ciliary muscle contracts and pulls the ciliary processes and zonule anteriorly. This movement relaxes the suspensory ligament and allows the elastic lens to round up and shorten its focal length.

Lens

The lens is a biconvex, transparent, solid, elastic structure which lies between the iris and the vitreous body. It is enclosed in a glassy, elastic capsule. It contains no blood vessels.

The **anterior surface** of the lens is less curved than the posterior. Its central part is opposite the pupil, and lateral to this, the margin of the iris is in contact with the lens. Further laterally, the lens and iris are separated from each other by the aqueous humour in the posterior chamber. The **posterior surface** of the lens fits into the hyaloid fossa. The equator of the lens is a blunt margin that forms one boundary of the zonular spaces. ◑ The lens becomes tougher and less elastic with age. This accounts for the decreased ability to focus on near objects. It also becomes less transparent and more opaque, a condition known as cataract.

Dissection 12.6 provides instructions on how to study the capsule of the lens and the lens.

See Clinical Applications 12.1, 12.2, 12.3, and 12.4 for the practical implications of the anatomy discussed in this chapter.

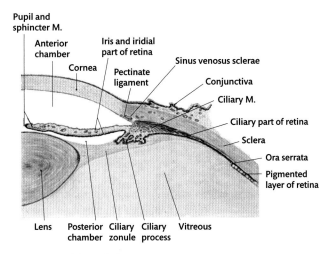

Fig. 12.8 Section through the anterior part of the eyeball.

DISSECTION 12.6 Lens

Objective

I. To study the lens and the capsule of the lens.

Instructions

1. Incise the anterior surface of the lens with a sharp knife, and apply a little pressure to the margin with the finger and thumb. This will extrude the body of the lens and allow the capsule to be studied separately.

2. Compress the body of the lens between the finger and thumb, and note that the central part (nucleus) is firmer than the remainder. The lens is made up of a number of concentric laminae, which can be easily peeled off after the lens has been hardened in alcohol.

CLINICAL APPLICATION 12.1 Corneal reflex

Testing for the corneal or blink reflex is part of neurological examination. It is especially useful in patients with head injury to assess the integrity of the brainstem. Stimulation of the cornea of one eye with a wisp of cotton causes both eyelids to blink. This reflex blink protects the eye from foreign bodies. Stimulus of the cornea of one side causes a direct (same side) and consensual (opposite side) blink response.

The afferent (sensory) limb of the reflex arc is mediated through the nasociliary branch of the ophthalmic division of the trigeminal nerve, which supplies the cornea. The efferent (motor) limb is through the temporal and zygomatic branches of the facial nerve which supply the orbicularis oculi. An absent corneal reflex may be due to sensory neuropathy affecting the trigeminal nerve, a lesion in the seventh cranial nerve, or a brainstem injury. Failure to blink on one side indicates seventh nerve palsy on that side. Failure to blink on both sides usually indicates a sensory loss of the tested side.

CLINICAL APPLICATION 12.2 Corneal transplant

Corneal transplant, or keratoplasty, is a procedure where diseased corneal tissue is surgically removed and replaced by healthy donor corneal tissue harvested from a recently deceased individual. Corneal transplants can be 'penetrating' when the whole thickness of the cornea is replaced, or 'lamellar' when the graft involves only a few layers of the cornea. The fact that the cornea is avascular, devoid of lymphatics, and has relatively few antigen-presenting cells makes it immunologically privileged and less likely to be rejected than other organ transplants.

CLINICAL APPLICATION 12.3 Central retinal vessel occlusion

Obstruction of either the central retinal artery or the vein can result in acute-onset loss of vision due to ischaemia of the retina. Sometimes, only a branch of the vessel may be occluded, resulting in patchy loss of vision.

Study question 1: what is the branching pattern of the central retinal artery? (Answer: the artery divides into superior and inferior branches, and each of these, in turn, divides into nasal and temporal divisions.)

Study question 2: the central retinal artery is typically an end artery. What does this mean? (Answer: end arteries are the sole supply of arterial blood to a territory. They do not anastomose with other arteries. As such, if

an end artery is occluded, there is complete deprivation of blood to the area supplied by it.)

Increased pressure in the subarachnoid space tends to compress the central vein of the retina and cause distension of its tributaries in the retina. These distended veins can be seen with the ophthalmoscope.

The central artery of the retina and its branches are blood vessels which can be examined in the living, and signs of vascular pathology can be observed first hand. You should take every opportunity to use an ophthalmoscope and examine the normal retina and blood vessels.

CLINICAL APPLICATION 12.4 Convergence–accommodation reflex

Failure to bring both eyes to focus on an object leads to double vision. To test this, hold up your finger about 30 cm from your nose, and look past it at a distant object (do not focus on the finger). In this situation, the finger appears double and out of focus. Now slowly bring your eyes to focus on the finger. The two images move together and come into focus as a single object.

The ability to change focus from distant objects to near objects is dependent on convergence and accommodation. Convergence occurs when the two medial recti work together and ensure that the image of the finger falls on corresponding parts of the two retinae. Accommodation occurs when the ciliary muscles contract, the ciliary zonule and lens are brought forward, the suspensory ligament of the lens is relaxed, and the lens becomes more spherical, bringing the near object to focus on the retina.

The two actions are linked together in the **convergence–accommodation reflex** and are associated with constriction of the pupil.

CHAPTER 13
Organs of hearing and equilibrium

Introduction

The ear contains the auditory apparatus and the organs for balance and equilibrium. It is readily divisible into three parts: the external ear, the middle ear, and the internal ear.

The **external ear** consists of the auricle and the external acoustic meatus. The auricle collects the sound waves, and the external acoustic meatus transmits them medially to the tympanic membrane. The tympanic membrane separates the external ear from the middle ear. The **middle ear** is a narrow air-filled chamber, also known as the **tympanic cavity**. It lies between the tympanic membrane and the lateral wall of the internal ear. The pressure in the tympanic cavity is maintained at atmospheric pressure by the communication of the cavity with the nasal part of the pharynx through the auditory tube. Three small auditory ossicles—the **malleus**, **incus**, and **stapes**—lie in the middle ear and stretch across it from the tympanic membrane to the lateral wall of the internal ear. They transmit the vibrations of the tympanic membrane to the internal ear. The **internal ear** consists of a complex system of communicating cavities—the **bony labyrinth**—situated in the dense part of the petrous temporal bone. Suspended in the bony labyrinth is a similarly shaped, but narrower complex of membranous tubes and sacs—the **membranous labyrinth**—on which the sensory nerve fibres of the vestibulocochlear nerve end [Fig. 13.1].

The external ear

Review the parts of the auricle described in Chapter 4.

Dissection 13.1 provides instructions on how to dissect the external acoustic meatus.

External acoustic meatus

The external acoustic meatus runs medially and slightly forwards. It is almost exactly in line with the internal acoustic meatus, and their shadows are superimposed in a true lateral radiograph of the skull. The external acoustic meatus is approximately 24 mm long. The lateral one-third of it is cartilaginous, and the medial two-thirds is bony. The tympanic membrane lies obliquely, so that the anterior wall and floor are longer than the posterior wall and roof. The diameter of the external acoustic meatus is not uniform; the narrowest point—the **isthmus**—is about 5 mm from the tympanic membrane. The vertical diameter is greatest at the lateral end, and the anteroposterior diameter is greatest at the medial end. The meatus is slightly curved with an upward convexity [Fig. 13.1].

➲ All these points should be kept in mind when attempting to remove a foreign body from the meatus.

➲ The bony part of the meatus is absent in the newborn, and the tympanic membrane is much nearer the surface and more oblique than in the adult.

The skin of the cartilaginous portion contains many **ceruminous glands** and hair follicles. The

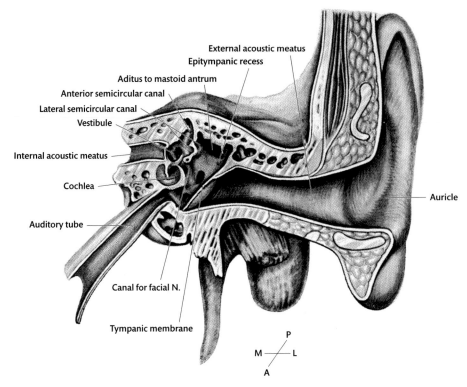

Fig. 13.1 The parts of the ear (semi-diagrammatic). The mucous membrane lining the middle ear cavity and auditory tube is shown in blue. M = medial; L = lateral; A = anterior; P = posterior.

DISSECTION 13.1 External acoustic meatus

Objective

I. To study the external acoustic meatus.

Instructions

1. Remove the anterior wall of the cartilaginous part of the external acoustic meatus with a knife or scissors.

2. Pass a probe into the bony part of the meatus to determine its length, and using the probe as a guide, cut away the anterior wall of the bony part of the meatus (tympanic bone). Take care not to injure the tympanic membrane.

hairs are directed laterally and prevent the entry of small objects into the meatus. In the bony part of the canal, the skin is thin and tightly adherent to the periosteum. It has no hairs and few, if any, glands and continues as a very delicate layer over the lateral surface of the tympanic membrane.

Tympanic membrane

The tympanic membrane is shaped like an elliptical disc. It is stretched across the medial end of the external acoustic meatus and forms the greater part of the lateral wall of the middle ear cavity. It slopes obliquely downwards, forwards, and medially, and its lateral surface is deeply concave. The point of maximum convexity on the medial surface is called the **umbo** [Figs. 13.2, 13.3]. The tympanic membrane is made up of a taut fibrous layer with a thickened margin. The thickened membrane is inserted into the tympanic groove on a ring-like ridge of the tympanic bone at the medial end of the meatus [Fig. 13.4]. The **handle of the malleus** is attached to the medial surface of the tympanic membrane, and the lower end reaches the umbo. Close to the upper edge of the membrane, the lateral process of the malleus projects laterally, causing the membrane to bulge into the meatus.

Above the lateral process of the malleus, the ring and groove for the margin of the tympanic membrane are replaced by a shallow depression—the **tympanic notch**. At the tympanic notch, the

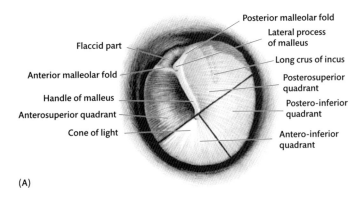

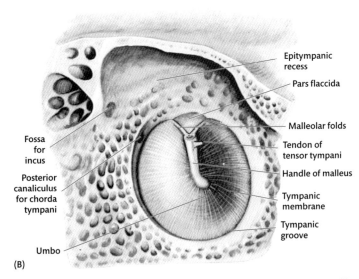

Fig. 13.2 (A) Left tympanic membrane seen from the lateral side. The four arbitrary quadrants are indicated by solid lines and the handle of the malleus. (B) The left tympanic membrane and epitympanic recess seen from the medial side. The head and neck of the malleus have been removed.

thickened edge of the tympanic membrane leaves the bone and passes to the lateral process of the malleus, forming the anterior and posterior **malleolar folds** [Fig. 13.2B]. Between these folds and the margin of the tympanic notch lies the less tense, **flaccid part** of the membrane, which differs from the rest in not having a well-defined fibrous layer.

When the tympanic membrane is examined in the living, its surface appears highly polished, and a cone of reflected light extends antero-inferiorly from the tip of the handle of the malleus. The malleolar folds can be seen as two lines outlining the flaccid part, and the **long process of the incus** (the intermediate auditory ossicle) can be seen dimly through the membrane, parallel and posterior to the handle of the malleus.

Dissection 13.2 provides instructions on dissection of the middle ear cavity.

Middle ear

Introduction to middle ear cavity

The narrow middle ear cavity, together with the tympanic membrane, is known as the tympanum. It is lined with mucous membrane and is filled with air. It communicates anteriorly with the nasopharynx through the auditory tube [Fig. 13.6], and posteriorly through the mastoid antrum [Fig. 13.7] with the mastoid air cells—small air-filled cavities in the mastoid process.

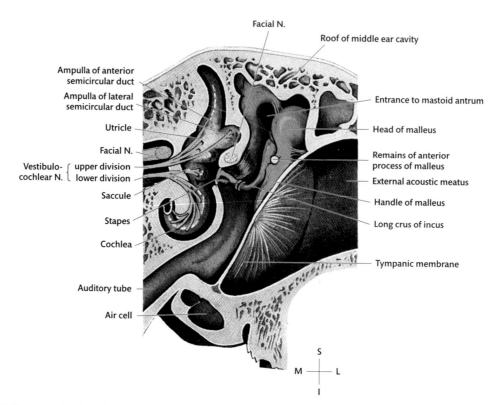

Facial N.

Roof of middle ear cavity

Ampulla of anterior semicircular duct

Ampulla of lateral semicircular duct

Utricle

Facial N.

Vestibulo-cochlear N. { upper division / lower division

Saccule

Stapes

Cochlea

Auditory tube

Air cell

Entrance to mastoid antrum

Head of malleus

Remains of anterior process of malleus

External acoustic meatus

Handle of malleus

Long crus of incus

Tympanic membrane

S
M ─┼─ L
I

Fig. 13.3 Coronal section through the left tympanic cavity, viewed from the front (semi-diagrammatic). L = lateral; M = medial; S = superior; I = inferior.

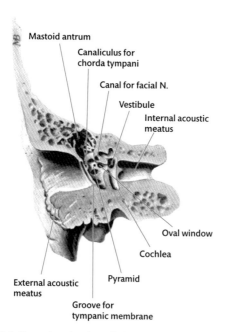

Mastoid antrum

Canaliculus for chorda tympani

Canal for facial N.

Vestibule

Internal acoustic meatus

Oval window

Cochlea

External acoustic meatus

Pyramid

Groove for tympanic membrane

Fig. 13.4 Coronal section through the right temporal bone, seen from in front. The posterior wall of the middle ear cavity is seen.

The vertical and anteroposterior diameters of the middle ear cavity are each approximately 15 mm; the width varies from 6 mm above to 4 mm below,

and is even less in the middle where the medial and lateral walls bulge into the cavity [Fig. 13.3]. The part of the cavity superior to the tympanic membrane is called the **epitympanic recess** [Figs. 13.1, 13.2B, 13.5].

Boundaries of the middle ear cavity

The middle ear cavity has a roof, a floor, posterior, anterior, medial, and lateral walls. The **roof** or **tegmental wall** of the tympanic cavity is the thin bone **tegmen tympani**, which separates the cavity from the middle cranial fossa [Fig. 13.3]. The **floor** or **jugular wall** is narrow. It is formed by a thin plate of bone which separates the cavity from the jugular fossa. It contains the superior bulb of the jugular vein. ➲ Chronic inflammation of the middle ear may spread through the tegmen to the meninges of the brain, or through the floor to the jugular vein, and lead to thrombosis (clotting) of the blood in the vein and spread of infection through the bloodstream.

The **posterior** or **mastoid wall** [Figs. 13.4, 13.7] has a series of openings in it: (1) above is the opening or **aditus** which leads from the epitympanic recess into the mastoid antrum; (2) inferiorly, close to the

DISSECTION 13.2 Middle ear cavity

Objectives

I. To open into the middle ear cavity. **II.** To identify the parts of the ossicles seen after removing the roof. **III.** To identify the openings of the auditory tube, the aditus of the mastoid antrum, and the semicanal for the tensor tympani.

Instructions

1. Strip the dura mater from the floor of the middle cranial fossa as far anteriorly as the mandibular nerve. The greater petrosal nerve will be found emerging from the anterior surface of the petrous temporal bone and running anteromedially inferior to the trigeminal ganglion.

2. The cavity of the middle ear is separated from the middle cranial fossa by a thin layer of bone—the **tegmen tympani**. It lies parallel and slightly lateral to the greater petrosal nerve.

3. Force a small aperture in the tegmen tympani with the point of a rigid knife or seeker. Slip a strong probe through the aperture under the tegmen, and lever it up. Break it away, first in an anteromedial, and then in a posterolateral, direction towards the junction of the transverse and sigmoid sinuses. Keep the probe close to the tegmen to avoid damage to the contents of the middle ear cavity.

4. Remove the broken edges of the tegmen, and expose the cavity of the middle ear. Avoid injury to the parts of the auditory ossicles which extend superiorly.

5. Attempt to pass a blunt seeker into the anteromedial part of the cavity, and slide it anteromedially till it appears through the pharyngeal opening of the auditory tube.

6. Explore the middle ear cavity.

7. The upper part of the posterior (mastoid) wall of the middle ear cavity has an opening—the **aditus**. This opening links the middle ear with the mastoid antrum and the mastoid air cells. Make an attempt to find the aditus [Fig. 13.3].

8. Identify the rounded head of the malleus articulating with the incus, and the short crus of the incus which passes posteriorly towards the posterior wall of the cavity [Fig. 13.5].

9. Inferior to the head of the malleus, note the sloping tympanic membrane and the handle of the malleus lying in it.

10. Identify the thin tendon which passes from the malleus to the medial wall of the middle ear. This is the tendon of the **tensor tympani** which turns nearly 90 degrees at the medial wall to become continuous with the muscle belly.

11. The muscle runs in a semicanal, superomedial to the auditory tube. Break through the thin wall of this canal, and expose the muscle [Fig. 13.5].

12. Immediately superior to the attachment of the tendon to the malleus, the chorda tympani nerve [Fig. 13.3] runs across the medial surface of the tympanic membrane and the malleus, forming a narrow ridge. Identify it.

13. Look for the long crus of the incus which passes inferiorly to the stapes, which is not visible at this stage.

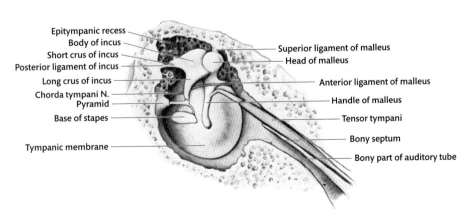

Fig. 13.5 Left tympanic membrane and auditory ossicles, seen from the medial side. Note the auditory tube and the tensor tympani in its semicanal.

Epitympanic recess
Body of incus
Short crus of incus
Posterior ligament of incus
Long crus of incus
Chorda tympani N.
Pyramid
Base of stapes
Tympanic membrane

Superior ligament of malleus
Head of malleus
Anterior ligament of malleus
Handle of malleus
Tensor tympani
Bony septum
Bony part of auditory tube

medial wall, is a small conical projection called the **pyramid** [Fig. 13.4] with an opening on the apex. The pyramid contains the **stapedius muscle**. The stapedius tendon exits through the aperture on the apex of the pyramid and passes to the stapes; (3) lateral to the pyramid, there is an opening through which the **chorda tympani branch** of the facial nerve enters the middle ear [Fig. 13.4].

The **anterior** or **carotid wall** is narrow, because the medial and lateral walls converge anteriorly. Three features are present on the anterior wall: (1) superiorly, the opening of the semicanal for the tensor tympani; (2) the orifice of the auditory tube in an intermediate position [Fig. 13.5]; (3) inferiorly, a plate of bone which separates the middle ear cavity from the carotid canal [Fig. 13.6]. The semicanals for the tensor tympani and the auditory tube are separated by a bony septum. This septum is continued posteriorly on the medial wall of the middle ear as a shelf-like projection—the **processus cochleariformis**. The posterior end of this projection forms a pulley, around which the tendon of the tensor tympani turns laterally through 90 degrees to run to the malleus [Fig. 13.5].

The **medial** or **labyrinthine wall** separates the middle ear from the internal ear. It is almost entirely bony [Fig. 13.7]. The cochlea of the internal ear forms a bulge—the **promontory** on the medial wall. Two small apertures are seen in relation to the promontory: (1) the **fenestra vestibuli**, or oval window, lies above the promontory and is filled by the base of the stapes [Fig. 13.3]; (2) the **fenestra cochleae**, or round window, lies below the promontory and is closed by the delicate **secondary tympanic membrane**. These two apertures lead into the cavity of the bony labyrinth. Movements of the stapes generate pressure waves to the fluid in the bony labyrinth (perilymph). Since fluid is incompressible, movements of the stapes result in corresponding movements of the secondary tympanic membrane, which thus prevents damping of the stapedial oscillations. The **sinus tympani** is a depression between and behind the two windows. The facial nerve and the lateral semicircular canal, enclosed in the bone, produce parallel ridges on the superior aspect of the medial wall. These bony ridges extend posteriorly into the aditus and the mastoid antrum [Fig. 13.7].

The **lateral wall** of the middle ear cavity is formed by the tympanic membrane.

Mucous membrane of the middle ear cavity

The thin delicate lining of the walls of the tympanic cavity also covers the auditory ossicles and is continuous with the lining of the auditory tube, mastoid

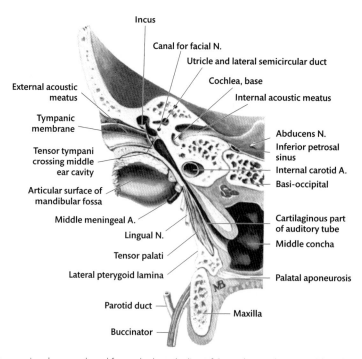

Fig. 13.6 An oblique coronal section passing downwards and forwards along the line of the auditory tube, viewed from behind. The mandible and muscles of mastication have been removed, leaving the branches of the mandibular nerve on the lateral aspect of the tensor palati.

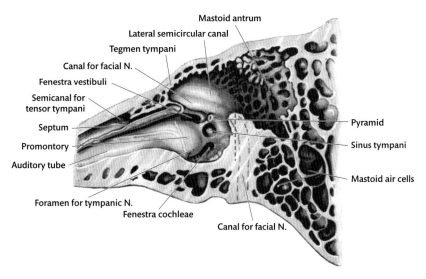

Labels on figure:
Mastoid antrum
Lateral semicircular canal
Tegmen tympani
Canal for facial N.
Fenestra vestibuli
Semicanal for tensor tympani
Septum
Promontory
Auditory tube
Foramen for tympanic N.
Fenestra cochleae
Canal for facial N.
Pyramid
Sinus tympani
Mastoid air cells

Fig. 13.7 Vertical section through the left middle ear cavity and auditory tube to show the medial wall of the middle ear cavity. The auditory ossicles have been removed. The position of the posterior wall of the middle ear cavity is shown by the red line.

antrum, and mastoid air cells. The middle ear cavity contains: (1) the auditory ossicles—malleus, incus, and stapes; (2) the tendon of the stapedius and tensor tympani muscles; and (3) the chorda tympani nerve and the tympanic plexus of nerves. All these structures are covered by the mucous membrane.

➔ The tympanic cavity and the cavity of the auditory tube may become blocked when the mucous membrane swells during inflammation. Once blocked, the air in the cavity is absorbed by surrounding blood vessels, leading to a fall in the pressure and hearing loss because the tympanic membrane cannot vibrate freely.

Auditory ossicles

These three small bones form a chain which extends from the tympanic membrane on the lateral wall of the middle ear cavity to the oval window on the medial wall. The malleus is attached to the tympanic membrane, the stapes to the oval window, and the incus is slung between the two [Fig. 13.5].

Malleus

The **head of the malleus** is the rounded upper part of the bone which lies in the epitympanic recess. The slender **manubrium**, or handle, is attached to the tympanic membrane.

Incus

The **body of the incus** lies in the epitympanic recess and articulates with the head of the malleus. It has a **long crus** which projects inferiorly and articulates with the head of the stapes, and a **short crus** which extends posteriorly and is attached to the bone by a ligament.

Stapes

The stapes is shaped like a stirrup. It has a head which articulates with the long crus of the incus, and an oval foot piece, or **base**, which is attached to the oval window (fenestra vestibuli) by an elastic **annular ligament**.

Movements of the ear ossicles

When the tympanic membrane and the handle of the malleus vibrate, the head of the malleus imparts a rotatory movement to the incus around the axis of its short crus. This moves the long crus of the incus which, in turn, imparts the same movement to the stapes.

Tympanic muscles

There are two muscles in the tympanic cavity—the stapedius and the tensor tympani.

Stapedius

The **stapedius** is placed within the pyramid and the canal which curves inferiorly from it on the posterior wall of the tympanic cavity. Its tendon enters the middle ear through an opening on the apex of the pyramid. It is inserted into the posterior surface of the neck of the stapes [Fig. 13.5]. **Nerve supply**: the facial nerve. **Action**: it prevents excessive movements of the stapes.

➲ Paralysis of the stapedius leads to uninhibited movement of the stapes and increased sensitivity to sounds (hyperacusis).

Tensor tympani

The tensor tympani takes origin from the superior surface of the cartilaginous part of the auditory tube and the adjacent parts of the greater wing of the sphenoid and petrous temporal bone (see Fig. 3.7 to get an understanding of the origin). It passes posterolaterally in the semicanal, superior to the bony part of the auditory tube. In the middle ear cavity, it turns laterally through 90 degrees on the processus cochleariformis and is inserted on the superior part of the handle of the malleus [Fig. 13.5]. **Nerve supply**: the mandibular nerve, through fibres which traverse the otic ganglion. **Actions**: it tenses the tympanic membrane, increases its medial convexity, and restricts its movement. It prevents wide excursions of the ear ossicles and damage to the inner ear from loud sounds.

Chorda tympani nerve

The chorda tympani arises from the facial nerve in the temporal bone, a short distance above the stylomastoid foramen [Fig. 13.8]. It ascends in a bony canaliculus to the posterior wall of the middle ear cavity and enters the cavity through the posterior wall. In the tympanic cavity, the chorda tympani runs forwards across the medial surface of the upper part of the tympanic membrane and the neck of the malleus [Fig. 13.5]. It leaves the middle ear through the petrotympanic fissure [see Fig. 15.8], runs antero-inferiorly, medial to the spine of the sphenoid, and joins the lingual nerve a short distance inferior to the skull [Fig. 13.8].

The chorda tympani carries taste fibres from the anterior two-thirds of the tongue, and preganglionic parasympathetic fibres to the submandibular ganglion. The parasympathetic fibres innervate the submandibular and sublingual salivary glands and the glands in the anterior two-thirds of the tongue.

Mastoid antrum and mastoid air cells

The mastoid antrum is an air-filled extension from the middle ear cavity. It lies posterior to the epitympanic recess and communicates with it through an opening—the **aditus ad antrum**—on the posterior wall of the middle ear [Fig. 13.7]. Mastoid air cells are numerous small cavities lined with mucous membrane, located in the petromastoid part of the temporal bone. They are interconnected and open into the posterior wall of the mastoid antrum. In the adult, the mastoid antrum is 1.5 cm medial to the **suprameatal triangle** (the small triangular area on the surface of the skull, immediately posterosuperior to the bony external acoustic meatus). In the child, the mastoid antrum is more superficial.

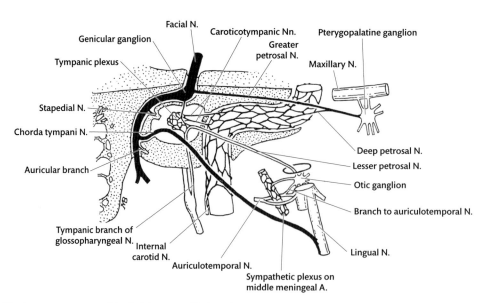

Fig. 13.8 The intrapetrous course of the facial nerve and its branches.

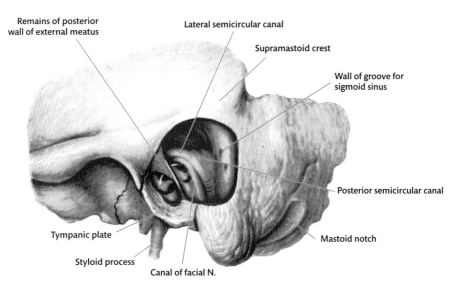

Remains of posterior wall of external meatus

Lateral semicircular canal

Supramastoid crest

Wall of groove for sigmoid sinus

Posterior semicircular canal

Mastoid notch

Tympanic plate

Styloid process

Canal of facial N.

Fig. 13.9 Dissection of the mastoid antrum and petromastoid part of the temporal bone from the lateral side. The arrow passes from the mastoid antrum into the tympanic cavity through the aditus.

The walls of the antrum are formed by parts of the temporal bone. The tegmen tympani forms the **roof**. The **floor** and **posterior wall** are formed by the mastoid process and have the openings of the mastoid air cells in them. The sigmoid venous sinus lies close to the posterior wall and may be separated from it only by a thin plate of bone [Figs. 13.9, 13.10 13.11]. The jugular bulb may have the same close relation to the floor. ➲ Infections of the antrum may involve both the sigmoid sinus and the internal jugular vein in septic thrombosis, and may spread along their tributaries to form an abscess in the adjacent part (cerebellum) of the brain. The **medial wall** of the antrum is the petrous temporal bone. The bony ridge produced by the lateral semicircular canal in the medial wall of the tympanic cavity extends posteriorly into the medial wall of the mastoid antrum [Fig. 13.9].

The ridge on the medial wall of the middle ear produced by the **facial nerve** in its bony canal does not reach the antrum but turns inferiorly (at the aditus) into the bone which separates the middle ear cavity from the mastoid air cells and the inferior part of the antrum [Fig. 13.9]. The facial nerve descends vertically in this bone to emerge at the stylomastoid foramen [Fig. 13.7].

Auditory tube

The auditory, or pharyngotympanic tube consists of bony and cartilaginous parts. The cartilaginous part is approximately 2.5 cm long and is described with the pharynx.

The **bony part** is approximately 1.5 cm long. It is widest at its junction with the middle ear cavity, and narrowest where it joins the cartilaginous part, posteromedial to the spine of the sphenoid. The bony part lies between the petrous and tympanic parts of the temporal bone, below the semicanal for the tensor tympani, lateral to the internal carotid artery in the carotid canal [Figs. 13.1, 13.5, 13.6, 13.7, 13.10, 13.11].

Using the instructions given in Dissection 13.3, dissect the mastoid antrum, mastoid air cells, and the middle ear cavity.

Intrapetrous parts of the facial and vestibulocochlear nerves

The facial and vestibulocochlear nerves have already been traced to the internal acoustic meatus [Chapter 8]. These nerves should now be followed into the petrous temporal bone. The vestibulocochlear nerve ends in the internal ear. The facial nerve follows an angulated course through the petrous bone to emerge at the stylomastoid foramen on the inferior surface of the temporal bone.

Dissection 13.4 provides instructions on dissecting the intrapetrous part of the facial nerve.

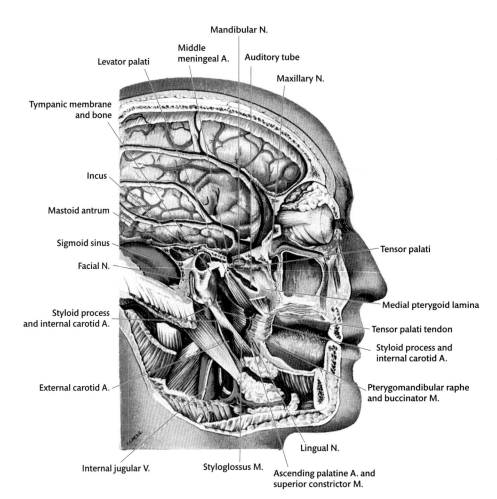

Mandibular N.

Middle meningeal A.

Levator palati

Auditory tube

Maxillary N.

Tympanic membrane and bone

Incus

Mastoid antrum

Sigmoid sinus

Facial N.

Styloid process and internal carotid A.

External carotid A.

Tensor palati

Medial pterygoid lamina

Tensor palati tendon

Styloid process and internal carotid A.

Pterygomandibular raphe and buccinator M.

Lingual N.

Internal jugular V.

Styloglossus M.

Ascending palatine A. and superior constrictor M.

Fig. 13.10 Dissection of the auditory tube and mastoid antrum from the lateral side. Note the continuity of the mastoid antrum, middle ear cavity, and auditory tube.

Facial nerve

The facial nerve runs laterally through the internal acoustic meatus, anterosuperior to the vestibulocochlear nerve. Here it is joined by the **nervus intermedius**. At the lateral extremity of the meatus, it enters the facial canal in the bone and continues laterally for a short distance to the **genicular ganglion** [Figs. 13.8, 13.12]. Medial to the ganglion, the nerve lies anterosuperior to the vestibule of the internal ear and superior to the base of the cochlea [Fig. 13.3]. At the genicular ganglion, the facial nerve gives off the **greater petrosal nerve** [Fig. 13.8].

At the genicular ganglion, the facial nerve turns abruptly backwards and runs posteriorly in the upper part of the medial wall of the middle ear, immediately superior to the oval window and the pyramid. It turns inferolaterally below the aditus

to descend through the bone between the middle ear cavity anteriorly and the mastoid antrum and air cells posteriorly. In the vertical part of its course, the facial nerve gives off: (1) the nerve to the stapedius; (2) the chorda tympani; and (3) small branches to the auricular branch of the vagus [Figs. 13.7, 13.8, 13.9].

Vestibulocochlear nerve

The vestibulocochlear nerve is postero-inferior to the facial nerve in the internal acoustic meatus. At the lateral end of the meatus, the vestibulocochlear nerve splits into the cochlear and vestibular parts. Each of these parts divides into a number of small branches which pass through foramina in the lateral part of the meatus, to supply the membranous labyrinth of the internal ear [Figs. 13.3, 13.12].

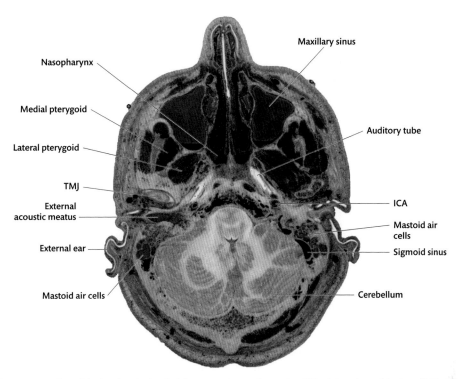

Maxillary sinus

Nasopharynx

Medial pterygoid

Lateral pterygoid

TMJ

External
acoustic meatus

External ear

Mastoid air cells

Auditory tube

ICA

Mastoid air
cells

Sigmoid sinus

Cerebellum

Fig. 13.11 Transverse section of the head at the level of the external acoustic meatus. ICA = internal carotid artery; TMJ = temporomandibular joint.

Image courtesy of the Visible Human Project of the US National Library of Medicine.

DISSECTION 13.3 Mastoid antrum, mastoid air cells, and middle ear cavity

Objectives

I. To open the mastoid antrum and mastoid air cells. **II.** To remove the tympanic membrane and study the middle ear cavity from the lateral aspect.

Instructions

1. Remove all the soft parts, including the periosteum, from the lateral surface of the mastoid temporal bone, and identify the suprameatal triangle and the supramastoid crest. With a fine chisel, remove the cortical bone from the suprameatal triangle. Extend the bone removal anteromedially, parallel with the posterior wall of the external acoustic meatus, until the mastoid antrum is opened.

2. Remove the spongy bone from the mastoid area until the compact bone, posterior and medial to it, is exposed. This process exposes the **mastoid air cells** and mastoid antrum. The extent of the mastoid air cells and antrum is variable.

3. Identify the structures which cause projections on the bony walls of the aditus and antrum, particularly the canal for the facial nerve, the sigmoid sinus, and the ridge produced by the lateral semicircular canal [Fig. 13.9].

4. Cut away the posterior and superior walls of the external acoustic meatus up to the level of the roof of the mastoid antrum.

5. Remove the tympanic membrane. Try to identify the chorda tympani nerve at its posterosuperior margin and the handle of the malleus.

6. Examine the long crus of the incus, the position of the stapes, and the stapedius tendon.

7. Review the medial wall of the middle ear cavity [Figs. 13.3, 13.7].

DISSECTION 13.4 Facial nerve

Objective

I. To expose the intrapetrous part of the facial nerve.

Instructions

1. Identify the **arcuate eminence** on the anterior surface of the petrous temporal bone (in the middle cranial fossa). It marks the position of the **anterior semicircular canal**.

2. On the posterior surface of the petrous temporal bone (posterior cranial fossa), identify the internal acoustic meatus and the nerves entering it.

3. Place a chisel horizontally across the upper part of the internal acoustic meatus and, with a sharp tap from a hammer, attempt to break off the superior part of the petrous temporal bone. Frequently, the bone breaks along the canal for the facial nerve, through parts of the anterior and lateral semicircular canals, and removes the roof of the internal acoustic meatus.

4. Chip away any extra pieces of bone to expose the facial nerve as far as the aditus.

5. Note the sharp bend—the **genu**—of the facial nerve and the swelling on it at this point—the **genicular ganglion**.

6. Identify the greater petrosal nerve which arises from the genicular ganglion.

7. Trace the facial nerve, as it turns posteriorly into the medial wall of the middle ear cavity. Follow it posteriorly above the fenestra vestibuli, till it turns inferiorly in the medial wall of the aditus.

8. Turn to the inferior surface of the skull, and identify the facial nerve as it emerges at the stylomastoid foramen.

9. Place the edge of a chisel across the lateral margin of the foramen, and attempt to split the bone along the line of the vertical part of the facial nerve with a sharp tap. If it splits satisfactorily, the posterior canaliculus for the chorda tympani and the entire length of the canal for the facial nerve will be exposed. If not, complete the exposure with bone forceps.

10. Note the position of the vertical part of the facial nerve in relation to the middle ear cavity, mastoid air cells, and antrum.

11. Finally, break away one wall of the pyramid and expose the stapedius.

The internal ear

The internal ear consists of a series of communicating bony spaces (the **bony labyrinth**) in the petrous temporal bone, and a series of smaller membranous tubes and sacs—the **membranous labyrinth**—within the bony labyrinth. The membranous labyrinth is filled with a clear fluid—the **endolymph**. It is separated from the walls of the bony labyrinth by a space which contains a similar fluid—the **perilymph**—and some delicate connective tissue. The cochlear portion of the inner ear is concerned with hearing. The vestibular portion is concerned with maintaining equilibrium. It records the direction of gravity acting on the head, and rotational movements of the head.

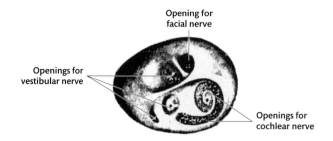

Fig. 13.12 Lateral end of the left internal acoustic meatus showing the openings in the bone for passage of facial, vestibular, and cochlear nerves.

Objective

I. To expose the bony and membranous labyrinths.

Instructions

1. Free the facial nerve from its canal as far as the aditus, but retain its continuity with the greater petrosal nerve.

2. Using the chisel and hammer, cut more bone from the superior surface of the petrous temporal bone, till the level of the middle of the internal acoustic meatus is reached. (The bone should be cracked by sharp taps from a hammer, so as to avoid driving the chisel into the middle ear cavity and the ear ossicles.) As each flake of bone is removed, examine the holes in the bone produced by the semicircular canals, and try to see the semicircular ducts of the membranous labyrinth lying free within them.

3. Note also the branches of the vestibulocochlear nerve entering the bone at the lateral end of the meatus.

4. Identify the vestibule and cochlea [Fig. 13.13]. They are seen at the level of the middle of the internal acoustic meatus. The vestibule is the cavity lying immediately lateral to the internal acoustic meatus, between it and the medial wall of the middle ear. The cochlea lies anterolateral to the lateral end of the meatus.

5. The main features of the bony labyrinth are now exposed. It is desirable at each stage to establish the continuity of its various parts by passing a fine wire through each foramen that is exposed.

6. If time permits, a better dissection may be obtained by decalcifying an intact temporal bone in dilute acid for several weeks, and then dissecting it carefully with a sharp knife.

Using the instructions given in Dissection 13.5, expose the bony and membranous labyrinths.

Bony labyrinth

The bony labyrinth is divided into three parts: (1) a small chamber called the **vestibule**; (2) a coiled tube—the **cochlea**—anterior to the vestibule; and (3) three **semicircular canals**, superior and posterior to the vestibule [Fig. 13.13A]. The vestibule, cochlea, and semicircular canals communicate freely with each other and are lined throughout by a delicate endosteum [Fig. 13.13B].

Vestibule

The vestibule is a small, ovoid bony chamber about 5 mm long, placed between the lateral end of the internal acoustic meatus and the medial wall of the middle ear. The three semicircular canals open into its superior and posterior aspects through five openings [Fig. 13.13B, red asterisks]. Two tubes within the cochlea—the **scala vestibuli** and **scala tympani**—open into the anterior aspect of the vestibule [Fig. 13.13B, green and blue asterisk]. The **oval window**, or **fenestra vestibuli**, lies on the lateral wall of the vestibule and is closed by the base of the stapes. The round window, or fenestra cochleae, lies on the inferior aspect of the vestibule and is closed by the secondary tympanic

membrane [Figs. 13.13A, 13.13B]. In the posterior part of the medial wall of the vestibule is the mouth of a small canal—the **aqueduct of the vestibule**—which passes to the posterior surface of the petrous temporal bone and opens between the bone and the dura mater. [Figs. 13.13A, 13.13B, 13.4].

Semicircular canals

The three semicircular canals—anterior, posterior, and lateral—open into the vestibule. Each of the three canals forms more than half a circle and has a swelling—the **ampulla**—at one end. The canals are oriented such that each canal forms one of three adjacent sides of an obliquely set cube. The anterior and posterior canals lie in approximately vertical planes, and their adjoining ends meet in a common limb—**crus commune** [Fig. 13.13B]. The crus commune opens into the vestibule. As such, the three canals have five (not six) points of entry into the vestibule. The **ampullae** of the anterior and lateral semicircular canals lie at the anterior ends.

The **anterior canal** is at right angles to the long axis of the petrous temporal bone and produces the **arcuate eminence** on the anterior surface of that bone. The **posterior canal** is postero-inferior to the anterior canal and lies almost parallel to the posterior surface of the petrous temporal bone

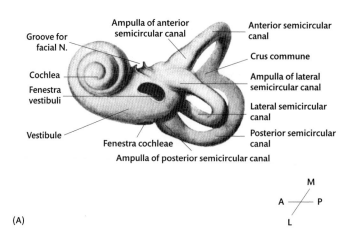

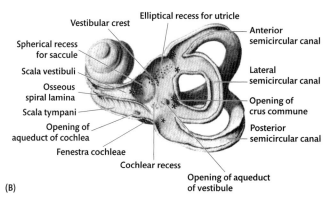

Fig. 13.13 Left bony labyrinth, viewed from the lateral side. (A) External surface. (B) Inner aspect. Red asterisks = opening of semicircular canals into vestibule. Green asterisk = opening of the scala vestibuli into the vestibule. Blue asterisk = opening of the scala tympani into the round window.

(deep to the slit for the aqueduct of the vestibule). The **lateral canal** is nearly horizontal but slopes a little anterosuperiorly in the angle between the opposite ends of the other two canals. Its most lateral part produces a bulge in the medial wall of the tympanic cavity, the aditus, and the mastoid antrum.

The semicircular canals of one inner ear are mirror images of those in the other ear. As such, the two lateral canals lie in the same plane, and the anterior canal of one side is parallel to the posterior canal of the other.

Cochlea

The cochlea is shaped like a tube coiled around a central pillar—the **modiolus**. The modiolus points anterolaterally. The cochlea has two-and-a-half turns and rapidly diminishes in diameter towards its apex. It has the appearance of a spiral

lying on its side [Figs. 13.13A, 13.13B]. It lies anterior to the vestibule, with its base directed towards the lateral end of the internal acoustic meatus. The large first turn produces the bulge of the **promontory** on the medial wall of the middle ear cavity [Figs. 13.7, 13.13A].

The **modiolus** is thick at its base where it abuts on the internal meatus, but rapidly tapers towards the apex, forming the internal wall of the cochlear tube. Winding spirally round the modiolus, like the thread of a screw, is a thin, narrow plate of bone (the **spiral lamina**) which partially divides the cochlear tube into two canals [Fig. 13.13B]. A canal known as the **spiral canal** runs in the base of the spiral lamina and lodges the sensory **spiral ganglion** of the cochlea.

The cells of the spiral ganglion are bipolar neurons. They send their peripheral processes through minute canals in the spiral lamina to the sensory

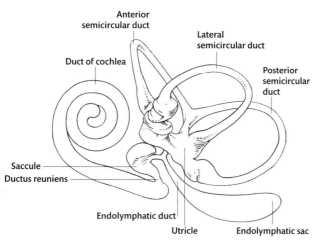

Fig. 13.14 Diagrammatic representation of the right membranous labyrinth.

Labels in figure:
Anterior semicircular duct
Lateral semicircular duct
Duct of cochlea
Posterior semicircular duct
Saccule
Ductus reuniens
Endolymphatic duct
Utricle
Endolymphatic sac

organ of the cochlea. The central processes of the neurons run in a number of minute longitudinal canals in the modiolus and emerge at its base as the cochlear part of the vestibulocochlear nerve.

The central part of the bony cochlea, between the spiral lamina and the lateral wall, contains a part of the membranous labyrinth—the **duct of the cochlea**. The membranous cochlear duct separates the remainder of the space within the cochlea into the **scala tympani** and **scala vestibuli** [Fig. 13.13B]. These two perilymph-filled tubes run parallel to, and on either side of, the cochlear duct, and are continuous with each other at the apex of the cochlea around the blind end of the cochlear duct—the **helicotrema**.

The scala vestibuli is continuous with the vestibule at the base of the cochlea. The scala tympani ends on the round window (fenestra cochleae), which is covered by the **secondary tympanic membrane** [Fig. 13.13B, blue asterisk]. Pressure waves generated in the scala vestibuli, by movements of the stapes, are transferred through the scala vestibuli and the scala tympani.

The scala tympani is also continuous with the **aqueduct of the cochlea**, which passes through a canal in the bone—the **cochlear canaliculus** [Fig. 13.13B].

Membranous labyrinth

The membranous labyrinth consists of: (1) the duct of the cochlea which lies in the bony cochlea; (2) the utricle and saccule—two small membranous sacs which lie in the vestibule; and (3) three membranous tubes—the semicircular ducts—which lie in the semicircular canals [Figs. 13.3, 13.14]. The saccule and utricle are joined to each other by a narrow tube through the root of the **endolymphatic duct**. The saccule is continuous with the base of the cochlear duct through the **ductus reuniens**. The utricle has the membranous semicircular ducts opening into it.

The **cochlear duct** lies in the cochlear part of the bony labyrinth. Pressure waves generated in the scala vestibuli by movements of the stapes are transferred through the scala vestibuli and the scala tympani. The cochlear duct with its sensory organ lies between the scala vestibuli and tympani and is sensitive to these changes in pressure. The cochlear duct is innervated by the cochlear division of the vestibulocochlear nerve.

The **semicircular ducts** lie in the semicircular canals of the bony labyrinth. They are considerably narrower than the canals and are situated against the peripheral bony walls of the canals. They open into the utricle and have ampullae in the same position as the ampullae of the canals. The **ampullae** of the ducts contain specialized folds of lining epithelium—the **crista ampullaris**. The crista is surmounted by hair cells embedded in a gelatinous **cupula** and is the sensory organ of the duct. It records movements which result from rotation of the head in the plane of the duct. The ampullae are so arranged that, in any parallel pair of semicircular ducts, rotation of the head causes the endolymph to flow in the same direction. It moves towards the ampulla in one canal, and away from the ampulla in the other opposite canal. The crista ampullaris is innervated by the vestibular part of the vestibulocochlear nerve.

The **utricle** occupies a depression in the superior wall of the vestibule, and the smaller **saccule** lies antero-inferior to it [Fig. 13.13B]. The endolymphatic duct unites the utricle and saccule and passes through the aqueduct of the vestibule to end as a dilated **endolymphatic sac**, external to the dura mater. The utricle and saccule each have an area of thickened epithelium in their walls known as the **macula**. The macula has hair cells on which are a number of concretions of calcium salts—the **statoconia**. The macula of the utricle lies in a horizontal plane, and that of the saccule lies in a vertical plane. They record the direction of the gravitational field relative to the head. Both maculae are innervated by the vestibular part of the vestibulocochlear nerve.

See Clinical Applications 13.1, 13.2, 13.3, and 13.4 for the practical implications of the anatomy discussed in this chapter.

CLINICAL APPLICATION 13.1 Tympanic membrane perforation and myringotomy

Perforation of the tympanic membrane can occur as a result of trauma or even spontaneously, when there is infection in the middle ear cavity (**otitis media**). Most often, these perforations heal spontaneously. However, large perforations may require repair. The temporalis fascia is often used as graft for repair of tympanic membrane perforations.

In some instances, it may be necessary to surgically incise the tympanic membrane (**myringotomy**) to relieve pressure built up within the middle ear cavity.

Study question 1: name the structure a surgeon must be careful to avoid during incision of the tympanic membrane. What precaution should be taken to avoid this? (Answer: the chorda tympani. The surgeon should stay away from the upper third of the tympanic membrane to avoid injury to the chorda tympani nerve.)

CLINICAL APPLICATION 13.2 Otitis media

Otitis media is inflammation within the middle ear cavity. It could be the result of an acute infection and could resolve spontaneously or with antibiotics. Acute otitis media is common in children, often beginning as an upper respiratory tract infection with a blocked nose. It presents with fever and severe earache, often leading to rupture of the tympanic membrane and ear discharge.

Study question 1: explain the anatomical basis for upper respiratory tract infections leading on to otitis media. (Answer: the mucosa of the nasopharynx is continuous with that of the middle ear cavity through the auditory tube. Infections can spread from the nasopharynx to the middle ear cavity through the tube. Oedema and blockage of the auditory tube can further increase the risk of infection.) **Chronic otitis media** refers to long-term damage of the middle ear mucosa due to repeated infection and inflammation. It is invariably associated with a perforated tympanic membrane, repeated episodes of ear discharge, and conductive hearing loss. An invasive, non-cancerous epithelial growth can occur within the middle ear—**cholesteatoma**—and cause extensive bone damage.

CLINICAL APPLICATION 13.3 Mastoiditis

Mastoiditis is inflammation of the mucosa lining the mastoid antrum and air cells. The mucosa of the middle ear is continuous with the mucosa of the mastoid antrum, and infections can spread from one cavity to the other. Surgery for chronic otitis media with mastoiditis aims to remove diseased tissue and repair the tympanic membrane to restore hearing. The common approach to the mastoid antrum is through its lateral wall—the suprameatal triangle.

Study question 1: discuss the important relations of the mastoid antrum. (Answer: the vertical course of the facial nerve lies along the anterior wall of the mastoid antrum. The cranial cavity lies just above the roof. The sigmoid venous sinus lies posterior to the antrum at a variable distance, depending on the pneumatization of the mastoid process.)

CLINICAL APPLICATION 13.4 Facial nerve lesions

Clinically, it is possible to differentiate injuries to the facial nerve at different sites along its course. (1) When the facial nerve is affected at, or distal to, the stylomastoid foramen, the patient will show only signs of paralysis of the facial muscles on that side. (2) When the facial nerve is affected in the brain, in the internal acoustic meatus, or at the level of the genicular ganglion, in addition to paralysis of facial muscles, the patient will also have loss of taste on the anterior two-thirds of the corresponding half of the tongue (due to destruction of fibres in the chorda tympani) and hyperacusis (due to destruction of the nerve to the stapedius). Secretions of the submandibular and sublingual glands and lacrimal, nasal, palatine, and oral glands will be diminished (due to damage to the secretomotor fibres in the greater petrosal and chorda tympani nerves). An injury in the internal acoustic meatus is also likely to involve the vestibulocochlear nerve.

CHAPTER 14
The parotid region

Parotid gland

The parotid gland lies below the external acoustic meatus, between the mandible in front and the sternocleidomastoid behind. It is the largest salivary gland and produces serous secretions. It has a very irregular shape because during development, it does not grow within a well-defined capsule, as does the submandibular gland, but invades the fascia of this region. It becomes disseminated through the fascia and encloses the structures which traverse the fascia.

Shape and position of the parotid gland

The parotid gland is shaped like an inverted pyramid, with the base directed superiorly and the apex directed inferiorly. It has lateral or superficial, anteromedial, and posterolateral surfaces [Figs. 14.1, 14.2, 14.3, 14.4].

The upper end of the parotid gland is grooved by the external acoustic meatus and is wedged between it and the back of the temporomandibular joint. The auriculotemporal nerve and the superficial temporal vessels pierce the gland just behind the joint [see Fig. 4.6].

The lower end of the gland lies between the sternocleidomastoid and the angle of the mandible, on the posterior belly of the digastric [see Fig. 6.6]. It extends into the carotid triangle. It is pierced by the cervical branch of the facial nerve and the two branches of the retromandibular vein. It is separated from the submandibular gland by the stylomandibular ligament. Note the close proximity of the parotid and submandibular glands in Fig. 6.1.

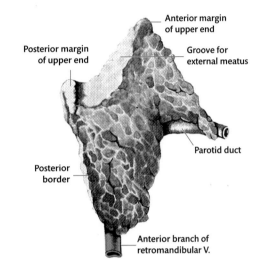

Fig. 14.1 Parotid gland, lateral surface.

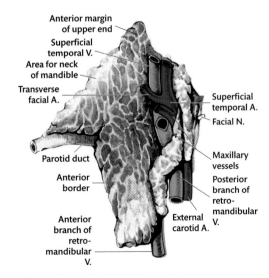

Fig. 14.2 Parotid gland, anteromedial surface.

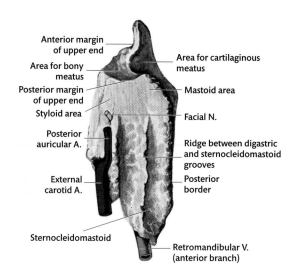

Anterior margin of upper end
Area for bony meatus
Posterior margin of upper end
Styloid area
Posterior auricular A.
External carotid A.
Sternocleidomastoid

Area for cartilaginous meatus
Mastoid area
Facial N.
Ridge between digastric and sternocleidomastoid grooves
Posterior border
Retromandibular V. (anterior branch)

Fig. 14.3 Parotid gland, posteromedial surface.

the posterior belly of the digastric. The stylohyoid muscle and styloid process lie medial to the parotid [Fig. 14.5].

A part of the cervical fascia is thickened, deep to the gland, to form the **stylomandibular ligament**. This ligament passes from the styloid process of the temporal bone to the posterior border of the ramus of the mandible and separates the parotid from the submandibular gland.

A portion of this superficial part of the gland is often detached from the rest of the gland and forms the **accessory parotid gland** [see Fig. 4.6].

Branches of the facial, great auricular, and auriculotemporal nerves; the external carotid, superficial temporal, and transverse facial arteries; and the retromandibular vein traverse the substance of the parotid gland. All of these have been seen already, and their position should be reviewed.

Parotid duct

The lateral or superficial surface of the gland is covered by skin, superficial fascia, branches of the great auricular nerve, and the platysma. The deep surface of the parotid is very irregular and is divided into anteromedial and posteromedial surfaces. The anteromedial surface is related to the posterior margin of the ramus of the mandible, the masseter, and the medial pterygoid [Fig. 14.2]. The part of the gland deep to the ramus of the mandible is the **deep lobe**. The posteromedial surface of the parotid gland is related to, and grooved by, the mastoid process, the sternocleidomastoid muscle, and

The parotid duct is a thick-walled tube formed within the gland by the union of the ductules which drain its lobules. It appears at the anterior border of the gland on the surface of the masseter, approximately a finger-breadth below the zygomatic arch. It runs anteriorly across the masseter, below the accessory parotid gland, accompanying the zygomatic branches of the facial nerve. The duct hooks medially over the anterior border of the masseter and can be felt there by rolling it against

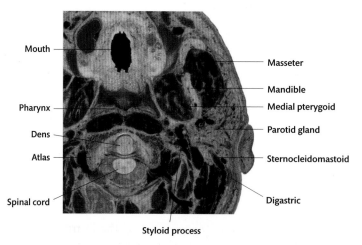

Mouth
Pharynx
Dens
Atlas
Spinal cord

Masseter
Mandible
Medial pterygoid
Parotid gland
Sternocleidomastoid
Digastric

Styloid process

Fig. 14.4 Horizontal section through the head, showing the parotid gland.
Image courtesy of the Visible Human Project of the US National Library of Medicine.

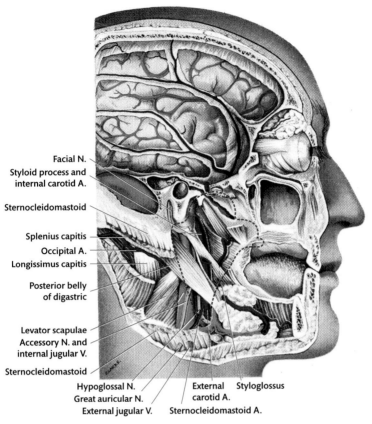

Facial N.
Styloid process and
internal carotid A.

Sternocleidomastoid

Splenius capitis
Occipital A.
Longissimus capitis

Posterior belly
of digastric

Levator scapulae
Accessory N. and
internal jugular V.

Sternocleidomastoid

Hypoglossal N.
Great auricular N.
External jugular V.

External
carotid A.
Sternocleidomastoid A.

Styloglossus

Fig. 14.5 Dissection of the head to show the structures deep to the parotid gland. The outline of the parotid gland is shown by the red dotted line.

the muscle, with the jaw clenched. The duct pierces the buccal pad of fat, the buccopharyngeal fascia, and the buccinator muscle to open into the vestibule of the mouth, opposite the second upper molar tooth [see Figs. 4.6, 4.8; Figs. 14.1, 14.2].

Structures within the parotid gland

A number of important structures lie within the parotid gland.

1. The **external carotid artery** enters and leaves the gland on its deep surface. It gives off the **posterior auricular artery** immediately before entering the gland, and divides into the **maxillary** and **superficial temporal arteries** where it emerges behind the neck of the mandible. Within the gland, the superficial temporal artery gives off the **transverse facial** and **middle temporal arteries** [Figs. 14.2, 14.3].

2. The **retromandibular vein** is formed in the parotid by the union of the superficial temporal and maxillary veins. It is joined by the middle temporal and transverse facial veins. It divides into anterior and posterior branches at the lower end of the gland [Fig. 14.2].

3. The **facial nerve** enters the posteromedial surface of the gland, close to the stylomastoid foramen [Fig. 14.3], and divides into five terminal branches in the gland. The branches radiate forwards, superficial to the artery and the vein, and emerge from the anteromedial surface close to the anterior border of the gland. Within the gland, branches of the facial nerve receive communicating branches from the great auricular and auriculotemporal nerves.

4. The **parotid lymph nodes** are embedded in the gland, especially near its superficial surface. The superficial nodes drain the auricle, the anterior part of the scalp, and the upper part of the face. The deeper nodes drain the external acoustic meatus, middle ear, auditory tube, nose, palate, and deeper parts of the cheek. Both groups drain to the cervical lymph nodes [see Fig. 9.18].

Using the instructions given in Dissection 14.1, identify and clean the structures within the parotid gland.

Objectives

I. To identify and trace the facial nerve and its branches in the parotid gland.   **II.** To expose the external carotid artery and retromandibular vein in the gland.

Instructions

1. Expose the surface of the parotid gland, and follow its duct to the buccinator muscle.

2. Follow one of the branches of the facial nerve back through the gland to the trunk of the nerve, and then trace the other branches forwards through it. Look for communicating branches from the auriculotemporal nerve which are relatively large.

3. Trace the trunk of the facial nerve to the stylomastoid foramen, and find the posterior auricular branch and the branch to the posterior belly of the digastric and the stylohyoid. These branches are given off deep to the gland.

4. Find and trace the posterior auricular artery.

5. Expose the retromandibular vein and the external carotid artery by removing more of the gland.

6. Remove the remainder of the gland piecemeal, and expose the structures which surround it, retaining as far as possible the structures which pass through it.

Vessels and nerves of the parotid gland

The blood supply to the parotid gland is from the adjoining vessels. Sensory nerve fibres reach it through the **great auricular** and **auriculotemporal** nerves, and post-ganglionic parasympathetic secretory fibres come from the otic ganglion through the auriculotemporal nerve. The preganglionic parasympathetic fibres to the parotid gland reach the otic ganglion through its lesser petrosal branch of the glossopharyngeal nerve [see Fig. 13.8]. Sympathetic post-ganglionic fibres reach the gland through the plexus on the external carotid or middle meningeal arteries [see Fig. 15.7].

Facial nerve

The seventh cranial nerve—the facial nerve—leaves the brain at the lower border of the pons [see Fig. 24.2], passes with the vestibulocochlear (eighth cranial) nerve into the internal acoustic meatus, and emerges from the temporal bone at the stylomastoid foramen [see Figs. 3.6, 3.9]. It runs a complicated course through the petrous part of the temporal bone [see Fig. 13.8]. After emerging through the stylomastoid foramen, the facial nerve curves anteriorly and enters the posteromedial surface of the parotid gland. Before entering the gland, it gives off the posterior auricular nerve (to the occipital belly of occipitofrontalis and the auricular muscles) and

a small branch which divides to supply the posterior belly of the digastric and the stylohyoid muscle. In the gland, it divides into its main branches—temporal, zygomatic, buccal, marginal mandibular, and cervical [see Fig. 4.7]. The temporal and zygomatic can sometimes be felt on the zygomatic arch.

See Clinical Applications 14.1 and 14.2 for the practical implications of the anatomy discussed in this chapter.

CLINICAL APPLICATION 14.1 Parotid tumour

A 45-year-old woman presented with a complaint of a mass below the lobule of her right ear. The mass was not painful, and she had noticed it inadvertently while washing her face about a week ago. On examination, the mass was mobile, non-tender, firm, and solitary. The overlying skin, oral cavity, oropharynx, and neck revealed no changes. Further tests were done, and a T2-weighted magnetic resonance axial image (MRI) showed a neoplastic mass lesion in the right parotid gland [Fig. 14.6].

The mass was found to be a benign pleomorphic adenoma, and a superficial parotidectomy was planned to remove the lesion.

Study question 1: what one structure within the parotid gland requires special attention to ensure that it is not damaged during surgical removal of the mass? (Answer: the facial nerve.)

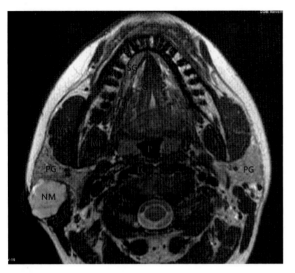

Fig. 14.6 T2-weighted axial image at the level of the parotid gland. Asterisks = mandibular alveolus; G = genioglossus; H = hyoglossus; P = pharynx; PG = parotid gland; PT = palatine tonsils; LC = longus colli; M = masseter; MP = medial pterygoid; SCM = sternocleidomastoid; SG = sublingual gland. A neoplastic mass lesion (NM) is seen in the right parotid gland.

CLINICAL APPLICATION 14.2 Auriculotemporal syndrome or gustatory sweating

Auriculotemporal syndrome, or gustatory sweating, is redness and sweating of the side of the face in response to a salivatory stimulus of either smell or taste of food. It could follow parotid gland surgery (or other surgery involving the capsule of the parotid gland) and is said to be the result of aberrant connections occurring between the secretomotor fibres destined for the parotid gland and the sweat glands of the face. It is also known as Frey's syndrome.

CHAPTER 15
The temporal and infratemporal regions

Introduction to the temporal region

Begin your study of the temporal region by revising the details given in Chapter 4. The temporal region is bound superiorly and posteriorly by the superior temporal line, anteriorly by the zygomatic bone, and inferiorly and laterally by the zygomatic arch [see Fig. 3.4]. It is separated inferiorly from the infratemporal fossa by the infratemporal crest on the sphenoid. The main content of the temporal fossa is the temporalis muscle and its vessels and nerves. The temporalis is covered by the temporal fascia.

Temporal fascia

The temporal fascia is a strong, glistening membrane stretched over the temporal fossa and the temporalis muscle. Superiorly, it is attached to the superior temporal line on the lateral aspect of the skull. Inferiorly, it splits into two. The superficial layer is attached to the upper margin of the zygomatic arch. The deep layer passes medial to the arch to become continuous with the fascia deep to the masseter. The two layers are separated from each other by a little fat.

Muscles of mastication

The masseter, temporalis, medial and lateral pterygoids are the muscles of mastication. They share a common embryological origin—the first pharyngeal arch—and are supplied by the mandibular division of the trigeminal nerve.

Prior to studying the temporal and infratemporal fossae, examine the masseter muscle on the side of the jaw.

Masseter

The masseter is a thick quadrate muscle of mastication which covers the lateral aspect of the ramus and coronoid process of the mandible [see Fig. 4.8]. It takes origin from the inferior margin and deep surface of the zygomatic arch, from the tubercle of the zygoma posteriorly to the junction of the zygomatic arch with the zygomatic process of the maxilla anteriorly. It is inserted into the lateral surface of the ramus and coronoid process of the mandible [Fig. 15.1]. The deep fibres run vertically, and the superficial fibres run postero-inferiorly [see Figs. 4.8, 4.10].

Nerve supply: the mandibular division of the trigeminal nerve. The nerve enters the deep surface of the masseter by passing through the mandibular notch, immediately anterior to the capsule of the temporomandibular joint. **Actions**: it raises the mandible and clenches the teeth. Its superficial

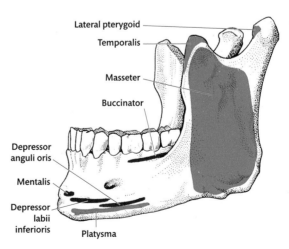

Fig. 15.1 Muscle attachments on the superficial surface of the mandible. Red = origins; blue = insertions.

DISSECTION 15.1 Temporalis

Objective

I. To expose the temporalis by turning down the zygomatic arch.

Instructions

1. Divide the zygomatic arch anterior and posterior to the attachment of the masseter, and turn it down with that muscle. Divide the neurovascular bundle which enters the deep surface of the muscle, immediately anterior to the temporomandibular joint, and any fibres of the temporalis that may join the masseter.

2. Strip the masseter from the surface of the mandible as far as the angle, but leave it attached there.

3. Expose the temporalis.

fibres help to protract the mandible. Acting alternately, the two muscles (right and left) move the chin from side to side, producing a grinding movement of the teeth.

Dissection 15.1 provides instructions on dissection of the temporalis.

Temporalis

The temporalis is a fan-shaped muscle. It takes origin from the lateral side of the skull below the inferior temporal line (medial wall of the temporal fossa [see Fig. 4.10]) and from the temporal fascia. It converges towards the coronoid process of the mandible, the anterior fibres descending vertically and the posterior fibres running almost horizontally forwards. It forms a tendon on its superficial surface, which is inserted into the apex and anterior margin of the coronoid process and the anterior margin of the ramus. The deeper muscular fibres are attached to the medial side of the coronoid process and extend down to the junction of the anterior border of the ramus and the body of the mandible, behind the third mandibular molar tooth [Figs. 15.1, 15.2B]. Some of the superficial fibres may join the masseter and pass with it to the ramus of the mandible.

Nerve supply: deep temporal branches of the mandibular nerve. **Actions**: the temporalis raises the mandible, and its horizontal posterior fibres retract the mandible after protraction.

Introduction to the infratemporal region

The infratemporal fossa lies inferior to the zygomatic arch and the infratemporal surface of the greater wing of the sphenoid [see Fig. 3.6]. It is bound by the ramus and angle of the mandible laterally, the lateral pterygoid plate medially, the posterior aspect of the maxilla anteriorly, and the tympanic plate, mastoid, and styloid process of the temporal bone posteriorly.

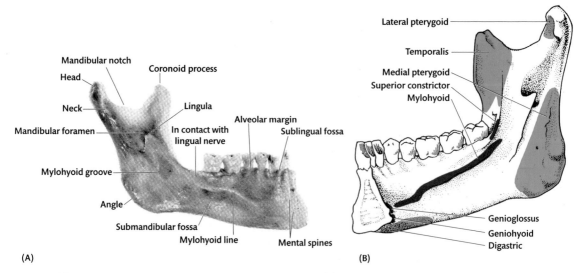

Fig. 15.2 (A) The medial surface of the mandible. The third molar is missing. (B) Muscle attachments to the medial surface of the mandible. Red = origins; blue = insertions.

Superficial contents of the infratemporal fossa

Using the instructions given in Dissection 15.2, expose the superficial contents of the infratemporal fossa.

Lateral pterygoid muscle

The lateral pterygoid muscle arises by two heads. The smaller **upper head** takes origin from the infratemporal ridge and infratemporal surface of the greater wing of the sphenoid medial to it. The **lower head** takes origin from the lateral surface of the lateral pterygoid plate. The muscle narrows, as it passes posteriorly, and is inserted into the front of the neck of the mandible and the articular disc of the temporomandibular joint through its capsule [Figs. 15.1, 15.2B, 15.3].

Nerve supply: the mandibular nerve. **Actions**: acting together, the two muscles protrude the mandible and depress the chin, by drawing the head of the mandible and the disc forwards onto the articular tubercle. When one muscle acts alone, the head of the mandible on that side is drawn forwards, and the mandible pivots around the opposite joint so that the chin is swung towards the opposite side.

Medial pterygoid muscle

The medial pterygoid muscle also has two heads of origin which embrace the lower head of the lateral pterygoid [Fig. 15.3]. The **superficial head** is small and takes origin from the maxillary tuberosity. The **deep head** forms nearly the whole muscle and takes origin from the medial surface of the lateral pterygoid plate. The two heads unite inferior to the anterior part of the lateral pterygoid and pass downwards, backwards, and laterally, to be inserted into the ramus of the mandible between the mandibular foramen and the angle of the mandible [Fig. 15.2B]. Its fibres are nearly parallel to the superficial fibres of the masseter.

Nerve supply: the mandibular nerve. **Actions**: it (1) raises the mandible; (2) helps in protraction;

183

DISSECTION 15.2 Superficial dissection of the infratemporal fossa

Objectives

I. To expose the contents of the infratemporal fossa.
II. To identify and trace the first two parts of the maxillary artery. **III.** To identify branches of the maxillary nerve.

Instructions

1. Using a hammer and chisel, make an oblique cut on the mandible from the mandibular notch to the point where the anterior margin of the ramus meets the body of the mandible. Separate the coronoid process from the mandible. Take care not to injure the **buccal nerve** and artery which lie close to the lowest tendinous fibres of the temporalis.

2. Turn the coronoid process and the temporalis upwards, and separate the muscle fibres from the lower part of the temporal fossa by blunt dissection [see Fig. 15.3].

3. Find the **deep temporal vessels and nerves** which ascend between the muscle and the skull.

4. Make a horizontal cut through the neck of the mandible and another immediately above the mandibular foramen [Fig. 15.2]. The position of the mandibular foramen can be determined by sliding the handle of a knife between the ramus of the mandible and the subjacent soft parts, and pressing down till it is arrested by the inferior alveolar nerve and vessels entering the foramen. (While making the second cut, cut halfway through the bone with a saw, and complete the division with bone forceps. Remove the pieces of bone, and expose the underlying muscles, vessels, and nerves.)

5. Remove the fat and parts of the pterygoid plexus of veins which obscure your view.

6. Identify the pterygoid muscles and parts of the maxillary vessels [Fig. 15.3].

7. Identify the maxillary artery, and follow it anterosuperiorly till it disappears medially. Carefully remove the fat from the region just superior to this.

8. The maxillary nerve may be seen passing towards the inferior orbital fissure to continue as the infra-orbital nerve [Fig. 15.4].

9. Find the two branches of the maxillary nerve in this region: (1) the **zygomatic nerve** which passes through the inferior orbital fissure; and (2) the **posterior superior alveolar nerve**, which divides into branches that descend and disappear into small holes in the posterior surface of the maxilla.

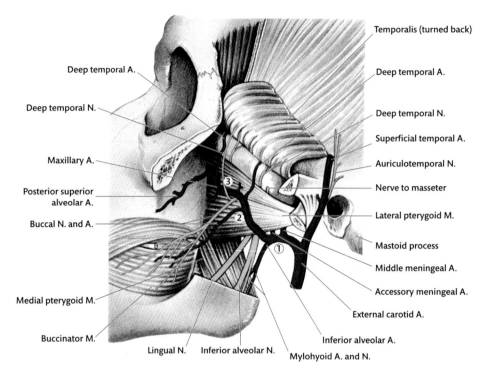

Temporalis (turned back)

Deep temporal A.

Deep temporal A.

Deep temporal N.

Deep temporal N.

Superficial temporal A.

Auriculotemporal N.

Maxillary A.

Nerve to masseter

Posterior superior
alveolar A.

Lateral pterygoid M.

Buccal N. and A.

Mastoid process

Middle meningeal A.

Accessory meningeal A.

Medial pterygoid M.

External carotid A.

Buccinator M.

Inferior alveolar A.

Lingual N.   Inferior alveolar N.

Mylohyoid A. and N.

Fig. 15.3 Dissection of the infratemporal fossa. 1 = first part of maxillary artery; 2 = second part of maxillary artery; 3 = third part of maxillary artery.

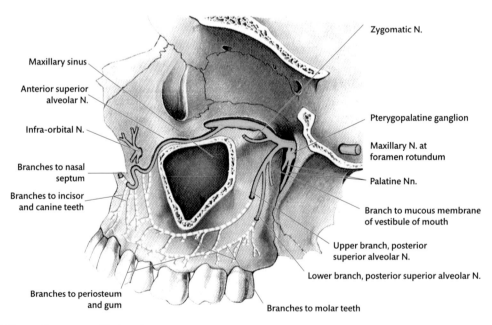

Zygomatic N.

Maxillary sinus

Anterior superior
alveolar N.

Pterygopalatine ganglion

Infra-orbital N.

Maxillary N. at
foramen rotundum

Branches to nasal
septum

Palatine Nn.

Branches to incisor
and canine teeth

Branch to mucous membrane
of vestibule of mouth

Upper branch, posterior
superior alveolar N.

Lower branch, posterior superior alveolar N.

Branches to periosteum
and gum

Branches to molar teeth

Fig. 15.4 The maxillary nerve and its branches.

and (3) moves the chin to the opposite side. The two medial pterygoid muscles acting alternatively produce a grinding movement, similar to the action of the superficial fibres of the masseter.

Maxillary artery

The maxillary artery is a branch of the external carotid artery. It arises posterior to the neck of the mandible [Fig. 15.3]. The first part of the maxillary artery runs horizontally forwards between the neck of the mandible and the sphenomandibular ligament [p. 186], on the lower border of the lateral pterygoid muscle. The second part runs anterosuperiorly, superficial to the lower head of the lateral pterygoid muscle and deep to the insertion of the temporalis. The third part turns medially, between the two heads of the lateral pterygoid, enters the pterygomaxillary fissure, and ends in the pterygopalatine fossa in a number of branches. The second part of the artery often lies between the two pterygoid muscles and bends laterally between the heads of the lateral pterygoid muscle before entering the pterygopalatine fossa [see Fig. 3.5; Fig. 15.3].

During its course, the artery gives branches to the external acoustic meatus, middle ear, muscles of the infratemporal fossa, skull bones and dura mater, and arteries which accompany the nerves in the infratemporal and pterygopalatine fossae.

The **inferior alveolar** branch of the maxillary artery descends with the inferior alveolar nerve, enters the mandibular foramen, and runs through the mandibular canal to supply the lower teeth, gums, and mandible. It gives off the **mental artery** which supplies the skin over the chin and lower lip. It also gives off the mylohyoid artery which runs with the mylohyoid nerve in the mylohyoid groove [see Fig. 6.6; Fig. 15.2B]. The corresponding veins drain into the pterygoid venous plexus.

Pterygoid venous plexus and maxillary vein

The numerous veins of the infratemporal fossa are difficult to dissect, since they form a dense plexus—the **pterygoid venous plexus**—around the lateral pterygoid muscle. Veins corresponding to the branches of the maxillary artery open into this network. The pterygoid plexus is drained posteriorly by one or two short, wide maxillary veins. The maxillary veins enter the parotid gland and drain into the retromandibular vein, posterior to the neck of the mandible [see Fig. 14.2].

Communications of the pterygoid venous plexus

The pterygoid venous plexus has widespread communications with all the surrounding veins, but particularly with: (1) the **cavernous sinus** by an emissary vein which runs through the foramen ovale or the sphenoidal emissary foramen; and (2) the **facial vein**, through the deep facial vein which runs posteriorly on the buccinator muscle, deep to the masseter and the ramus of the mandible. ⊃ Infectious material from the face can reach the cavernous sinus through these communications.

Temporomandibular joint

The temporomandibular joint is a synovial joint formed by the articulation between the head of the mandible, and the mandibular fossa and the articular tubercle of the temporal bone. These two articular surfaces are separated by an articular disc which completely divides the joint cavity into upper and lower parts [Fig. 15.5].

The **fibrous capsule** of the joint is attached to the margins of the articular area on the temporal bone and around the neck of the mandible. Laterally, it is thickened to form a triangular band—the **lateral ligament**. The base of the lateral ligament is attached to the zygomatic process of the temporal bone and the zygomatic tubercle, and the apex is attached to the lateral side of the neck of the mandible. The **articular disc** is an oval plate of dense fibrous tissue which is fused with the fibrous capsule around its periphery. It is more

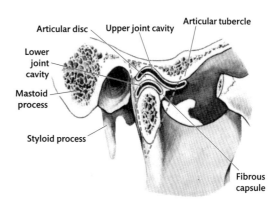

Fig. 15.5 Section through the temporomandibular joint. Dotted lines represent the position of the lateral ligament.

DISSECTION 15.3 The temporomandibular joint

Objective

I. To open the temporomandibular joint and study its interior.

Instructions

1. Remove the lateral ligament, and expose the disc and the two separate synovial cavities within the joint.

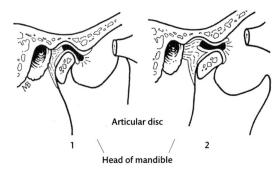

Articular disc

Head of mandible

Fig. 15.6 Diagrams to show the changing relationship between the head of the mandible and the temporal bone when the mouth is being opened. (1) The mouth is closed. (2) When the mouth is opened: (i) the head of the mandible and the articular disc slide forwards on to the articular tubercle; and (ii) the head of the mandible rotates on the disc.

tightly bound to the mandible than to the temporal bone. The upper surface of the disc is concavo-convex to fit the articular tubercle and the mandibular fossa. Its lower surface is concave and fits the head of the mandible [Fig. 15.5].

Using the instructions given in Dissection 15.3, open the temporomandibular joint.

The fibrous capsule and the lateral ligament are the only proper ligaments of the joint. The sphenomandibular and stylomandibular ligaments also connect the mandible to the skull but add little, if anything, to the strength of the joint. The integrity of the joint is maintained principally by the muscles of mastication. As with any joint maintained mainly by muscles, the temporomandibular joint is easily dislocated.

The **sphenomandibular ligament** is a long, membranous band which passes from the spine of the sphenoid to the lingula and lower margin of the mandibular foramen. It lies superficial to the medial pterygoid muscle. At the lower part, it is pierced by the mylohyoid vessels and nerve. (This ligament is of considerable developmental interest, as it is the remnant of the first branchial arch cartilage, the superior part of which gives rise to the malleus.)

Movements of the temporomandibular joint

Movements at the temporomandibular joint are elevation, depression, protraction, retraction, and side-to-side grinding movements of the jaw.

When the jaw is **depressed** to open the mouth wide, two separate movements—sliding and rotatory movements—take place: (1) the articular disc and the head of the mandible slide forwards on the articular surface of the temporal bone, and the

head of the mandible comes to lie inferior to the articular tubercle.; (2) at the same time, the head of the mandible rotates on the lower surface of the articular disc in the lower joint cavity [Fig. 15.6]. The latter movement alone is capable of permitting simple chewing movements over a small range, without separating the lips. (The rotatory movement can be confirmed by placing a forefinger on the head of the mandible, immediately in front of the tragus, while making chewing movements.) When the mouth is opened wide, the head of the mandible swings forwards and downwards. (Confirm that the finger on the head of the mandible slips into the mandibular fossa vacated by the head, and that the mouth cannot be closed while the finger remains in the fossa.) The axes for the small and wide rotatory movements is different. In small movements, the axis is through the head of the mandible; in wider-range movements, the axis is through the mandibular foramen. By being on the axis, the vessels and nerves entering the mandible are not stretched when the mouth is opened wide. Muscles causing depression of the jaw are the lateral pterygoid and the digastric acting on a fixed hyoid bone.

Elevation of the jaw closes the mouth. It is brought about by the temporalis, masseter, and medial pterygoid.

Protraction of the jaw is the movement of pulling the jaw forwards. In protraction, the head of the mandible and the articular disc slide forwards on the temporal articular surface on both sides, but the mouth is not opened. The lateral pterygoid protracts the jaw. The medial pterygoid and the superficial fibres of the masseter also protract the jaw, but less effectively.

The reverse movement to protraction is **retraction** which is brought about by the posterior fibres of the temporalis. When these movements alternate on the two sides by the muscles of opposite sides acting alternately, a grinding movement is produced as the chin swings from side to side.

Deeper contents of the infratemporal fossa

Using the instructions given in Dissection 15.4, complete the deep dissection of the infratemporal fossa.

Middle meningeal artery

The **middle meningeal artery** arises from the maxillary artery at the lower border of the lateral pterygoid muscle. It ascends between the two roots of the auriculotemporal nerve and enters the skull through the foramen spinosum [Figs. 15.3, 15.7]. It is posterolateral to the mandibular nerve and lies on the lateral surface of the tensor palati muscle and the auditory tube. Its intracranial course is described in Chapter 8.

The **accessory meningeal** and **anterior tympanic arteries** arise either from the middle meningeal artery or from the maxillary artery. The accessory meningeal artery enters the skull through the foramen ovale, and the anterior tympanic enters the middle ear through the petrotympanic fissure, close to the chorda tympani nerve.

Mandibular nerve

The mandibular branch of the trigeminal nerve arises from the trigeminal ganglion in the cranium and leaves the skull through the foramen ovale. In the foramen ovale, it is joined by the motor root of the trigeminal nerve.

Immediately below the skull, it lies between the lateral pterygoid muscle and the tensor palati which separates it from the auditory tube [see Fig. 3.7]. It divides almost immediately into anterior (predominantly motor) and posterior (predominantly sensory) divisions [Figs. 15.7, 15.8].

Branches of the trunk

The **meningeal branch** arises from the trunk of the nerve and enters the skull through the foramen spinosum. It supplies the dura mater and skull and sends a filament to the middle ear.

The **nerve to the medial pterygoid** arises from the trunk and runs forwards into the deep surface of the muscle. At its origin, it lies close to the otic ganglion.

187

DISSECTION 15.4 Deep dissection of the infratemporal fossa

Objectives

I. To identify and trace the auriculotemporal nerve.
II. To identify and trace the middle meningeal artery.

Instructions

1. Separate the two heads of the lateral pterygoid muscle, avoiding injury to the buccal nerve between them.

2. Carefully detach the upper head from the capsule of the temporomandibular joint and remove it piecemeal from the infratemporal fossa. Take care not to damage the deep temporal nerves which pass between the lateral pterygoid and the skull.

3. Separate the lower head of the lateral pterygoid from the lateral pterygoid lamina, and strip it posteriorly from the underlying structures, leaving the buccal nerve intact.

4. Disarticulate the head of the mandible from the articular disc, and remove it with the lower head of the lateral pterygoid. Take care not to damage the **auriculotemporal nerve** which curves round the medial and posterior surfaces of the joint capsule.

5. Expose the underlying structures.

6. Identify the middle meningeal artery, and trace it to the foramen spinosum. Note the two roots of the auriculotemporal nerve which surround the artery close to the skull.

7. Identify the origin of the auriculotemporal nerve from the mandibular nerve, and trace it posteriorly.

8. Expose the other branches of the mandibular nerve— inferior alveolar, lingual, and buccal [Fig. 15.7]. Identify the chorda tympani nerve joining the lingual nerve. Trace the chorda tympani towards the spine of the sphenoid.

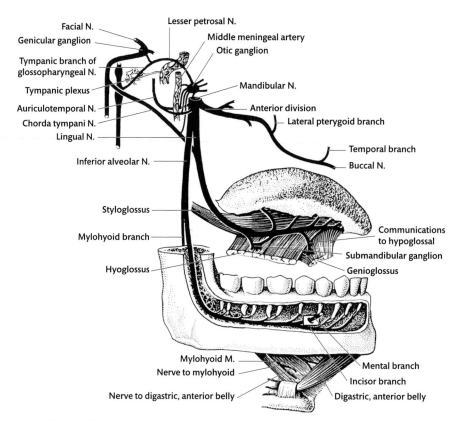

Fig. 15.7 Distribution of the mandibular nerve. Note the sympathetic filaments to the otic ganglion and the tympanic plexus from the middle meningeal and internal carotid arteries.

Branches of the anterior division

Buccal nerve

The large sensory branch—the **buccal nerve**—passes between the two heads of the lateral pterygoid and runs antero-inferiorly to the surface of the buccinator muscle, often piercing the lowest fibres of insertion of the temporalis on the deep surface of the ramus of the mandible [Fig. 15.3]. On the buccinator, it forms a plexus with the buccal branch of the facial nerve (motor to the buccinator) and is sensory to the entire thickness of the cheek—from the skin to the mucous membrane.

Nerve to the lateral pterygoid

The nerve to the lateral pterygoid runs with the buccal nerve and enters the muscle as it passes between the heads of the lateral pterygoid.

Deep temporal nerves

The two deep temporal nerves—anterior and posterior—pass into the temporal fossa between the skull and the lateral pterygoid, grooving the bone to enter the deep surface of the temporalis [Figs. 15.3, 15.7, 15.8].

Nerve to the masseter

The nerve to the masseter arises with the posterior deep temporal nerve. It runs laterally between the skull and the lateral pterygoid muscle (immediately anterior to the capsule of the temporomandibular joint) and enters the deep surface of the masseter by passing through the mandibular notch. It gives one or two twigs to the temporomandibular joint [Fig. 15.8].

Branches of the posterior division

Auriculotemporal nerve

The **auriculotemporal nerve** arises by two roots which surround the middle meningeal artery. They unite posterior to the artery, run backwards lateral to the spine of the sphenoid, and hook around the posterior surface of the neck of the mandible. Here the nerve turns superiorly in contact with the parotid gland and crosses the root of the zygomatic process of the temporal bone with the superficial temporal artery [Figs. 15.7, 15.8]. The nerve carries post-ganglionic parasympathetic secretomotor fibres from the otic ganglion to the parotid gland. (Preganglionic fibres reach the otic ganglion

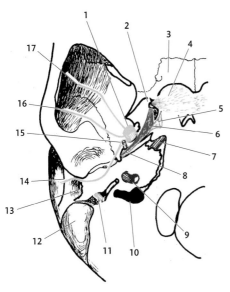

Fig. 15.8 A diagrammatic representation of the external surface of the base of the skull to show the position of some of the nerves and blood vessels and of the tensor veli palatini. Red = arteries and muscle. Green = tendon and auditory tube. 1 = mandibular nerve; 2 = pterygoid hamulus; 3 = horizontal plate of palatine bone; 4 = palatine aponeurosis (tendon of tensor veli palatini); 5 = pharyngeal opening of auditory tube; 6 = tensor veli palatini; 7 = internal carotid artery in upper part of foramen lacerum; 8 = chorda tympani nerve; 9 = internal carotid artery; 10 = jugular foramen; 11 = facial nerve; 12 = mastoid process; 13 = external acoustic meatus; 14 = auriculotemporal nerve; 15 = middle meningeal artery; 16 = nerve to masseter; 17 = deep temporal nerve to temporalis.

through the lesser petrosal branch of the glossopharyngeal nerve.)

The auriculotemporal nerve gives the following **branches**: (1) slender filaments to the posterior part of the capsule of the temporomandibular joint; (2) one or two thick branches to the parotid gland—these sensory nerves mingle with branches of the facial nerve in the substance of the gland; and (3) cutaneous branches to the auricle and temple [see Fig. 4.7].

Inferior alveolar nerve

The inferior alveolar nerve is the largest branch of the posterior division. It runs vertically downwards with the inferior alveolar artery between the medial and lateral pterygoid muscles. The nerve and artery each give off a mylohyoid branch and then enter the mandibular foramen. In the body of the mandible, the inferior alveolar nerve and artery give branches to the teeth and gums, and send a branch (the **mental nerve** and **artery**) through the mental foramen to supply the skin of the chin

and the mucous membrane of the lower lip [see Fig. 4.7; Figs. 15.3, 15.7, 15.8].

The **mylohyoid nerve** contains the only motor fibres present in the posterior division. It pierces the sphenomandibular ligament and runs antero-inferiorly in a groove on the medial aspect of the mandible to the digastric triangle, inferior to the mylohyoid muscle. In the triangle, it is joined by the submental artery and supplies the mylohyoid muscle and the anterior belly of the digastric [see Fig. 6.6].

Lingual nerve

The lingual nerve arises from the posterior division of the mandibular nerve and curves antero-inferiorly on the medial pterygoid muscle to reach the medial surface of the mandible, in front of the inferior alveolar nerve. It passes between the mandible and the mucous membrane covering it, just inferior to the last molar tooth and above the posterior fibres of the mylohyoid muscle [Figs. 15.2A, 15.3, 15.7]. Its further course will be described in Chapter 16. The lingual nerve is sensory to the mucous membrane of the anterior two-thirds of the tongue and to the adjacent part of the floor of the mouth and gum.

The lingual nerve gives no branches in the infratemporal fossa but is joined by the chorda tympani branch of the facial nerve, deep to the lateral pterygoid muscle [Fig. 15.7]. It may send a communicating branch to the inferior alveolar nerve.

Chorda tympani

The chorda tympani is a slender branch of the facial nerve. It arises from the facial nerve on the posterior wall of the middle ear cavity, runs anteriorly across the lateral wall of that cavity (on the tympanic membrane), and leaves the tympanic cavity through the petrotympanic fissure. It then grooves the medial side of the spine of the sphenoid, running antero-inferiorly to join the posterior surface of the lingual nerve [see Figs. 13.5, 13.8; Fig. 15.7]. It contains sensory and preganglionic parasympathetic fibres. The sensory fibres arise from the taste buds on the anterior two-thirds of the tongue. The preganglionic fibres synapse in the submandibular ganglion and supply the submandibular and sublingual glands.

Using the instructions given in Dissection 15.5, dissect the otic ganglion and tensor palati muscles.

Otic ganglion

The otic ganglion is a minute collection of parasympathetic nerve cells which lies between the mandibular nerve and the tensor palati, immediately below the foramen ovale [Fig. 15.7]. It is one of the four parasympathetic ganglia of the head. A number of different fibres pass through the otic ganglion, but only the preganglionic parasympathetic fibres synapse in the ganglion.

Connections of the otic ganglion

The preganglionic parasympathetic fibres to the otic ganglion run in the lesser petrosal nerve, a branch of the glossopharyngeal nerve [Fig. 15.7]. Post-ganglionic parasympathetic fibres (secretomotor fibres) arise from the cells of the ganglion and pass to the parotid gland in the auriculotemporal nerve.

Other nerves traverse the ganglion but have no functional connection with it. They are: (1) motor fibres to the tensor palati and tensor tympani muscles from the nerve to the medial pterygoid muscle; (2) sympathetic fibres from the plexus on the middle meningeal artery, for distribution through the branches of the ganglion; and (3) sensory fibres from the glossopharyngeal and trigeminal nerves for distribution through the branches of the ganglion.

Tensor palati (tensor veli palatini)

The tensor palati is a thin, triangular muscle which takes origin from the scaphoid fossa at the root of the medial pterygoid lamina, and the posteromedial margin of the greater wing of the sphenoid as far posteriorly as the spine of the sphenoid and the auditory tube [see Figs. 3.6, 3.7]. It lies immediately medial to the foramina ovale and spinosum in the uppermost part of the lateral wall of the pharynx and will be seen later [see Fig. 6.5].

Maxillary nerve

The maxillary nerve will be completely dissected at a later stage, but its course and some of its branches can be seen now.

Dissection 15.6 provides instructions on dissecting the branches of the maxillary nerve in the orbit.

The maxillary nerve is the second of the three divisions of the trigeminal nerve. It arises from the trigeminal ganglion in the cranium and passes forwards on the side of the body of the sphenoid, at the lower border of the cavernous sinus, to the **foramen rotundum** [see Fig. 8.14]. It emerges from the foramen rotundum into the upper part of the pterygopalatine fossa and curves laterally through the pterygomaxillary fissure to enter the infratemporal fossa. In the infratemporal fossa, it turns sharply forwards into the infra-orbital groove as the **infra-orbital nerve** (Fig. 15.4; see Fig. 19.7). Confirm this course in a dried skull by passing a bristle through the foramen rotundum into the infra-orbital groove.

Branches of the maxillary nerve

The maxillary nerve gives off the following branches: (1) a **meningeal** branch which arises near the origin of the nerve; (2) in the pterygopalatine fossa, two **ganglionic** branches which pass inferiorly to join the pterygopalatine ganglion [Fig. 15.4]; (3) the **posterior superior alveolar nerve** which arises in the infratemporal fossa and divides into two branches which descend over the posterior surface of the maxilla. They supply the gum and the mucous membrane of the cheek and then enter the canals in the bone. In the canals, they run forwards above the tooth sockets and form a plexus with the superior alveolar branches of the infra-orbital nerve. They give dental branches to the molar teeth. Within the bone, these nerves run with corresponding branches of the maxillary artery; (4) the **zygomatic nerve** which arises close to the foramen rotundum and enters the orbit through the inferior orbital fissure. It gives a delicate branch to the lacrimal nerve, pierces the periosteum, and divides into **zygomaticotemporal** and **zygomatico-facial** branches. These pass forwards in the periosteum of the lateral wall of the orbit and pierce the zygomatic bone to reach the skin of the temple (zygomaticotemporal nerve) and face (zygomaticofacial nerve) [see Fig. 4.7; Fig. 15.4]; and (5) the **infra-orbital nerve** which is a continuation of the maxillary nerve in the infra-orbital groove and canal. It emerges through the infra-orbital foramen onto the face, deep to the orbicularis oculi. It divides into sensory branches to the upper lip, nose, and lower eyelid. The infra-orbital nerve is accompanied by the corresponding vessels [see Fig. 4.7].

About the middle of the floor of the orbit, the infra-orbital nerve gives off the **anterior superior alveolar nerve**, which descends through the anterior wall of the maxilla and joins the plexus formed by the posterior superior alveolar nerves. The anterior superior alveolar nerves supply branches to the upper first molar, premolars, canine, and incisor teeth. They also supply the adjacent gum and send branches to the maxillary

DISSECTION 15.7 Mandibular canal

Objective

I. To expose the inferior alveolar nerve and vessels in the mandibular canal.

Instructions

1. Expose the mandibular canal by removing the outer table of the mandible with a chisel and bone forceps.
2. Identify the inferior alveolar vessels and nerve.

sinus and to the mucous membrane of the antero-inferior part of the nose [Fig. 15.4].

A middle superior alveolar nerve is described in 30 per cent of individuals.

Structures within the mandibular canal

Dissection 15.7 provides instructions on exposing the contents of the mandibular canal.

The mandibular canal is traversed by the inferior alveolar vessels and nerve, which give dental branches to the roots of the lower teeth and gingival branches of the adjacent gum.

The mental nerve and artery arise from the inferior alveolar nerve and artery in the canal and emerge through the mental foramen.

See Clinical Applications 15.1 and 15.2 for the practical implications of the anatomy discussed in this chapter.

CLINICAL APPLICATION 15.1 Clinical testing of the trigeminal nerve

There are several ways to test the integrity of the trigeminal nerve clinically.

1. Testing sensations of pain, temperature, and touch over the forehead, prominence of the cheek, and chin.

   Study question 1: using your knowledge of the nerve supply of the face, explain why, while testing the integrity of the trigeminal nerve, one must be careful not to include the skin over the angle of the mandible. (Answer: the skin over the angle of the mandible is not supplied by the trigeminal nerve. It is supplied by the great auricular nerve from the cervical plexus. The trigeminal nerve is distributed through its three divisions to the skin of the rest of the face and anterior scalp.)

2. Testing the corneal reflex.

   Study question 2: explain why in facial palsy, the corneal reflex is impaired. (Answer: the corneal reflex is impaired in facial

palsy because the efferent limb of the reflex is through the branches of the facial nerve that supply the orbicularis oculi.)

3. Inspection of jaw movement. Look for deviation of the jaw when the mouth is opened.

   Study question 3: to which side does the mandible deviate if the trigeminal nerve is paralysed, and why? (Answer: deviation of the jaw is to the affected side because of the unopposed action of the pterygoid muscles of the normal side.)

4. Testing the jaw jerk. The jaw jerk is elicited by tapping the chin while the mouth is held loosely open. A positive response is jerking of the jaw upwards by the masseter muscle.

   Study question 4: which part of the trigeminal nerve carries proprioceptive impulses from the muscles of mastication? (Answer: the mandibular division.)

CLINICAL APPLICATION 15.2 Dislocation of the temporomandibular joint

The temporomandibular joint may be dislocated by a side blow to the chin when the mouth is open or in fractures of the mandible. Sometimes it is dislocated with excessive stretching of the lateral pterygoid in yawning or when opening the mouth to take a big bite. The head of the mandible slips anteriorly out of the mandibular fossa—**anterior dislocation**—and the person is un-able to close the mouth. It is reduced with downward and backward pressure on the lower molars, to disengage the head of the mandible and slip it back in place.

Posterior dislocation is rare and usually results from a frontal blow to the chin.

Table 15.1 provides an overview of the movements of the mandible.

Table 15.1 Movements of the mandible

Movement	Muscles	Nerve supply
Elevation of chin (closing the mouth)	Masseter	Mandibular
	Medial pterygoid	Mandibular
	Temporalis (anterior part)	Mandibular
Depression of chin (opening the mouth)*	Lateral pterygoid	Mandibular
	Digastric (hyoid fixed)	Mandibular and facial
	Geniohyoid (hyoid fixed)	C. 1 ventral ramus
	Mylohyoid (hyoid fixed)	Mandibular
Protraction	Lateral pterygoid	Mandibular
	Medial pterygoid	Mandibular
	Masseter (superficial part)	Mandibular
Retraction*	Temporalis (posterior part)	Mandibular
	Digastric (hyoid fixed)	Mandibular and facial
Chewing—a side-to-side grinding movement	Medial and lateral pterygoids and masseter	Mandibular
	Temporalis (all parts), masseter (deep part)	Mandibular

* During depression and retraction of the jaw, the hyoid is fixed by the action of infrahyoid muscles. Nerve supply: ansa cervicalis.

CHAPTER 16
The submandibular region

Introduction

The submandibular region lies between the body of the mandible and the hyoid bone. The superficial part includes the submental and digastric triangles which have been dissected already. Its deeper parts, now to be dissected, include the root of the tongue and the floor of the mouth [Fig. 16.1].

Dissection 16.1 provides instructions on exposing the submandibular region.

Digastric muscle

The digastric muscle has two bellies—the **anterior** and **posterior** bellies [Chapter 6]. The anterior

belly of the digastric takes origin from the lower border of the mandible, close to the mandibular symphysis. The posterior belly arises from the floor of the mastoid notch on the medial side of the mastoid process. The two bellies are united by an intermediate tendon at the upper border of the hyoid bone. The tendon passes through a short, strong loop of fibrous tissue which binds it down to the hyoid bone at the junction of the body with the greater horn. It allows the hyoid bone to slide backwards and forwards on the tendon [see Figs. 6.2A, 6.4, 6.7, 15.2B, 18.2].

The **anterior belly** is covered by deep fascia and is overlapped by the submandibular gland [Fig. 6.1]. The **posterior belly** is deep to the mastoid process, the lower part of the parotid gland, angle of the mandible, facial vein, and the

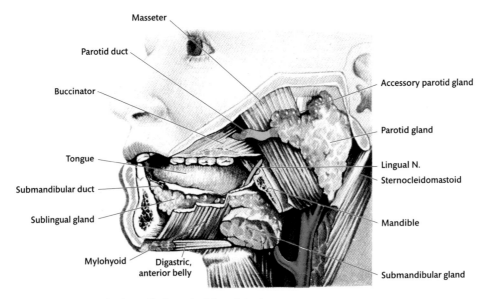

Fig. 16.1 Dissection of the parotid, submandibular, and sublingual glands.

Objective

I. To mobilize the mandible and open into the sub-mandibular region.

Instructions

1. Turn the trachea and oesophagus medially on the right. On the left, extend the neck and flex the head to the right.

2. Cut across the facial artery and vein at the lower border of the mandible, and detach the anterior belly of the digastric from the mandible. Turn the mandible upwards, and fix it with hooks.

3. Complete the exposure of the posterior belly of the digastric and of the stylohyoid muscles.

submandibular gland. It runs obliquely, superficial to the neurovascular bundle of the neck—the internal jugular vein, internal and external carotid arteries, spinal accessory, and hypoglossal nerve. The occipital artery runs posterosuperiorly on its deep surface and grooves the temporal bone, just medial to the origin of the muscle [Figs. 6.4, 6.6].

Nerve supply: the posterior belly of the digastric is supplied by the facial nerve, and the anterior belly by the mylohyoid nerve. **Actions**: if the hyoid bone is fixed, the digastric helps to depress the mandible. The chief action of both bellies, acting together, is to raise the hyoid bone (and hence the tongue) in swallowing. (It is not possible to swallow with the mouth open, because the digastric is already shortened.) Acting with the infrahyoid muscles, the digastric fixes the hyoid bone and forms a stable platform on which the tongue can move.

Stylohyoid muscle

The stylohyoid is a small slip of muscle which arises from the styloid process and descends along the upper border of the posterior belly of the digastric. Inferiorly, the tendon splits to surround the intermediate tendon of the digastric and is inserted into the hyoid bone at the junction of the body and greater horn [see Fig. 6.2]. **Nerve supply**: the facial nerve. **Action**: it helps to pull the hyoid upwards and backwards during swallowing [see Fig. 18.2].

DISSECTION 16.2 The submandibular region

Objectives

I. To study the submandibular gland and duct.
II. To identify and trace the facial artery in the sub-mandibular region. **III.** To expose the posterior border of the mylohyoid and hyoglossus. **IV.** To identify and trace the hypoglossal and lingual nerves. **V.** To identify the submandibular ganglion.

Instructions

1. Turn the submandibular gland posteriorly, and expose the mylohyoid muscle.

2. Note the deep part of the gland which hooks round the free posterior border of the mylohyoid muscle and runs forwards on its superior surface.

3. Dissect out the facial artery from the deep surface of the gland, and trace its branches in this region.

4. Identify the mylohyoid nerve on the mylohyoid muscle.

5. Turn the submandibular gland anteriorly, and identify the hypoglossal nerve lying on the hyoglossus muscle immediately superior to the greater horn of the hyoid bone.

6. At a higher level, identify the lingual nerve as it crosses the hyoglossus.

7. Identify the submandibular ganglion, which is suspended from the lingual nerve.

8. Identify the submandibular duct, which passes forwards from the deep part of the gland.

Using the instructions given in Dissection 16.2, dissect the submandibular region.

Submandibular gland

The submandibular salivary gland is about half the size of the parotid gland. It has a superficial and deep part. The **superficial part** is wedged between the body of the mandible and the mylohyoid muscle [see Fig. 9.1]. Anteriorly, the superficial part reaches the level of the mental foramen, and superiorly it reaches up to the mylohyoid line on the medial surface of the mandible. Posterior to the free margin of the mylohyoid, the **deep part** of the gland extends forwards, deep to the mucous membrane of the mouth [Figs. 16.2A, 16.3].

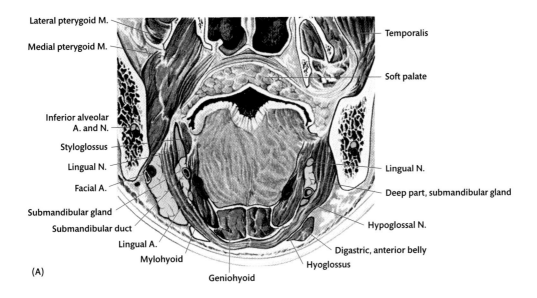

- Lateral pterygoid M.
- Medial pterygoid M.
- Temporalis
- Soft palate
- Inferior alveolar A. and N.
- Styloglossus
- Lingual N.
- Facial A.
- Lingual N.
- Deep part, submandibular gland
- Submandibular gland
- Submandibular duct
- Hypoglossal N.
- Lingual A.
- Mylohyoid
- Digastric, anterior belly
- Hyoglossus
- Geniohyoid

(A)

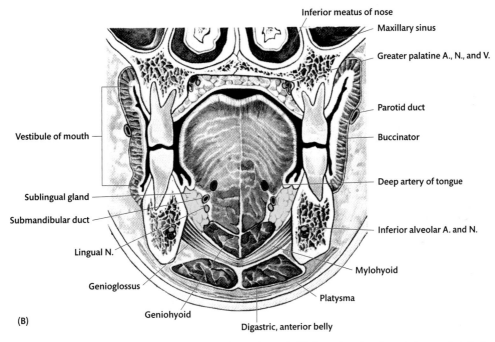

- Inferior meatus of nose
- Maxillary sinus
- Greater palatine A., N., and V.
- Parotid duct
- Vestibule of mouth
- Buccinator
- Deep artery of tongue
- Sublingual gland
- Submandibular duct
- Inferior alveolar A. and N.
- Lingual N.
- Mylohyoid
- Genioglossus
- Platysma
- Geniohyoid
- Digastric, anterior belly

(B)

Fig. 16.2 (A) Coronal section through the mouth, posterior to the molar teeth. (B) Coronal section through the mouth at the level of the second molar teeth.

The gland is loosely covered by the investing layer of the deep cervical fascia which ascends from the hyoid bone and splits to enclose it. The superficial layer of this fascia is attached to the inferior border of the mandible, and the thinner deep layer is attached to the mylohyoid line [see Fig. 15.2A]. Posteriorly, these layers fuse and form the stylomandibular ligament. This ligament separates the submandibular gland from the parotid gland.

Surfaces of the submandibular gland

The superficial part of the submandibular gland has three surfaces—inferolateral, lateral, and medial. The **inferolateral** surface is covered by: (1) the superficial fascia containing the platysma and the cervical branch of the facial nerve; (2) the deep fascia; and deep to this (3) the facial vein and a few **submandibular lymph nodes**. (Most of the lymph nodes lie in the groove between the submandibular gland and the mandible.) The **facial artery** grooves the posterosuperior part of this surface, then loops antero-inferiorly between the gland and the medial pterygoid muscle, and appears at the inferior margin of the mandible.

The **lateral** surface is related to the medial pterygoid, facial artery, and mandible [see Fig. 9.15].

The **medial** surface extends from the mylohyoid line inferiorly to the bellies of the digastric muscle. It is related to the mylohyoid, hyoglossus, hypoglossal, and lingual nerves and the submandibular ganglion. The posterior part of the medial surface is in contact with the pharynx. This surface is grooved by the facial artery.

The submandibular duct arises from the medial surface of the gland and passes anteriorly in the angle between the side of the tongue and mylohyoid.

The **deep part of the gland** is a thin, flat process which extends anteriorly on the lateral side of the duct [see Fig. 9.15; Figs. 16.2A, 16.3], superior to the mylohyoid. Figs. 16.4A and B are transverse sections through the head at the level of the submandibular glands.

Nerves and vessels of the submandibular gland

(1) The sensory nerves to the gland are carried by the lingual nerve. (2) The parasympathetic secretomotor supply is from the nerve cells in the **submandibular ganglion**. The preganglionic parasympathetic fibres to the ganglion come through the chorda tympani branch of the facial nerve and the lingual nerve. (3) The sympathetics are carried by a plexus on the facial artery.

The arterial supply to the submandibular gland is from several small branches of the facial and submental arteries.

Facial artery

The facial artery arises from the external carotid in the carotid triangle, immediately superior to the tip of the greater horn of the hyoid bone. It passes vertically upwards on the middle and superior constrictor muscles of the pharynx, under cover of the angle of the mandible and the digastric and stylohyoid muscles. It then turns forwards above these muscles and hooks round the posterosuperior part of the submandibular gland and the lower border of the mandible, to appear on the face at the antero-inferior angle of the masseter [see Figs. 4.6, 9.14, 9.15; Fig. 16.2A].

Branches in the neck

The branches of the facial artery in the neck include: (1) the **ascending palatine artery**; (2) the **tonsillar artery**, which ascends superficial to the styloglossus and pierces the superior constrictor to reach the palatine tonsil [see Fig. 9.15]; (3) small **glandular branches**, which pass to the submandibular gland; and (4) the **submental artery**, which arises between the submandibular gland and the mandible and runs forwards on the inferior surface of the mylohyoid muscle [see Fig. 6.1]. It

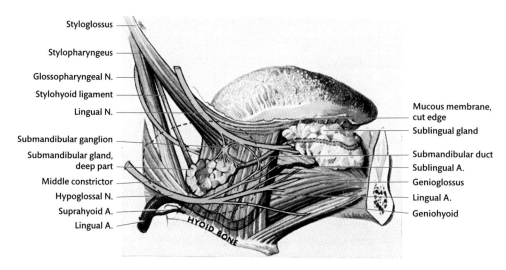

Fig. 16.3 Dissection of the submandibular region. Dotted red line = position of the superficial part of the submandibular gland.

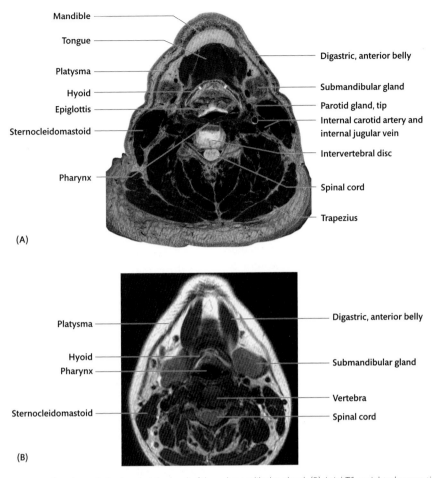

Mandible
Tongue
Platysma
Hyoid
Epiglottis
Sternocleidomastoid
Pharynx

Digastric, anterior belly
Submandibular gland
Parotid gland, tip
Internal carotid artery and internal jugular vein
Intervertebral disc
Spinal cord
Trapezius

(A)

Platysma
Hyoid
Pharynx
Sternocleidomastoid

Digastric, anterior belly
Submandibular gland
Vertebra
Spinal cord

(B)

Fig. 16.4 (A) Transverse section through the head at the level of the submandibular gland. (B) Axial T1-weighted magnetic resonance imaging (MRI) section at the level of the submandibular glands (SM).

Image A courtesy of the Visible Human Project of the US National Library of Medicine.

supplies the submandibular and sublingual glands and the adjacent muscles and skin.

Using the instructions given in Dissection 16.3, expose the mylohyoid muscle.

DISSECTION 16.3 Mylohyoid

Objective

I. To expose the mylohyoid muscle.

Instructions

1. Push the submandibular gland and the submental vessels posteriorly.

2. Cut the mylohyoid nerve, and turn the anterior belly of the digastric downwards.

3. Examine the attachments of the mylohyoid muscle.

Mylohyoid muscle

The mylohyoid is a thin sheet of muscle which takes origin from the mylohyoid line on the mandible. The fibres of the right and left muscles pass downwards, medially, and forwards and are inserted into a median fibrous raphe which extends from the mandible to the body of the hyoid bone. The most posterior fibres of the mylohyoid are inserted into the hyoid bone [see Fig. 6.1]. The two muscles together form a supporting sling under the tongue and separate the tongue from the submandibular region [Figs. 16.2A, 16.2B]. Each muscle has a free posterior border, around which the superficial and deep parts of the submandibular gland are continuous [see Fig. 6.6].

Nerve supply: the mylohyoid nerve. **Action**: it helps to raise the hyoid bone and tongue in swallowing and forms the muscular floor of the mouth.

DISSECTION 16.4 Further dissection of the submandibular region

Objectives

I. To identify the geniohyoid, genioglossus, styloglossus, and stylopharyngeus.   **II.** To identify and trace the vessels and nerves on the floor of the mouth.

Instructions

1. From the medial side, identify the cut edge of the mylohyoid muscle [see Fig. 17.3], and separate it from the overlying geniohyoid by sliding a blunt instrument backwards and forwards between them.

2. Find the plane of separation between the geniohyoid and genioglossus in the same way, and note that the fibres of the genioglossus radiate from the upper mental spine.

3. Pull the tongue away from the mandible, and cut carefully through the mucous membrane between it and the mandible. Strip the mucous membrane from the floor of the mouth and the mandible to expose the sublingual gland, the submandibular duct, the lingual nerve, the submandibular ganglion, the **hypoglossal nerve** [Fig. 16.3], and the **deep lingual vein**.

4. Make an opening into the submandibular duct, and pass a fine probe along it into the mouth.

5. Follow the **lingual nerve** posteriorly, and find its branches to the submandibular ganglion and the sublingual gland.

6. Note the proximity of the lingual nerve to the last molar tooth [Fig. 16.5].

7. Medial to the lingual nerve, hypoglossal nerve, and submandibular ganglion, clean the lateral surface of the hyoglossus muscle, with the styloglossus mingling with it posteriorly.

8. The **lingual artery** is deep to the hyoglossus but appears at its anterior margin. Identify the artery.

9. Confirm the continuity of the hypoglossal nerve and lingual artery and vein with the same structures in the neck.

10. Trace the styloglossus back to the styloid process. Find the stylohyoid ligament and the stylopharyngeus attached to it. Try to trace the ligament towards the lesser cornu of the hyoid bone, and follow the stylopharyngeus downwards.

11. Find the **glossopharyngeal nerve** as it curves round the **stylopharyngeus** and passes forwards deep to the hyoglossus.

12. Below the glossopharyngeal nerve, confirm the superior border of the middle constrictor muscle, and follow it to the hyoid bone and the stylohyoid ligament, lateral to the stylopharyngeus.

Dissection 16.4 provides instructions on further dissection of the submandibular region.

Hyoglossus

The hyoglossus is a flat, quadrate muscle which takes origin from the greater horn and body of the hyoid bone. Its fibres pass superiorly into the posterior half of the side of the tongue, interdigitating with the fibres of the styloglossus [Figs. 16.3, 16.6B].

Nerve supply: the hypoglossal nerve. **Actions**: it depresses the side of the tongue and assists the genioglossus to enlarge the oral cavity in sucking, when the hyoid bone is fixed by the infrahyoid muscles.

Styloglossus

The styloglossus is a long muscle which takes origin from the tip of the styloid process and the adjacent part of the stylohyoid ligament. It passes anteroinferiorly and is inserted into the whole length of the side of the tongue, intermingling with the fibres of the hyoglossus [see Fig. 6.6; Fig. 16.3].

Nerve supply: the hypoglossal nerve. **Action**: it pulls the tongue posterosuperiorly in swallowing.

Geniohyoid

The geniohyoid muscle takes origin from the lower mental spine on the mandible and is inserted into the body of the hyoid bone [see Fig. 15.2B;

Fig. 16.6B]. The two muscles lie side by side on the superior surface of the mylohyoid and are almost horizontal in the resting position [Fig. 16.2].

Nerve supply: the first cervical ventral ramus through the hypoglossal nerve. **Action**: it pulls the elevated hyoid bone directly forwards, sliding the pulley on the taut intermediate tendon of the digastric. This increases the anteroposterior diameter of the pharynx to receive the bolus of food during swallowing.

Genioglossus

The genioglossus is a flat, fan-shaped muscle in contact with its fellow in the median plane. It arises from the upper mental spine of the mandible and spreads out into the tongue in a vertical plane. It is inserted into the paramedian part of the dorsum of the tongue from the tip of the tongue almost to the hyoid bone [see Fig. 18.2; Fig. 16.3].

Nerve supply: the hypoglossal nerve. **Actions**: the postero-inferior fibres of the two muscles, acting together, protrude the tongue. The muscles also depress the central part of the tongue and increase the volume of the mouth, e.g. in sucking. The anterior fibres depress the tip of the tongue and retract it. ➲ If one muscle is active and the other is paralysed, the tip of the tongue deviates towards the paralysed side when protruded.

Hyoid bone

The hyoid bone is U-shaped and open posteriorly. It lies between the root of the tongue and the thyroid cartilage and forms a movable base for the tongue. It does not articulate with any other bone in the body but is held in position by the muscles and ligaments attached to it. It is connected to the mandible by the mylohyoid, geniohyoid, and anterior belly of the digastric; to the skull by the stylohyoid muscle, stylohyoid ligament, and posterior belly of the digastric; to the thyroid cartilage by the thyrohyoid muscle and thyrohyoid membrane; to the sternum by the sternohyoid; and to the scapula by the omohyoid.

The hyoid bone is raised by contraction of the digastric; pulled forwards by the geniohyoid; pulled posterosuperiorly by the stylohyoid; and depressed by the infrahyoid muscles. It is held fixed by contraction of these opposing muscles.

Submandibular duct

The submandibular duct emerges from the medial surface of the submandibular gland. It runs antero-superiorly in the angle between the mylohyoid and the side of the tongue. It opens on the floor of the mouth, beneath the anterior part of the tongue, on the top of the sublingual papilla, on the sublingual fold [see Fig. 17.2; Figs. 16.3, 16.5]. Examine these structures in the floor of your mouth. The wall of the duct is much thinner than that of the parotid gland and is not easily palpated.

At first, the submandibular duct lies on the hyoglossus, between the lingual nerve above and the hypoglossal nerve below, separated from the mylohoid muscle by the deep part of the submandibular gland. Further anteriorly, it passes on to the genioglossus and has the sublingual gland between it and the mylohyoid. The **lingual nerve** hooks round the inferior surface of the duct and runs upwards into the tongue, medial to the duct [Fig. 16.3]. ➲ **Sialolithiasis** is the formation of calculi (stones) within the salivary gland. If the calculus forms in a duct, then saliva will be trapped in the gland. This may cause painful swelling and inflammation of the gland.

Sublingual gland

The sublingual gland is the smallest of the large salivary glands (3 cm long). It lies on the mylohyoid between the mandible and the genioglossus muscle and forms the sublingual fold on the floor of the mouth [Figs. 16.1, 16.2B, 16.3, 16.5]. The lingual nerve and submandibular duct lie medial to it.

Ducts of the sublingual gland

Numerous small ducts (8–20) open into the mouth on the sublingual fold.

Vessels and nerves of the sublingual gland

The arterial supply to the sublingual gland is from the sublingual branch of the lingual artery. The nerve supply is from branches of the lingual nerve. The lingual nerve contains post-ganglionic parasympathetic fibres from the cells of the

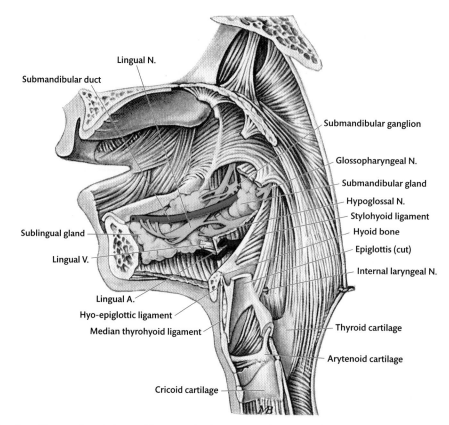

Fig. 16.5 Dissection of the mouth and pharynx. The tongue has been removed to expose the structures which lie between it and the mylohyoid muscle.

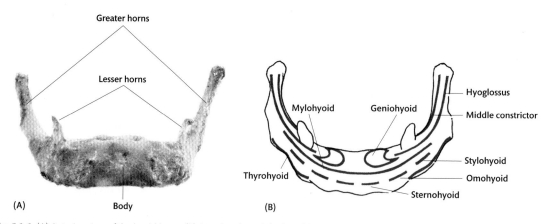

Fig. 16.6 (A) Anterior view of the hyoid bone. (B) Anterior view of the hyoid bone to show muscle attachments.

submandibular ganglion. It also contains sensory and post-ganglionic sympathetic fibres [Fig. 16.5].

Lingual nerve

The lingual nerve is a branch of the posterior division of the mandibular nerve. It descends between the ramus of the mandible and the medial pterygoid muscle [see Fig. 15.3]. It then turns forwards and enters the mouth by passing inferior to the lower border of the superior constrictor muscle of the pharynx [see Fig. 15.2B; Fig. 16.5]. It continues antero-inferiorly between the mucous membrane of the mouth and the body of the mandible, postero-inferior to the last molar tooth [Fig. 16.1]. In the submandibular region, the nerve lies close to the side of the tongue, crosses the styloglossus and the upper part of the hyoglossus, and hooks beneath the submandibular duct [Fig. 16.3]. ⊃ The lingual nerve is liable to be injured by clumsy extraction of the last molar tooth. It is also accessible to local anaesthetics at this point.

Branches of the lingual nerve

The lingual nerve: (1) communicates with the submandibular ganglion through two or more branches; (2) sends one or two branches to the hypoglossal nerve. These branches descend along the anterior border of the hyoglossus [Fig. 16.3]. It gives: (3) thin branches to the mucous membrane of the mouth and gums; (4) a few small branches to the sublingual gland; and (5) branches which pierce the substance of the tongue and run superiorly to supply the mucous membrane of the anterior two-thirds of the tongue.

Submandibular ganglion

The submandibular ganglion is one of the four parasympathetic ganglia in the head. It lies on the upper part of the hyoglossus muscle, inferior to the lingual nerve and superior to the submandibular duct. It is suspended from the lingual nerve by two short branches [Fig. 16.3]. The posterior of these branches carries preganglionic **parasympathetic nerve fibres** from the chorda tympani branch of the facial nerve. These nerves synapse on the cells of the ganglion. The anterior branch carries axons from the ganglion cells (post-ganglionic fibres) to the lingual nerve for distribution to the sublingual gland and to the glands in the anterior two-thirds of the tongue. From the inferior border of the submandibular ganglion, several small branches carry post-ganglionic fibres to the submandibular gland and duct and to the mucous membrane of the mouth.

Post-ganglionic **sympathetic fibres** reach the ganglion from the plexuses on the facial and lingual arteries, and supply the glands [Figs. 16.3, 16.5]. **Sensory fibres** from the lingual nerve also traverse the ganglion and are distributed through its branches.

Hypoglossal nerve

The hypoglossal nerve has already been traced to the posterior margin of the mylohyoid muscle

DISSECTION 16.5 Structures deep to the hyoglossus

Objectives

I. To identify and trace the lingual vessels deep to the hyoglossus. **II.** To expose the genioglossus, middle constrictor, and stylohyoid ligament.

Instructions

1. Detach the hyoglossus carefully from the hyoid bone, and turn it upwards without dividing the structures on its lateral surface.

2. Identify: (1) the lingual artery and its dorsal branches; (2) the lingual veins; (3) the posterior part of the genioglossus and the origin of the middle constrictor muscle of the pharynx; and (4) the attachment of the stylohyoid ligament.

[Chapter 6]. It can now be followed anteriorly with the deep lingual vein across the hyoglossus, between the hyoid bone and the submandibular duct. Anterior to the hyoglossus, the hypoglossal nerve pierces the genioglossus muscle and breaks up into branches to the muscles of the tongue [Fig. 16.3].

Branches of the hypoglossal nerve

The hypoglossal nerve supplies the styloglossus, hyoglossus, genioglossus, geniohyoid (C. 1 fibres), and intrinsic muscles of the tongue (all the tongue muscles, except the palatoglossus which is supplied by the vagus).

It communicates freely with the lingual nerve on the lateral surface of the hyoglossus and in the substance of the tongue. These communications transmit sensory nerve fibres from the muscles to the brainstem. For distribution of the first cervical nerve with the hypoglossal nerve, see ansa cervicalis [Chapter 6].

Using the instructions given in Dissection 16.5, dissect the structures deep to the hyoglossus.

Lingual artery

The lingual artery arises from the front of the external carotid artery, opposite the tip of the greater horn of the hyoid bone. It loops on the hyoid bone, runs anteriorly under cover of the hyoglossus, and ends by becoming the deep artery of the tongue [see Fig. 9.15; Fig. 16.3].

The initial segment lies deep to the skin, fasciae, and hypoglossal nerve, before passing deep to the hyoglossus. It gives off the **suprahyoid artery** which runs along the superior border of the hyoid bone, lateral to the hyoglossus. Deep to the hyoglossus, the artery gives off two or more **dorsal lingual branches**, which run posterosuperiorly to supply the substance of the tongue and end in the mucous membrane [Fig. 16.3].

At the anterior border of the hyoglossus, the lingual artery is crossed by branches of the hypoglossal nerve, the submandibular duct, and the lingual nerve. It gives off the **sublingual artery**, which runs anterosuperiorly to supply the sublingual gland and the neighbouring muscles [Fig. 16.3].

The lingual artery continues as the **deep artery of the tongue**, which enters the tongue about its middle and runs forwards to the tip, lying close to the mucous membrane of the ventral surface of the tongue. It is tortuous to allow for the elongation of the tongue when protruded. It sends numerous branches into the substance of the tongue [Fig. 16.3].

Veins of the tongue

The arrangement of the veins of the tongue is variable. The **deep lingual vein** is the principal vein of the tongue. It begins at the tip of the tongue and runs posteriorly near the median plane. It lies immediately deep to the mucous membrane on the inferior surface of the tongue and can be seen through it in life [see Fig. 17.1]. It descends along the anterior margin of the hyoglossus and crosses the superficial surface of that muscle below the hypoglossal nerve. Two venae comitantes run with the lingual artery and are joined by the dorsal lingual veins. All the veins unite at the posterior border of

the hyoglossus to form the **lingual vein**. The lingual vein either joins the facial vein or crosses the external and internal carotid arteries, to drain into the internal jugular vein [see Fig. 6.1].

Stylohyoid ligament

The stylohyoid ligament passes from the tip of the styloid process of the temporal bone to the lesser horn of the hyoid bone. It may be partly cartilaginous or ossified. Occasionally, it may contain muscle fibres [Figs. 16.3, 16.5].

It is of embryological interest as it represents the remnant of the cartilage of the second pharyngeal arch of the embryo. The remainder of the cartilage forms the stapes, the styloid process of the temporal bone, the lesser horn, and the upper part of the body of the hyoid bone. It corresponds to the sphenomandibular ligament of the first pharyngeal arch.

See Clinical Application 16.1 for the practical implications of the anatomy discussed in this chapter.

CLINICAL APPLICATION 16.1

Ranula

When the duct of a salivary gland is obstructed, the secretions will remain in the gland and develop into a retention cyst, with the gland itself becoming dilated. Such a retention cyst can be the result of minor trauma to the oral mucosa, resulting in fibrosis and scarring around the duct.

A **ranula** is a large, tense, bluish swelling in the floor of the mouth, to one side of the midline. It results from obstruction to drainage of the sublingual gland.

CHAPTER 17
The mouth and pharynx

The mouth

The mouth is the first part of the digestive tube. It is subdivided by the teeth and gums into the smaller external vestibule, which is deep to the lips and cheeks, and the larger mouth proper within the dental arch.

Vestibule of the mouth

The vestibule receives the ducts of the parotid glands and the mucous glands of the lips and cheeks. Superiorly and inferiorly, it is bound to the maxillae and mandible by the reflection of the mucous membrane from the lips and cheeks. Posteriorly, the vestibule communicates with the cavity of the mouth proper through the interval between the last molar teeth and the rami of the mandible. ➲ In paralysis of the facial muscles, the lips and cheeks fall away from the teeth and gums, and food tends to lodge in the vestibule.

Lips

The superficial structures in the lips have been examined [Chapter 4]. Each lip consists of a sheet of muscle covered externally by skin and internally by mucous membrane and connective tissue. The muscle layer is formed by the orbicularis oris and the various facial muscles which converge on it. The mucous membrane is continuous with the skin at the margins of the lips. In the midline, the mucous membrane forms a raised fold—the **frenulum**, between the lip and the jaw. Deep to

the mucous layer are numerous mucous **labial glands** with ducts which open into the vestibule of the mouth. Each lip has an **arterial arch** formed by the labial branches of the facial arteries [see Fig. 4.6].

The **lymph vessels** of the lower lip pass to the submandibular nodes; those of the upper lip pass to the submandibular and superficial parotid nodes.

Cheeks

The cheeks are directly continuous with the lips and have the same general structure. The principal muscle in the cheek is the **buccinator**. Posteriorly, the buccinator lies edge to edge with the superior constrictor muscle of the pharynx at the pterygomandibular raphe [see Fig. 6.5]. It is covered externally by the **buccopharyngeal fascia** and internally by the **pharyngobasilar fascia**.

There is a considerable amount of subcutaneous fat in the cheek, particularly in infants where the encapsulated **buccal pad of fat** is especially well formed. This pad of fat assists in sucking by increasing the rigidity of the cheek in the absence of teeth. Numerous **buccal glands** lie in the connective tissue beneath the mucosa, and four or five larger mucous **molar glands** lie external to the buccinator around the entry of the parotid duct. The **parotid duct** passes above the buccal pad of fat, pierces the buccinator and its fasciae, and enters the mouth opposite the second upper molar tooth [see Fig. 4.6].

Gums and teeth

The gums are composed of dense fibrous tissue covered with a smooth, vascular mucous membrane. They are attached to the alveolar margins of the jaws and the neck of the teeth. At the neck of the tooth, the fibrous tissue of the gum is continuous with the **periodontal membrane** which attaches the tooth to its socket.

In the adult, there are 16 **permanent teeth** in each jaw. On each side, from the midline, these are the two incisors, one canine, two premolars, and three molars. The complete **primary dentition** consists of ten teeth in each jaw—on each side, two incisors, one canine, and two molars. The first of these to erupt are the lower central incisors which erupt at approximately six months of age. The last milk teeth to erupt are the second milk molars at approximately two years of age. The first permanent tooth to erupt is the first molar. It erupts at approximately six years of age.

Floor of the mouth

The floor of the mouth is covered by mucous membrane. Laterally, this mucous membrane passes from the side of the tongue on to the mandible. Anteriorly, it stretches from one half of the mandible to the other, beneath the free anterior part of the tongue. In the midline, it forms a fold—the **frenulum of the tongue**—between the floor of the mouth and

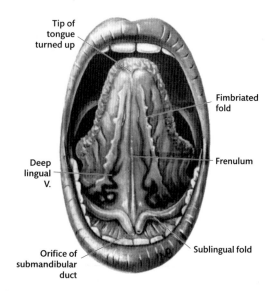

Fig. 17.1 The inferior surface of the tongue.

the inferior surface of the tongue. On both sides of the frenulum, the sublingual gland bulges upwards, forming the **sublingual fold** which ends anteriorly in the **sublingual papilla**. The submandibular duct opens on the apex of the papilla. The sublingual ducts open in a series of minute apertures on the top of the sublingual fold [see Fig. 17.1].

Roof of the mouth

The roof of the mouth is formed by the vaulted palate [Figs. 17.2, 17.3]. The anterior two-thirds of the palate is bony—the **hard palate**; the posterior

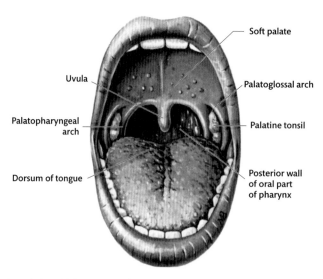

Fig. 17.2 The structures seen through the widely open mouth.

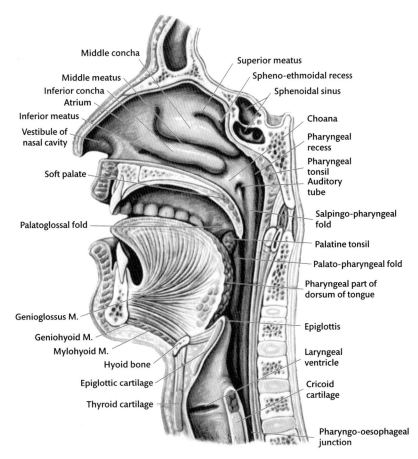

Middle concha
Middle meatus
Inferior concha
Atrium
Inferior meatus
Vestibule of
nasal cavity
Soft palate
Palatoglossal fold
Genioglossus M.
Geniohyoid M.
Mylohyoid M.
Hyoid bone
Epiglottic cartilage
Thyroid cartilage

Superior meatus
Spheno-ethmoidal recess
Sphenoidal sinus
Choana
Pharyngeal recess
Pharyngeal tonsil
Auditory tube
Salpingo-pharyngeal fold
Palatine tonsil
Palato-pharyngeal fold
Pharyngeal part of dorsum of tongue
Epiglottis
Laryngeal ventricle
Cricoid cartilage
Pharyngo-oesophageal junction

Fig. 17.3 Paramedian section through the nose, mouth, pharynx, and larynx.

third is made up of soft tissue—the **soft palate**. The soft palate has a free posterior margin from which hangs down the median **uvula**. A poorly marked median raphe, representing the line of embryological fusion between the two halves of the palate, extends from the incisive fossa to the uvula. The mucous membrane of the anterior part of the hard palate is thrown into three to four **transverse palatine folds**. The mucous membrane of the posterior part is comparatively smooth. By careful palpation with a finger or the tongue, feel the **pterygoid hamulus**, immediately posterior to the lingual surface of the third upper molar tooth.

Isthmus of the fauces

Posteriorly, the mouth narrows to join the pharynx at the isthmus of the fauces. The term fauces indicates the region where the mouth opens into the pharynx. It is bounded by the soft palate, the palatoglossal arches, and the dorsum of the tongue [Fig. 17.2].

Palatoglossal arch

The palatoglossal fold of mucous membrane covers the palatoglossus muscle. It passes antero-inferiorly from the soft palate to the posterior part of the side of the tongue [Fig. 17.2].

The pharynx

The pharynx is a wide muscular tube, about 12 cm long. It extends from the base of the skull above to the level of the body of the sixth cervical vertebra below [Fig. 17.3] where it is continuous with the oesophagus. The pharynx lies posterior to the nasal cavities and septum (**nasopharynx**), the mouth (**oropharynx**), and the larynx (**laryngopharynx**). It conducts air to and from the larynx, and food to the oesophagus. The oral part of the pharynx is common to both functions.

The pharynx is widest at the base of the skull, posterior to the orifices of the auditory tubes. From there, it narrows to the level of the palate (**pharyngeal isthmus**), widens again in the oral and laryngeal parts, and then rapidly narrows to the oesophagus.

The walls of the pharynx above the opening of the larynx are not in contact with each other and allow the passage of air through the mouth or nasal cavities to the larynx. Below the opening of the larynx, the anterior and posterior walls are in contact.

Position

The pharynx lies anterior to the prevertebral fascia. The pharyngeal venous plexus, the alar fascia, and a layer of loose areolar tissue lie between the pharynx and the prevertebral fascia and allow the pharynx to slide freely on it during swallowing. Lateral to the pharynx is the neurovascular bundle of the neck (common and internal carotid arteries, internal jugular vein, and vagus nerve) in the carotid sheath [Fig. 17.4], and the styloid process of the temporal bone and its muscles. The pharyngeal plexus of nerves ramifies on the pharynx and supplies it with motor and sensory fibres. Anteriorly, the pharynx opens into the nasal cavities, mouth, and larynx. The pharyngeal muscles are attached to structures in the lateral walls of these apertures.

Pharyngeal wall

The wall of the pharynx consists of five layers. From within out, they are the: (1) mucous membrane; (2) submucosa; (3) pharyngobasilar fascia; (4) pharyngeal muscles; and (5) buccopharyngeal fascia.

The **buccopharyngeal fascia** covers the external surfaces of the buccinator and the pharyngeal muscles. The **pharyngobasilar fascia** lines the internal surface of the pharyngeal muscles and attaches the pharynx to the base of the skull, the auditory tubes, and the lateral margins of the posterior nasal apertures (choanae). It also fills the gap in the pharyngeal wall above the free superior margin of the superior constrictor muscle [Fig. 17.5].

The muscles of the pharynx consist of the three constrictors—the superior, middle, and inferior constrictors— and the stylopharyngeus, salpingopharyngeus, and palatopharyngeus muscles [Fig. 17.5].

Using the instructions given in Dissection 17.1, dissect the muscles of the pharynx.

Pharyngeal plexus of veins

The pharyngeal plexus of veins lies on the posterior wall of the pharynx and receives blood from the pharynx and soft palate. Two or more veins drain from the plexus to each internal jugular vein. It also communicates with the pterygoid plexus and the cavernous sinuses.

Constrictor muscles of the pharynx

The three constrictor muscles—the superior, middle, and inferior constrictors—form a curved sheet on the posterior and lateral walls of the pharynx. They overlap each other from below upwards [Fig. 17.5]. They take origin from a series of bones and ligaments on the lateral wall and are inserted posteriorly into a median fibrous **raphe** which descends from the **pharyngeal tubercle** on the base of the skull to the oesophagus [see Fig. 9.5]. **Nerve supply**: the pharyngeal plexus of the glossopharyngeal and vagus nerves, with an additional supply to the inferior constrictor

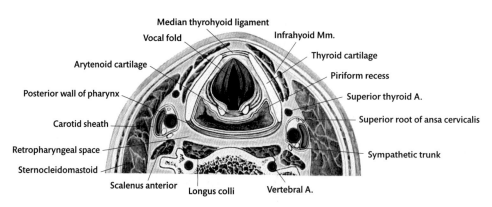

Median thyrohyoid ligament
Vocal fold
Infrahyoid Mm.
Arytenoid cartilage
Thyroid cartilage
Posterior wall of pharynx
Piriform recess
Superior thyroid A.
Carotid sheath
Superior root of ansa cervicalis
Retropharyngeal space
Sympathetic trunk
Sternocleidomastoid
Scalenus anterior
Longus colli
Vertebral A.

Fig. 17.4 Transverse section through the anterior part of the neck at the level of the upper part of the thyroid cartilage.

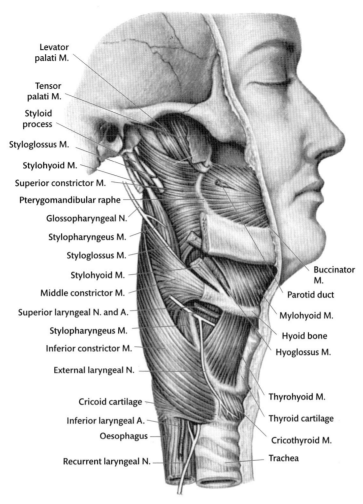

Levator palati M.
Tensor palati M.
Styloid process
Styloglossus M.
Stylohyoid M.
Superior constrictor M.
Pterygomandibular raphe
Glossopharyngeal N.
Stylopharyngeus M.
Styloglossus M.
Stylohyoid M.
Middle constrictor M.
Superior laryngeal N. and A.
Stylopharyngeus M.
Inferior constrictor M.
External laryngeal N.
Cricoid cartilage
Inferior laryngeal A.
Oesophagus
Recurrent laryngeal N.

Buccinator M.
Parotid duct
Mylohyoid M.
Hyoid bone
Hyoglossus M.
Thyrohyoid M.
Thyroid cartilage
Cricothyroid M.
Trachea

Fig. 17.5 Lateral view of the constrictors of the pharynx and associated muscles.

DISSECTION 17.1 Muscles of the pharynx

Objectives

I. To identify the three constrictors of the pharynx.
II. To identify and trace the stylopharyngeus muscle and glossopharyngeal nerve.

Instructions

1. On the right side, remove the buccopharyngeal fascia from the external surfaces of the pharyngeal muscles [Fig. 17.5].

2. Note the plexus of nerves and veins, and then remove them.

3. On the posterior surface of the pharynx at the level of the angle of the mandible, find the stylopharyngeus muscle entering the pharynx between the superior and middle constrictor muscles [Fig. 17.5].

4. Expose the glossopharyngeal nerve winding spirally round the posterior surface of the stylopharyngeus. Trace the branch to the stylopharyngeus. The nerve will be followed into the posterior part of the tongue later.

5. Find the upper border of the inferior constrictor. Turn this downwards, and expose the lowest fibres of the middle constrictor arching upwards from the hyoid bone.

6. On the left side, examine the interior of the pharynx, and strip off its mucous membrane to expose the pharyngeal muscles from the medial side [Fig. 17.6].

Objective

I. To expose the superior constrictor of the pharynx.

Instructions

1. On the right side, detach the medial pterygoid muscle from its origin, and turn it down. This exposes the full extent of the superior constrictor.

from the external and recurrent laryngeal nerves. **Actions**: see Swallowing, p. 215.

Dissection 17.2 provides instructions on dissection of the superior constrictor.

Superior constrictor

The superior constrictor lies in the wall of the nasal and oral parts of the pharynx. It arises from the lower part of the posterior margin of the medial pterygoid lamina, the pterygoid hamulus, the pterygomandibular raphe, the mandible near the posterior end of the mylohyoid line, and the mucous membrane of the mouth and side of the tongue. The fibres curve posteriorly to the median raphe. The upper fibres ascend to the pharyngeal tubercle [see Fig. 3.7]; the lower fibres descend internal to the middle constrictor. The stylopharyngeus muscle and glossopharyngeal nerve enter the pharynx between the superior and middle constrictors [Fig. 17.5].

The free **upper border** of the superior constrictor extends from the medial pterygoid lamina to the pharyngeal tubercle, leaving a gap between it and the skull. This gap is filled by the pharyngobasilar fascia, the tensor and levator palati muscles, and the auditory tube between them [Fig. 17.5]. The **auditory tube** and the **levator muscle** of the palate enter the pharynx above the superior margin of the superior constrictor, together with the ascending palatine artery. The **tensor palati** descends external to the upper part of the superior constrictor.

The **pterygomandibular raphe** is formed by the interlacing tendinous fibres of the superior constrictor and buccinator muscles. It extends from the pterygoid hamulus to the mandible near the posterior end of the mylohyoid line. The tendinous fibres run horizontally and are capable of separating and allowing the raphe to stretch when the mouth is opened [Fig. 17.5].

Middle constrictor

The middle constrictor is fan-shaped and takes origin from the greater and lesser horns of the hyoid bone, and the lower part of the stylohyoid ligament [Figs. 17.5, 17.6]. From this curved origin, the fibres fan out into the pharyngeal wall, the middle fibres running horizontally. The inferior part of the muscle passes deep to the inferior constrictor posteriorly but is separated from it laterally by a gap. The internal branch of the superior laryngeal nerve and the superior laryngeal artery pass through this gap to pierce the thyrohyoid membrane and enter into the pharynx [Fig. 17.5].

Inferior constrictor

The inferior constrictor takes origin from the side of the cricoid cartilage, the fascia covering the cricothyroid, and the oblique line on the thyroid cartilage [Fig. 17.5]. The part of the muscle arising from the thyroid cartilage is the **thyropharyngeus**, and that arising from the fascia over the cricothyroid and the cricoid cartilage the **cricopharyngeus**. Its fibres sweep posteriorly to the median raphe; the lowest fibres are horizontal, but the upper fibres ascend with increasing obliquity. The highest fibres almost reach the base of the skull, external to the other two constrictors. Inferiorly, the inferior constrictor overlaps the beginning of the oesophagus, the recurrent laryngeal nerve, and the inferior laryngeal artery [Fig. 17.5].

Interior of the pharynx

The pharynx is lined by mucous membrane, and the submucosa contains numerous mucous **pharyngeal glands** and nodules of lymph tissue. Aggregations of these **lymph follicles** form the pharyngeal, tubal, palatine, and lingual **tonsils**.

Nasopharynx

The nasal part of the pharynx, or nasopharynx, lies superior to the soft palate and is continuous inferiorly with the oral part, or oropharynx, through the narrow **pharyngeal isthmus** [Fig. 17.3].The opening of the nasal cavities into the nasopharynx is known as the **choana**. Each choana is oval in shape, approximately 2.5 cm high and 1.5 cm wide, and extends from the base of the skull to the posterior edge of the hard palate. They are separated from each other by the nasal septum [Fig. 17.3].

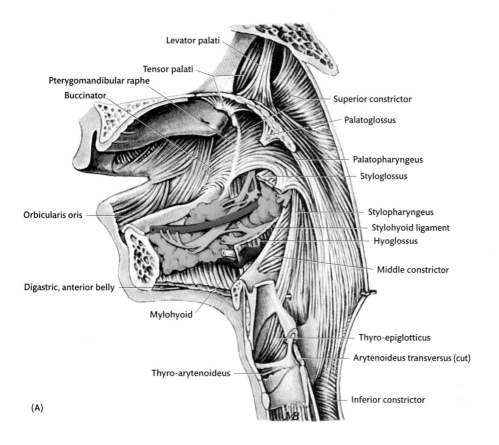

Levator palati

Tensor palati

Pterygomandibular raphe

Buccinator

Superior constrictor

Palatoglossus

Palatopharyngeus

Styloglossus

Orbicularis oris

Stylopharyngeus

Stylohyoid ligament

Hyoglossus

Middle constrictor

Digastric, anterior belly

Mylohyoid

Thyro-epiglotticus

Arytenoideus transversus (cut)

Thyro-arytenoideus

Inferior constrictor

(A)

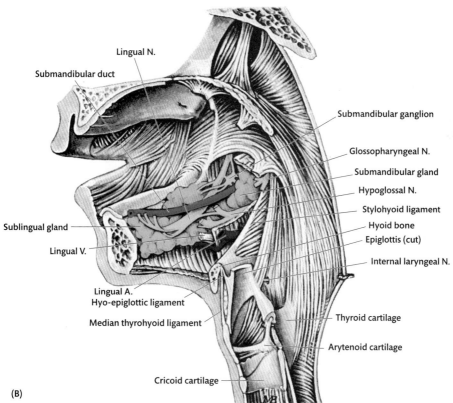

Lingual N.

Submandibular duct

Submandibular ganglion

Glossopharyngeal N.

Submandibular gland

Hypoglossal N.

Stylohyoid ligament

Sublingual gland

Hyoid bone

Lingual V.

Epiglottis (cut)

Internal laryngeal N.

Lingual A.

Hyo-epiglottic ligament

Median thyrohyoid ligament

Thyroid cartilage

Arytenoid cartilage

Cricoid cartilage

(B)

Fig. 17.6 (A) and (B) Structures lying adjacent to the mucous membrane of the mouth, pharynx, and larynx, seen from the medial side. The tongue has been removed to expose the structures which lie between it and the mylohyoid muscle.

The **roof** and **posterior wall** of the nasopharynx form a continuous curved surface. This surface extends over the inferior aspect of the sphenoid, the basilar part of the occipital bone, and the superior part of the longus capitis muscle. The **pharyngeal tonsil** bulges the mucous membrane into the cavity of the pharynx where the roof becomes continuous with the posterior wall [Fig. 17.3]. ↻ This lymph tissue is often enlarged in children—the adenoids.

It may be large enough to block the nasal part of the pharynx and give a 'nasal' quality to the voice.

The **pharyngeal orifice of the auditory tube** lies on the **lateral wall** of the pharynx, at the level of the inferior concha of the nose [Fig. 17.7]. It is bound superiorly and posteriorly by a firm, rounded **tubal ridge** around which lies the **tubal tonsil**. The slender **salpingopharyngeus muscle** descends from the tubal ridge into the lateral wall of the

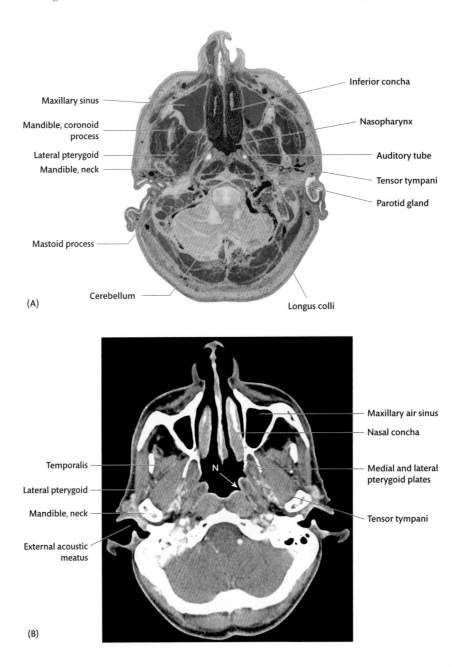

Fig. 17.7 (A) Transverse section of the head at the level of the nasopharynx. (B) Axial contrast computerized tomography (CT) through the head at the level of the nasopharynx. N = nasopharynx; arrow = opening of auditory tube.

Image A courtesy of the Visible Human Project of the US National Library of Medicine.

pharynx. It is covered by the salpingopharyngeal fold of mucous membrane. Posterior to the tubal ridge and the levator palati immediately behind it, the deep **pharyngeal recess** extends laterally, above the upper margin of the superior constrictor [Fig. 17.3]. The **pharyngeal isthmus** lies at the lower end of the nasopharynx, posterior to the palate. It is limited laterally by the **palatopharyngeal arches**.

➲ The nasopharynx can be illuminated by light reflected from a mirror introduced through the mouth. A view of the orifices of the auditory tubes, the side walls and roof of the nasopharynx, the choanae, and the posterior ends of the middle and inferior conchae can be obtained.

Salpingopharyngeus

This slender muscle arises by one or two slips from the inferior border of the pharyngeal end of the auditory tube. It descends in the salpingopharyngeal fold to join the palatopharyngeus.

Oropharynx

The oral part of the pharynx, or oropharynx, lies posterior to the palatoglossal arch. The posterior one-third of the dorsum of the tongue forms the anterior boundary [Figs. 17.2, 17.3]. Small, scattered collections of lymphocytes in the dorsum of the posterior third of the tongue give the pharyngeal part of the tongue its nodular appearance. These are the **lingual tonsil**. Immediately posterior to the tongue is the **epiglottis**—a curved, leaf-shaped plate of elastic cartilage covered with mucous membrane. The upper part of the epiglottis is posterior to the tongue and is readily visible through the mouth in children. Pull the epiglottis backwards to expose the **median glosso-epiglottic fold**—a median ridge of mucous membrane between the front of the epiglottis and the back of the tongue. On each side of this fold is a depression—the **epiglottic vallecula**. The **lateral glosso-epiglottic folds** are ridges of mucous membrane which form the lateral boundaries of the epiglottic valleculae. They extend from the margins of the epiglottis to the side walls of the pharynx at their junction with the tongue [see Fig. 18.1].

Palatine tonsils

The palatine tonsils are masses of lymphoid tissue which lie in the mucous membrane on the lateral walls of the oropharynx, between the palatoglossal and palatopharyngeal folds. They are deep to the angle of the mandible, between the back of the tongue and the soft palate. In children, they are larger than the fossae between the arches and, as such, bulge into the pharynx. They also extend superiorly into the soft palate and anteriorly lateral to the palatoglossal arch [Fig. 17.3].

The medial surface of the palatine tonsils is covered by mucous membrane which forms about 12 deep **tonsillar crypts**. Superiorly, the tonsil is bounded by a mucosal fold under which lies the **supratonsillar fossa**.

The lateral surface of the palatine tonsils is covered by a thin fibrous **capsule**. The capsule is attached to the pharyngobasilar fascia by loose areolar tissue. The superior constrictor of the pharynx and the facial artery lie further laterally [see Fig. 9.15; Fig. 17.8].

Vessels and nerves of the palatine tonsil

The main artery of the palatine tonsils is the **tonsillar branch of the facial artery** [see Fig. 9.15]. It pierces the superior constrictor and enters the inferior part of the lateral surface. One or more inconstant **veins** descend from the soft palate, lateral to the tonsillar capsule. They pierce the superior constrictor near the artery, and either end in the pharyngeal plexus or unite to form a single vessel which drains into the facial vein. ➲ These veins may be a source of troublesome bleeding at tonsillectomy, especially when they unite to form a single larger vein.

Efferent lymph vessels from the palatine tonsils pierce the superior constrictor and pass to nodes on the carotid sheath, including the jugulodigastric at the angle of the mandible and the posterior submandibular nodes. **Nerve supply**: sensory nerves are from the glossopharyngeal and lesser palatine nerves.

Lymphoid aggregations in the pharynx

Collections of lymphoid tissue in the pharynx form the pharyngeal and tubal tonsils in the nasopharynx, and the palatine and lingual tonsils in the oropharynx. These masses of lymph tissue form an almost complete ring in the wall of the pharynx where the nasal and oral cavities open into it. ➲ This tissue, like similar tissue in the small and large intestines, appears to be concerned with protection against ingested and inspired pathogens and is, no doubt, involved in the production of antibodies to invading organisms. The volume of this lymph tissue is normally much greater in children than in adults.

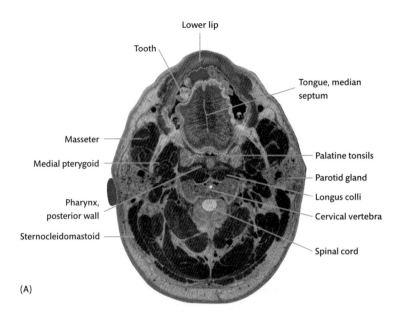

(A)

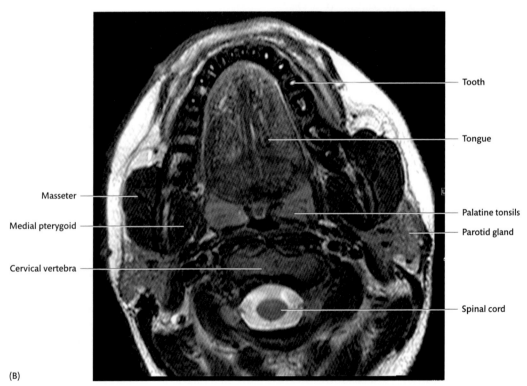

(B)

Fig. 17.8 (A) Transverse section through the oropharynx showing the palatine tonsils. (B) MRI image.

Image A courtesy of the Visible Human Project of the US National Library of Medicine.

Soft palate

The soft palate is a flexible, muscular flap which extends postero-inferiorly from the posterior edge of the hard palate. Laterally, it is attached to the lateral walls of the pharynx, and the **uvula** hangs down from the middle of its free posterior border. The lateral edge of the free border is continuous with the palatopharyngeal arch on each side [Fig. 17.2].

The soft palate acts as a flap valve. It can be raised and pulled posteriorly against the posterior pharyngeal wall, to shut off the nasopharynx from the oropharynx. This movement permits such actions as: (1) blowing a balloon or coughing, without air escaping through the nose; and (2) swallowing, without food and fluid regurgitating into the nose.

When the soft palate is pulled inferiorly against the posterior part of the tongue, it cuts off the mouth from the pharynx and permits respiration to continue during sucking or chewing, without danger of food or fluid entering the trachea. The uvula (somewhat like the nodules on the pulmonary and aortic valves [Vol. 2, p. 63]) helps to prevent the soft palate from being forced into the nasopharynx in coughing when the pressure difference between the nasopharynx and oropharynx is high, or into the mouth in sneezing when the pressure difference between the mouth and nasopharynx is high. When tensed, the soft palate assists the tongue in directing food and fluids towards the laryngeal part of the pharynx in swallowing.

Muscles of the soft palate

The soft palate is made up of a fold of mucous membrane enclosing parts of five pairs of muscles—the tensor palati, levator palati, palatoglossus, palatopharyngeus, and musculus uvulae. The musculus uvulae is an intrinsic muscle of the soft palate. Each of the remaining pairs of muscles form a sling between the muscles of the right and left, at the attachment to the **palatal aponeurosis**. The convex superior surface of the soft palate is continuous with the floor of the nasal cavities. Posteriorly, it abuts on the posterior pharyngeal wall. The **mucous membrane** of the oral surface is thick and has a layer of tightly packed **mucous glands**.

Tensor palati

The tensor palati takes origin from: (1) the scaphoid fossa at the base of the medial pterygoid lamina; (2) the spine of the sphenoid; (3) the auditory tube; and (4) the margin of the greater wing of the sphenoid. It passes downwards, anterior to the auditory tube, converges on a tendon, hooks around the **pterygoid hamulus** [see Fig. 15.8; Figs. 17.5, 17.6], and spreads out horizontally into the soft palate. In the soft palate, the tensor palati tendons of the two sides meet in the midline and form the **palatal aponeurosis** [see Fig. 13.6].

Anteriorly, this aponeurosis is attached to the palatine crests on the inferior surface of the hard palate and is thick and rigid. Posteriorly, it is thin. **Nerve supply**: mandibular division of the trigeminal nerve. **Action**: the tensor palati makes the anterior part of the soft palate rigid.

Musculus uvulae

The musculus uvulae take origin from the posterior nasal spine of the palatine bones and are inserted into the mucous membrane of the uvula. They lie on the superior surface of the palatal aponeurosis and run side by side in the midline. **Nerve supply**: the pharyngeal plexus formed by the glossopharyngeal and vagal nerves. **Actions**: the musculus uvulae shorten and tense the uvula.

Levator palati (levator veli palatini)

The levator palati arises from the medial side of the auditory tube and the adjacent part of the petrous temporal bone. It descends behind the auditory tube, medial to the free upper border of the superior constrictor muscle, and curves medially to join the opposite muscle. It is partially attached to the superior surface of the palatal aponeurosis. **Nerve supply**: the pharyngeal plexus formed by the glossopharyngeal and vagus nerves. **Action**: the two muscles acting together raise the palate symmetrically [Figs. 17.5, 17.6].

Palatoglossus

The **palatoglossus** is a small counterpart of the levator palati on the inferior surface of the palate. It takes origin from the inferior surface of the palatal aponeurosis, converges on the palatoglossal arch, and runs through the arch to merge with the muscles of the posterolateral part of the tongue [Figs. 17.3, 17.6]. **Nerve supply**: the pharyngeal plexus formed by the glossopharyngeal and vagus nerves. **Action**: the two muscles acting together draw the soft palate inferiorly onto the posterior part of the dorsum of the tongue.

Palatopharyngeus

The palatopharyngeus arises from the superior surface of the soft palate and the posterior margin of the hard palate. The fibres of the palatopharyngeus spread over the internal surface of the constrictors. Most of the muscle fibres converge on the palatopharyngeal arch and run inferiorly in it, on the internal surfaces of the constrictors of the pharynx. It is inserted into the posterior border of the lamina of the thyroid cartilage and fans out into the posterior pharyngeal wall [Fig. 17.6]. Superiorly, the palatopharyngeus is joined by the salpingopharyngeus, and inferiorly by the stylopharyngeus at the interval between the middle and superior constrictors. The superior margin of the palatopharyngeus passes almost horizontally backwards around the pharyngeal isthmus.

⬎ The part which surrounds the pharyngeal isthmus is greatly hypertrophied in persons with cleft palate, in an attempt to separate the oral and nasal parts of the pharynx.

Nerve supply: the pharyngeal plexus formed by the glossopharyngeal and vagus nerves. **Actions**: the main mass of the palatopharyngeus depresses the palate onto the posterior part of the dorsum of the tongue and prevents the soft palate from being forced into the nasal part of the pharynx when blowing against resistance through the mouth. The horizontal fibres, with those of the superior constrictor, narrow the pharyngeal isthmus. They also raise a ridge in the pharyngeal wall, against which the soft palate is elevated by the levator palati to separate the oropharynx and nasopharynx.

Vessels and nerves of the soft palate

The **ascending palatine branch of the facial artery** ascends on the lateral pharyngeal wall to the superior border of the superior constrictor, hooks over this border, and descends with the levator palati to the palate. This is the main arterial supply to the soft palate and is supplemented by the lesser palatine branches of the greater palatine artery.

The **lesser palatine** and **glossopharyngeal nerves** supply the mucous membrane. The tensor palati is supplied by the **mandibular nerve** through the otic ganglion. All the other muscles are supplied by the **pharyngeal plexus**—a glossopharyngeal/vagal complex.

Laryngopharynx

The laryngeal part of the pharynx, or laryngopharynx, lies posterior to the larynx. It decreases in width from above downwards, so that the **oesophageal orifice** is the narrowest part of the pharynx and lies opposite the inferior border of the cricoid cartilage [Fig. 17.3].

The **posterior** and **lateral walls** of the laryngopharynx are formed by the middle and inferior constrictor muscles, with the palatopharyngeus and stylopharyngeus on the inner aspect [Fig. 17.6].

The **anterior wall** is formed superiorly by: (1) the inlet of the larynx; and (2) the piriform recess which extends forwards on each side of the inlet. Inferiorly, the anterior wall is formed by: (3) the mucous membrane on the posterior surfaces of the arytenoid and cricoid cartilages [Fig. 17.9]. (The piriform recess lies medial to the thyroid cartilage and thyrohyoid membrane.) The interarytenoid muscles, the posterior crico-arytenoid muscles, and the attachment of the longitudinal muscles of the oesophagus lie in the anterior wall of the laryngopharynx [see Fig. 20.10].

Inlet of the larynx

The inlet of the larynx is an almost vertically placed opening. It is bound anterosuperiorly by the epiglottis, on each side by the aryepiglottic fold of mucous membrane, and inferiorly by the interarytenoid fold of mucous membrane [Fig. 17.9].

Each **aryepiglottic fold** is a thin fold that extends inferiorly from the margin of the epiglottis to the arytenoid cartilage. It contains the thin aryepiglottic muscle. Near the inferior end of the fold are two small pieces of cartilage which form the **corniculate** and **cuneiform tubercles** in its free edge [Fig. 17.9].

The **arytenoid cartilages** are paired three-sided cartilages placed side by side on the superior border of the lamina of the cricoid cartilage [see Fig. 20.3]. The interarytenoid fold of mucous membrane passes between them and forms the inferior boundary of the inlet. The interarytenoid fold encloses the muscles which pass between the posterior surfaces of the arytenoid cartilages [see Fig. 20.10].

Piriform recess

The deep piriform recess separates the aryepiglottic fold from the posterior surface of the lamina of the thyroid cartilage and the thyrohyoid membrane. It is lined with mucous membrane and ends as a blind sac inferiorly. Foreign bodies may lodge in this sac and pierce the mucous membrane.

Stylopharyngeus

The stylopharyngeus is the longest of the three styloid muscles. It arises from the medial surface of the

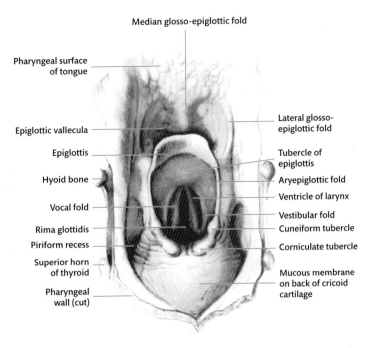

Median glosso-epiglottic fold

Pharyngeal surface of tongue

Epiglottic vallecula

Epiglottis

Hyoid bone

Vocal fold

Rima glottidis

Piriform recess

Superior horn of thyroid

Pharyngeal wall (cut)

Lateral glosso-epiglottic fold

Tubercle of epiglottis

Aryepiglottic fold

Ventricle of larynx

Vestibular fold

Cuneiform tubercle

Corniculate tubercle

Mucous membrane on back of cricoid cartilage

Fig. 17.9 Anterior wall of the laryngopharynx seen from above. The tongue and epiglottis are pulled forwards.

styloid process close to its root. It runs antero-inferiorly, between the internal and external carotid arteries, and passes obliquely through the pharyngeal wall between the superior and middle constrictor muscles [Fig. 17.5]. Within the pharynx, it blends with the anterior fibres of the palatopharyngeus and is inserted partly with it and partly into the lateral aspect of the epiglottis [Fig. 17.5]. **Nerve supply**: the glossopharyngeal nerve. **Actions**: it helps to raise the larynx and pulls the base of the epiglottis upwards and backwards during swallowing and speaking.

Using the instructions given in Dissection 17.3, dissect the pharynx.

Swallowing

Now that the walls of the pharynx have been seen from the inner medial aspect, it is possible to visualize the mechanism of swallowing.

In the first phase of swallowing, the mouth is closed, the tip of the tongue is raised against the hard palate, anterior to the bolus of food or fluid, and the bolus is squeezed posteriorly by pressing progressively more posterior parts of the tongue against the palate (intrinsic muscles of the tongue, mylohyoid, and styloglossus). As this movement

passes backwards, elevation of the posterior part of the tongue against the tensed anterior part of the soft palate (tensor palati) is achieved by raising the hyoid bone (digastric, stylohyoid). At the same time, the geniohyoid carries the hyoid bone anteriorly, and this increases the anteroposterior diameter of the oropharynx to receive the bolus. The middle and inferior constrictor muscles are simultaneously relaxed. At this stage, the superior constrictor muscle and horizontal fibres of the palatopharyngeus contract to draw the upper part of the posterior pharyngeal wall against the raised posterior part of the soft palate (levator palati). This movement effectively shuts off the nasopharynx from the oropharynx and prevents food or fluid from entering the nasopharynx.

The second phase of swallowing is very rapid. There is considerable elevation of the larynx and the attached inferior part of the pharynx, to the raised hyoid bone. (The hyoid bone is raised by the digastric, stylopharyngeus, and palatopharyngeus muscles.) This movement brings the thyroid cartilage within the concavity of the hyoid bone and approximates the arytenoid cartilages to the epiglottis, thus closing the laryngeal orifice. Contraction of the aryepiglottic muscles [see Fig. 20.10] may help to draw the epiglottis down on the arytenoid cartilages. More importantly, elevation of

Objective

I. To identify and trace the muscles and vessels of the pharynx.

Instructions

1. Remove the mucous membrane from the palatopharyngeal and palatoglossal arches and from the salpingopharyngeal fold, to expose the muscles within them [Figs. 17.3, 17.6]. (The palatoglossus and salpingopharyngeus are small and often difficult to display.)

2. Remove the mucous membrane, connective tissue, and pharyngobasilar fascia from the wall of the pharynx, anterior and posterior to the opening of the auditory tube.

3. Identify the levator palati, posterior to the auditory tube, and follow it into the palate.

4. The ascending palatine artery may be seen descending beside the levator palati to the palate.

5. Trace the tensor palati inferiorly, lateral to the medial pterygoid lamina [Fig. 17.6], by turning the cartilage of the auditory tube backwards.

6. Identify the superior constrictor, lateral to the levator palati. Expose its superior border, and remove the mucous membrane from the parts of its medial surface which are not covered by the palatal muscles.

7. Dissect out the palatine tonsil.

8. Uncover the anterior part of the superior constrictor muscle. This part is difficult to define, as some of its fibres sweep inferiorly into the tongue, and it is often partly covered by thin sheets of muscle fibres passing inferiorly from the palate, lateral to the tonsil.

9. Follow the palatopharyngeus upwards into the soft palate, stripping off the thick glandular mucous membrane from its inferior surface as far as the hard palate.

10. Identify the pterygoid hamulus with the tendon of the tensor palati spreading medially from its base, to form the palatal aponeurosis.

11. Identify the pterygomandibular raphe passing from the pterygoid hamulus to the mandible, and follow the superior constrictor anteriorly to the raphe.

12. Anterior to the pterygomandibular raphe, strip the mucous membrane from the internal surface of the buccinator, and identify its attachments.

13. Identify the opening of the parotid duct.

14. Identify the greater horn of the hyoid bone. Remove the mucous membrane from the medial surface of the middle constrictor, leaving the palatopharyngeus in position on its medial aspect.

15. Follow the **palatopharyngeus** to the posterior border of the lamina of the thyroid cartilage.

16. Anterior to the palatopharyngeus, identify the **stylopharyngeus** entering the pharynx between the middle and superior constrictor muscles. It spreads anteroposteriorly in such a manner that its posterior fibres are inserted with those of the palatopharyngeus, and the anterior fibres pass to the lateral aspect of the epiglottis.

17. Look for the internal laryngeal nerve entering the pharynx through the thyrohyoid membrane below the fibres of the stylopharyngeus [Fig. 17.6].

18. Find the **glossopharyngeal** nerve, anterolateral to the stylopharyngeus, where it enters the pharynx, and trace the nerve to the tongue.

19. Finally remove the mucous membrane from the medial surface of the inferior constrictor, the upper part of the oesophagus, and the piriform recess.

20. In the piriform recess, identify the medial surface of the thyroid cartilage and the thyrohyoid membrane with the superior laryngeal vessels and the internal laryngeal nerve piercing it.

the base of the **epiglottis** through its attachment to the thyroid cartilage, and by contraction of the stylopharyngeus, pushes the apex of the epiglottis against the bulging posterior surface of the tongue and tips it backwards over the closed laryngeal orifice. The bolus of food from the back of the tongue now slips onto the lingual surface of the epiglottis (which now faces superiorly) and is carried down by the contracting middle and inferior constrictor muscles. This is aided by the rapid downward displacement of the larynx and pharynx (brought about by the infrahyoid muscles) which follows immediately and reopens the laryngeal orifice.

The importance of elevation of the hyoid bone and of the digastrics in this movement is shown by the difficulty in swallowing with the mouth open when the digastrics cannot act effectively on the hyoid bone because they are already shortened.

DISSECTION 17.4 Auditory tube

Objective

I. To study the course of the auditory tube.

Instructions

1. Identify the groove for the cartilaginous part, and the bony part of the auditory tube on a dried skull [see Fig. 3.7].

2. Ascertain the direction of the cartilaginous part of the tube by passing a probe into its pharyngeal orifice. At first, it runs superiorly and then posterolaterally between the tensor and the levator palati muscles [see Figs. 13.6, 13.10, 15.8].

3. Note that the levator palati forms a rounded prominence, inferior to the opening of the auditory tube. Remove the mucous membrane from the mouth of the tube, and note that the superior and medial walls are formed by a folded plate of **cartilage**.

Auditory tube

Dissection 17.4 provides instructions on dissection of the auditory tube.

The auditory, or pharyngotympanic, tube connects the nasopharynx to the middle ear cavity. The tube is approximately 3.5 cm long. The bony, posterolateral 1.5 cm lies between the tympanic and petrous parts of the temporal bone and opens into the middle ear cavity. The cartilaginous anteromedial part lies in the groove between the petrous part of the temporal bone and the posterior border of the greater wing of the sphenoid.

The superior and medial walls of the pharyngeal opening of the tube are formed by a folded plate of **cartilage**. The inferolateral part of the tube is completed by dense fibrous tissue joining the edges of the cartilage. The tubal ridge is formed by the base of the cartilage plate. The lumen of the auditory tube is narrowest (**isthmus**) where the cartilaginous and bony parts meet, but it gradually increases in diameter from the isthmus to the pharyngeal orifice, which is the widest part of the tube. The tube functions to equalize the pressure in the middle ear with the atmospheric pressure.

Using the instructions given in Dissection 17.5, expose the otic ganglion from the medial side.

DISSECTION 17.5 Otic ganglion

Objective

I. To study the otic ganglion and mandibular nerve.

Instructions

1. If the otic ganglion has not yet been seen, free the opening of the auditory tube from the medial pterygoid lamina and turn it posteriorly.

2. Separate the cartilaginous part of the tube from the base of the skull and the tensor palati. This exposes the tensor tympani—a small slip of muscle arising from the petrous temporal bone, superomedial to the tube and passing posterolaterally with it.

3. Detach the tensor palati from the base of the skull, and turn it inferiorly.

4. Remove the layer of fascia which is exposed, and uncover the mandibular nerve with the otic ganglion on its anteromedial aspect.

5. Immediately posterior to the mandibular nerve lies the middle meningeal artery at the foramen spinosum.

6. Identify the branches of the mandibular nerve as far as possible from this aspect, and note the close relation to the pharyngeal wall.

7. Confirm this relation on the base of a macerated skull.

Carotid canal

The carotid canal lies in the petrous part of the temporal bone. It contains the internal carotid artery, the internal carotid plexus of sympathetic nerve fibres, and a plexus of veins. Its position and course can be seen best on a macerated skull.

Internal carotid artery

The part of the internal carotid artery in the carotid canal is approximately 2 cm long. At first, it ascends vertically, then bends anteromedially, and runs horizontally to the apex of the petrous temporal bone [Fig. 17.10]. It enters the foramen lacerum through its posterior wall, turns upwards,

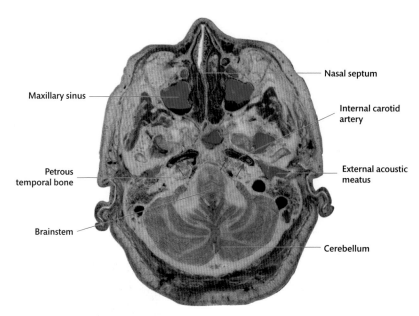

Labels on figure:
Maxillary sinus
Nasal septum
Internal carotid artery
Petrous temporal bone
External acoustic meatus
Brainstem
Cerebellum

Fig. 17.10 Transverse section through the petrous temporal bone showing the internal carotid artery in the carotid canal (red arrows). Image courtesy of the Visible Human Project of the US National Library of Medicine.

and pierces the dura mater in the middle cranial fossa. In the carotid canal, it lies anteromedial to the middle ear; inferior to the cochlea, greater petrosal nerve, and trigeminal ganglion [see Fig. 13.6]; and superior to the auditory tube.

Internal carotid nerve and plexus

The internal carotid nerve is a large branch of the superior cervical ganglion which enters the carotid canal. It forms the internal carotid plexus around the internal carotid artery. Secondary plexuses extend from it around the branches of the artery [see Fig. 13.8]. The internal carotid plexus consists mainly of post-ganglionic sympathetic fibres.

The internal carotid nerve supplies a large area. The deep petrosal branch of the internal carotid plexus joins the pterygopalatine ganglion and, through it, is distributed to the nose, palate, air sinuses, and pharynx. Branches of the internal carotid nerve also join the third, fourth, ophthalmic branch of the fifth, and sixth cranial nerves, and the ophthalmic artery to supply the contents of the orbit, the forehead, and the anterior part of the scalp.

See Clinical Applications 17.1, 17.2, and 17.3 for the practical implications of the anatomy discussed in this chapter.

CLINICAL APPLICATION 17.1 Blocking of the auditory tube

The auditory tube forms a route through which infections can pass from the nasopharynx to the middle ear cavity. It is readily blocked by infections, because the walls of its cartilaginous part lie in apposition. When the auditory tube is blocked, the residual air in the middle ear is absorbed into the blood vessels, causing a fall in pressure inside the middle ear cavity. When the block is associated with infection of the middle ear, there is an outpouring of fluid from the damaged mucous membrane, with an increase in pressure within the cavity. When the pressure in the middle ear cavity is either raised or lowered, free movement of the tympanic membrane is impeded and hearing is affected. With raised pressure, the normally concave tympanic membrane bulges into the external acoustic meatus—a feature readily confirmed with an otoscope.

CLINICAL APPLICATION 17.2 Cancer, oral mucosa

A 58-year-old man presented with a swelling in the right side of the vestibule of his mouth. Clinical examination led to suspicion of cancer of the oral mucosa, and a computerized tomogram (CT) was done. The images revealed a neoplastic mass of the buccal mucosa [Fig. 17.11].

Study question 1: study the image, and identify the structures marked 1, 2, 3, 4, and 5. (Answer: 1 = vestibule of the mouth in the unaffected side; 2 = masseter; 3 = facial vein; 4 = mandible; 5 = sublingual gland.)

Study question 2: state the sensory nerves, motor nerves, arteries, and lymph nodes likely to be involved. (Answer: sensory nerves = inferior alveolar and its mental branch; motor nerve = facial nerve; arteries = inferior alveolar branch of the maxillary artery, inferior labial branch of the facial artery; lymph nodes = submental and submandibular lymph nodes.)

Cancer of the oral mucosa is very common in India. Chewing tobacco mixed with betel leaves, areca nut (pan masala), and lime shell is one of the main risk factors for this cancer.

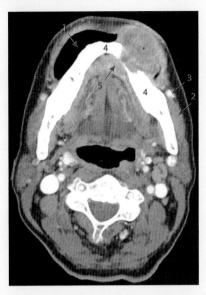

Fig. 17.11 Computerized tomogram of the head showing a neoplastic growth in the buccal mucosa (asterisk).

CLINICAL APPLICATION 17.3 Hypopharyngeal diverticula

Inferior constrictor fibres arising from the cricoid cartilage (the cricopharyngeus) form two bands. The upper fibres run obliquely backwards and upwards to the median raphe. The lower fibres run transversely to encircle the pharynx. An area of intrinsic weakness exists between the two bands—the Killian's triangle. Hypopharyngeal diverticula—protrusion of the mucosa through the muscle layers—commonly occurs through this part of the pharyngeal wall.

Hypopharyngeal diverticula can also occur above the cricopharyngeus (between the cricopharyngeus and thyropharyngeus) or below the cricopharyngeus (between the cricopharyngeus and oesophagus).

CHAPTER 18
The tongue

Introduction

The tongue is a mobile organ which bulges upwards from the floor of the mouth. Its posterior part forms the anterior wall of the oropharynx [see Figs. 17.2, 17.3]. It is covered by stratified squamous epithelium and consists mainly of skeletal muscle, interspersed with a little fat and numerous glands.

The tongue is separated from the teeth by a deep **alveololingual sulcus**. This sulcus is filled by the palatoglossal fold, posterior to the last molar tooth. The sulcus partly undermines the lateral margins of the tongue and extends beneath its free anterior third. The smooth mucous membrane in the alveololingual sulcus passes from the root of the tongue across the floor of the mouth to the internal aspect of the mandible and becomes continuous superiorly with that on the gum. Internal to the sulcus, the **root of the tongue** contains the muscles which connect the tongue to the hyoid bone and mandible, and transmits the nerves and vessels which supply it [see Fig. 17.1].

Dorsum of the tongue

The dorsum of the tongue extends from the tip of the tongue to the anterior surface of the epiglottis. It is arbitrarily divided into an anterior palatine part and a posterior pharyngeal part by a V-shaped sulcus—the **sulcus terminalis**. The apex of the sulcus terminalis points posteriorly and is marked by a pit—the **foramen caecum**. A shallow median groove extends from the tip of the tongue to the foramen caecum [Fig. 18.1].

The thick mucous membrane of the palatine part is rough due to the presence of papillae. In the pharyngeal part, the covering mucosa is smooth, thin, and finely nodular in appearance, due to the presence of the underlying **lymphoid follicles**—the lingual tonsil. Posteriorly, the lingual mucous membrane is continuous with that on the anterior surface of the epiglottis over the median and lateral glosso-epiglottic folds and the valleculae of the epiglottis [Fig. 18.1].

Lingual papillae

There are three types of lingual papillae—**circumvallate papillae**, **fungiform papillae**, and **filiform papillae**. The largest of these are the 7–12 **circumvallate papillae**, which lie immediately anterior to the sulcus terminalis. Each has the shape of a short cylinder, sunk into the surface of the tongue, with a deep trench surrounding it. The opposing walls of the trench have numerous taste buds.

Fungiform papillae are smaller and more numerous than circumvallate papillae. They are seen as bright red spots principally on the tip and margins of the living tongue, but also scattered over the remainder of the dorsum. Each fungiform papilla is attached by a narrow base and expands into a rounded, knob-like free extremity. Most of them carry taste buds.

Filiform papillae are numerous minute, pointed projections which cover all of the palatine part of the dorsum and the margins of the tongue. They are in rows parallel to the sulcus terminalis posteriorly, but transverse anteriorly.

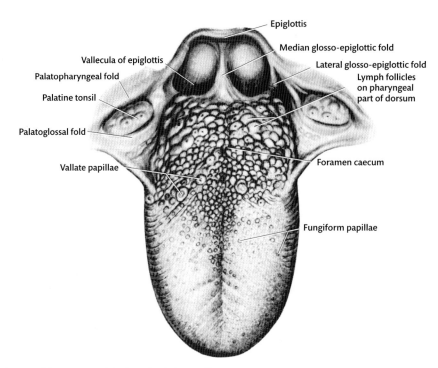

Epiglottis

Median glosso-epiglottic fold

Vallecula of epiglottis

Lateral glosso-epiglottic fold

Palatopharyngeal fold

Lymph follicles
on pharyngeal
part of dorsum

Palatine tonsil

Palatoglossal fold

Vallate papillae

Foramen caecum

Fungiform papillae

Fig. 18.1 The dorsum of the tongue, epiglottis, and palatine tonsils.

On the sides of the tongue, anterior to the lingual attachment of the palatoglossal arch, are five short, vertical folds of mucous membrane—the **foliate papillae**.

Inferior surface of the tongue

The inferior surface and sides of the tongue are covered by smooth, thin mucous membrane. In the midline, anteriorly the mucosa is raised into a sharp fold which joins the inferior surface of the tongue to the floor of the mouth. This is the **frenulum of the tongue** [see Fig. 17.1]. On the tongue, on each side of the frenulum is the deep lingual vein, which is seen through the mucous membrane in the living subject. Lateral to the deep lingual vein is a fringed **fimbriated fold** of mucous membrane. On each side of the frenulum, on the floor of the mouth, is the **sublingual papilla**, with the opening of the submandibular duct on it. Passing posterolaterally from the sublingual papilla

is the rounded **sublingual fold** (which contains the sublingual gland and the submandibular duct) and has the openings of the ducts of the sublingual gland [see Fig. 17.1].

Muscles of the tongue

The tongue is divided into two halves by a median fibrous septum. The muscles of each half consist of an extrinsic and an intrinsic group. The extrinsic muscles take origin from parts outside the tongue and can move the tongue and change its shape. The intrinsic muscles are solely inside the tongue and can only change its shape.

The extrinsic muscles of the tongue are the genioglossus, hyoglosssus, styloglossus [Chapter 16], and palatoglossus [Chapter 17]. The intrinsic muscles are the superior longitudinal, inferior longitudinal, vertical, and transverse muscles.

Using the instructions given in Dissection 18.1, trace the extrinsic muscles of the tongue.

DISSECTION 18.1 Extrinsic muscles of the tongue

Objective

I. To identify and trace the extrinsic muscles of the tongue.

Instructions

1. On the cut surface of the tongue, identify the genioglossus and geniohyoid. Confirm their attachments and position [Fig. 17.3].

2. On the right side, separate the buccinator, pterygomandibular raphe, and superior constrictor from their attachments to the mandible, and turn the remainder of the body of the mandible downwards to expose the lateral surface of the tongue. Avoid injury to the lingual nerve and the palatoglossus muscle.

3. Remove the remainder of the mucous membrane from the lateral surface of the tongue, and follow the extrinsic muscles into its substance.

Extrinsic muscles of the tongue

The extrinsic muscles of the tongue have been described in Chapters 16 and 17 [Fig. 18.2].

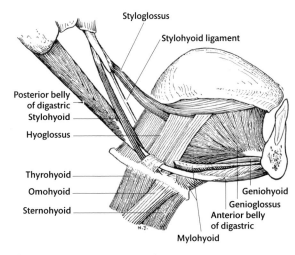

Fig. 18.2 The extrinsic muscles of the tongue.

Movements of the tongue

The posterior part of the tongue is attached to the hyoid bone. Hence the muscles which move the hyoid bone also move this part of the tongue [Chapter 16].

The **hyoglossus** and **genioglossus muscles** enter the tongue from below. The hyoglossus runs vertically along the lateral side of the tongue. The genioglossus is in a paramedian position. Both muscles depress the tongue [see Fig. 14.6; Fig. 18.2]. The genioglossus is fan-shaped when seen in sagittal section [see Fig. 17.3]. Its posterior fibres pull the tongue forwards and help to protrude it (as does the geniohyoid). Its anterior fibres depress and retract the tip of the tongue.

The **palatoglossus** and **styloglossus** enter the lateral part of the tongue from above. The palatoglossus passes almost transversely and is continuous with the intrinsic transverse fibres. The styloglossus runs anteriorly along the lateral margin [Fig. 18.2]. Both muscles can elevate the posterior part of the tongue. The styloglossus also retracts the tongue. The palatoglossus draws the palate down onto the tongue, narrows the isthmus of the fauces, and helps to isolate the mouth from the pharynx.

The **superior longitudinal muscle** lies close to the dorsum of the tongue. It curls the tip of the tongue upwards and rolls it posteriorly. The **inferior longitudinal muscle** lies in the lower part of the tongue, one on either side of the genioglossus [Fig. 18.3]. It curls the tip of the tongue inferiorly and act with the superior muscle to retract and widen the tongue.

The **transverse muscle fibres** lie inferior to the superior longitudinal muscle and run from the septum to the margins of the tongue between the vertical fibres of the genioglossus, hyoglossus, and intrinsic vertical muscles [see Fig. 17.8]. They narrow the tongue and increase its height.

The **vertical muscle fibres** run inferolaterally from the dorsum. They flatten the dorsum, increase the transverse diameter, and tend to roll up the margins. Acting with the transverse muscles, they increase the length of the tongue and assist with protrusion.

The actions given above represent only a few of the possible movements. Many other complex

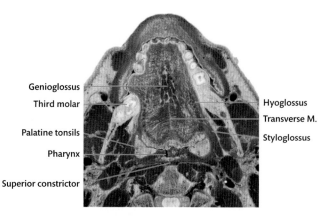

Genioglossus

Third molar

Palatine tonsils

Pharynx

Superior constrictor

Hyoglossus

Transverse M.

Styloglossus

Fig. 18.3 Horizontal section through the tongue and pharynx.
Image courtesy of the Visible Human Project of the US National Library of Medicine.

movements are produced by combinations of these muscles acting together. The tongue is bilaterally symmetrical, and unilateral action of any one muscle or group of muscles will cause the tongue to deviate from the midline. ➲ When one side of the tongue is paralysed, attempts to protrude the tongue result in the tip of the tongue deviating to the paralysed (stationary) side.

Septum of the tongue

The median fibrous septum of the tongue is best seen in a transverse section. It is strongest posteriorly where it is attached to the hyoid bone and is separated from the mucous membrane of the dorsum by the superior longitudinal muscle [see Figs. 16.2B, 17.8].

Glands of the tongue

Small serous and mucous glands lie between the muscle fibres deep to the mucous membrane of the pharyngeal surface, tip, and margins. Small serous glands lie near the vallate papillae and open into their trenches. Mucous and serous glands lie on the inferior surface of the tongue near its tip—the **anterior lingual gland**.

Nerves of the tongue

The sensory supply to the mucous membrane varies, depending on the type of sensation and location on the tongue. In the anterior two-thirds of the tongue, general sensation is carried by (1) the **lingual nerve**, and (2) taste sensation is carried by the **chorda tympani** branch of the facial nerve. (The chorda tympani runs with the lingual nerve in the mouth [see Fig. 15.7].) In the posterior one-third of the tongue, (3) the **glossopharyngeal** nerve carries taste and general sensation. The glossopharyngeal nerve also carries sensations from the circumvallate papillae. (4) Small branches of the internal laryngeal branch of the superior laryngeal nerve supply a small area of the tongue adjacent to the epiglottis.

The lingual and glossopharyngeal nerves also carry parasympathetic secretomotor fibres to the glands in the substance of the tongue.

The motor supply to the muscles of the tongue is from the **hypoglossal nerve** which innervates all the intrinsic and extrinsic muscles of the tongue, except the palatoglossus. (The palatoglossus is innervated by the vagus.)

Vessels of the tongue

The main **arteries** supplying the tongue are branches of the lingual artery. The deep artery of the tongue supplies the anterior part, and the dorsales linguae arteries supply the posterior part. The **deep lingual vein** and other veins are described in Chapter 16.

Lymph vessels of the tongue

These vessels cannot be dissected, but they are important because cancer of the tongue is common and it spreads through lymph vessels.

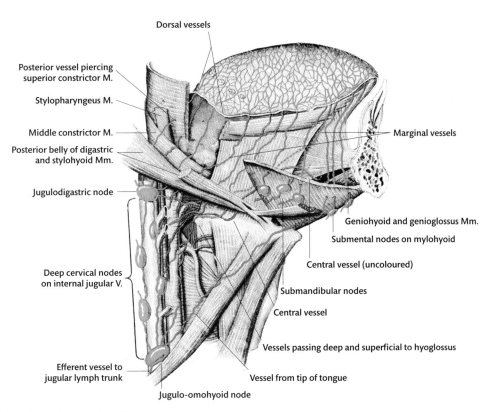

Dorsal vessels

Posterior vessel piercing superior constrictor M.

Stylopharyngeus M.

Middle constrictor M.

Posterior belly of digastric and stylohyoid Mm.

Jugulodigastric node

Deep cervical nodes on internal jugular V.

Efferent vessel to jugular lymph trunk

Jugulo-omohyoid node

Marginal vessels

Geniohyoid and genioglossus Mm.

Submental nodes on mylohyoid

Central vessel (uncoloured)

Submandibular nodes

Central vessel

Vessels passing deep and superficial to hyoglossus

Vessel from tip of tongue

Fig. 18.4 Lymph vessels and nodes of the tongue.

Lymph vessels from the tongue drain into the **jugulodigastric** and **jugulo-omohyoid** deep cervical lymph nodes. The lymph from the anterior part of the tongue (in front of the circumvallate papilla) drains through two sets of lymph vessels—the marginal and central vessels. Lymph from the posterior part drains through the dorsal lymph vessels. Lymph from the marginal vessels may pass through the **submental nodes** or **submandibular** nodes [Fig. 18.4]. Lymph from the median and paramedian tissue may cross the midline and drain bilaterally.

See Clinical Application 18.1 for the practical implications of the anatomy discussed in this chapter.

Table 18.1 provides an overview of the movements of the tongue.

225

CLINICAL APPLICATION 18.1 Gag reflex

Accidently touching the back of the tongue or the mucosa over the palatoglossal arch (for example while brushing one's teeth) could stimulate the gag reflex. The **gag reflex** results in reflex contraction of the pharyngeal muscles, soft palate, and isthmus of the fauces. In extreme cases, it is accompanied by retching and vomiting. The afferent limb for the reflex is through the glossopharyngeal nerve. The efferent limb is through the pharyngeal plexus—the vagus and glossopharyngeal.

Table 18.1 Movements of the tongue

Movement	Muscles	Nerve supply
Tip		
Elevation	Superior longitudinal*	Hypoglossal
Depression	Inferior longitudinal* and genioglossus	Hypoglossal
Retraction	Genioglossus (anterior fibres) and longitudinal muscles*	Hypoglossal
Turning to one side	Longitudinal* of that side with protrusors of opposite side	Hypoglossal and C. 1
Body		
Widening	Longitudinal* and vertical*	Hypoglossal
Heightening	Longitudinal* and transverse*	Hypoglossal
Shortening	Longitudinal*	Hypoglossal
Elongation	Transverse* and vertical*	Hypoglossal
Depression of median part	Genioglossus	Hypoglossal
Depression of edges	Hyoglossus	Hypoglossal
Depression of all	Lowering of hyoid bone [Table 9.2]	
Elevation	Elevation of hyoid bone [Table 9.2]	
	Styloglossus	Hypoglossal
	Mylohyoid	Trigeminal
	Palatoglossus	Pharyngeal plexus
Protrusion in the midline	Geniohyoid†	Ventral ramus C. 1
	Genioglossus (posterior fibres)†	Hypoglossal
	Vertical*	Hypoglossal
	(Transverse*)	Hypoglossal
Protrusion to one side	Action of above muscles on opposite side ± retractors of same side	
Retraction	Longitudinal*	Hypoglossal
	Styloglossus	Hypoglossal

* Intrinsic muscles.† These muscles help to maintain the patency of the airway when lying supine.

CHAPTER 19
The cavity of the nose

Cavity of the nose

Each nasal cavity is approximately 5 cm in height and 5–7 cm in length. It is narrow transversely, measuring approximately 1.5 cm at the floor and only 1–2 mm at the roof. The width is further reduced by the conchae, which project into the cavity from the lateral wall [Figs. 19.1, 19.2, 19.3].

The oval anterior apertures, or nostrils (**nares**), open on the inferior surface of the external nose. The posterior apertures, or **choanae**, open into the nasopharynx and face postero-inferiorly [Fig. 19.3]. The **vestibule of the nose** [Fig. 19.1] lies immediately above the nostril. It is lined with skin from which stout hairs or vibrissae project, forming a coarse filter.

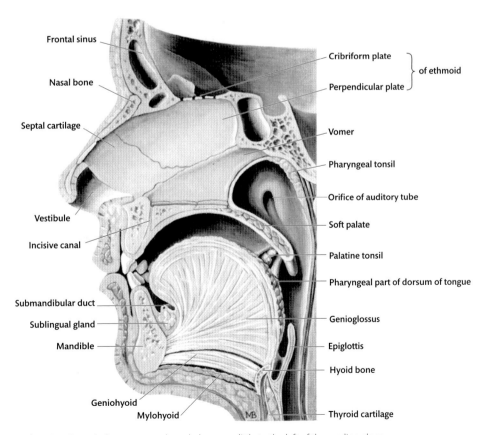

Fig. 19.1 Sagittal section through the nose, mouth, and pharynx, a little to the left of the median plane.

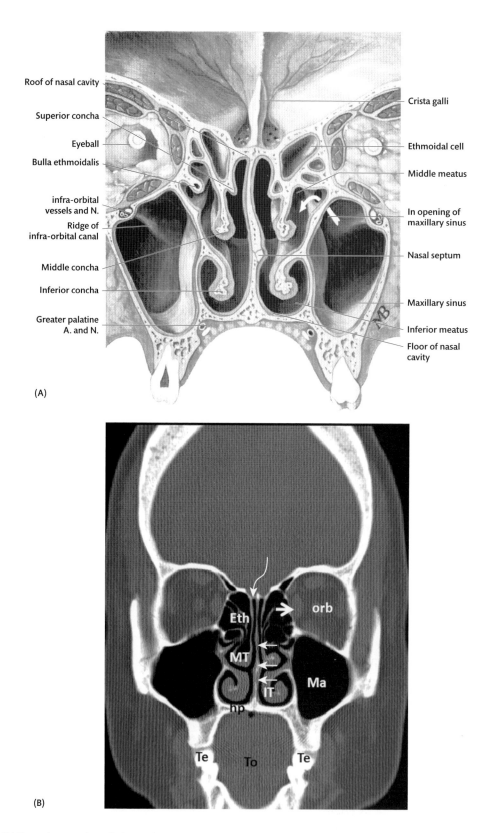

Roof of nasal cavity

Superior concha

Eyeball

Bulla ethmoidalis

infra-orbital
vessels and N.

Ridge of
infra-orbital canal

Middle concha

Inferior concha

Greater palatine
A. and N.

Crista galli

Ethmoidal cell

Middle meatus

In opening of
maxillary sinus

Nasal septum

Maxillary sinus

Inferior meatus

Floor of nasal
cavity

(A)

Eth

orb

MT

Ma

IT

hp

Te   To   Te

(B)

Fig. 19.2 (A) Coronal section through the nasal cavities, paranasal sinuses, and orbits, seen from behind. (B) Computerized tomogram through the nasal cavity. Eth = ethmoid; hp = hard palate; IT = inferior turbinate (concha); Ma = maxillary antrum; MT = middle turbinate (concha); orb = orbit; Te = teeth; To = tongue. Curved arrow = cribriform plate of the ethmoid. Thick arrow = medial wall of the orbit. Thin arrow = nasal septum.

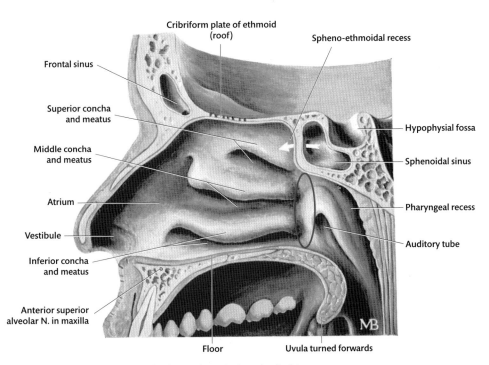

Cribriform plate of ethmoid (roof)

Spheno-ethmoidal recess

Frontal sinus

Superior concha and meatus

Middle concha and meatus

Atrium

Vestibule

Inferior concha and meatus

Anterior superior alveolar N. in maxilla

Hypophysial fossa

Sphenoidal sinus

Pharyngeal recess

Auditory tube

Floor

Uvula turned forwards

Fig. 19.3 Sagittal section through the nose and palate to show the lateral wall of the nose.

Septum of the nose

The nasal septum divides the nose into two narrow parts. It is seldom exactly in the midline but bulges to one or other side. Immediately above the nostril, the septum is slightly concave where it forms the medial wall of the vestibule of the nose. The skin of this part carries a number of stiff hairs or vibrissae. The remainder of the septum is covered with mucous membrane which is tightly adherent to the underlying periosteum and perichondrium (**mucoperiosteum** and **mucoperichondrium**, respectively). The lower, larger area of the septum is the **respiratory region**. The upper third is the **olfactory region** because its epithelium contains olfactory nerve cells. The respiratory mucous membrane is thick, spongy, and highly vascular. It contains numerous mucous glands and is capable of swelling to a considerable thickness when the vascular spaces in it are filled with blood. It also contains many arteriovenous anastomoses which increase the flow of blood through it to warm the air passing over it. The olfactory mucous membrane is more delicate and is yellowish in the fresh state [Figs. 19.1, 19.2].

Using the instructions given in Dissection 19.1, remove the mucous membrane and expose the components of the nasal septum.

DISSECTION 19.1 Nasal septum

Objective

I. To identify the bony and cartilaginous components of the nasal septum.

Instructions

1. Strip the mucous membrane off the nasal septum, and expose: (1) the vomer; (2) the perpendicular plate of the ethmoid; (3) the septal cartilage; and (4) small parts of the maxillary, palatine, nasal, and sphenoid bones. The relative positions of these parts are shown in Fig. 19.1.

2. Note that the anterior angle of the septal cartilage is blunt and rounded, and does not reach the point of the nose. The point of the nose is formed by the greater alar cartilages.

3. Remove the septum piecemeal from the mucous membrane, taking care not to damage the structures in that mucous membrane.

Components forming the septum

The septum is formed mainly by the perpendicular plate of the ethmoid, vomer, and septal cartilage [Fig. 19.1].

Nerves of the septum

The **nasopalatine nerve** is a long, slender nerve on the deep surface of the mucous membrane of the septum. It enters the nasal cavity from the pterygopalatine ganglion through the sphenopalatine foramen with the sphenopalatine branch of the maxillary artery. It runs medially across the roof of the nasal cavity, and then antero-inferiorly on the septum, in a groove on the surface of the vomer. On reaching the floor of the nasal cavity, it runs through the incisive canal and median incisive foramen with its fellow from the opposite side, and supplies the mucous membrane in the anterior part of the hard palate.

The medial **posterosuperior nasal branches** of the pterygopalatine ganglion, together with small branches from the nerve of the pterygoid canal, supply the posterosuperior parts of the septum. They are too small to be dissected easily.

The medial nasal branches of the **anterior ethmoidal nerve** run on the anterosuperior part of the nasal septum as far as the vestibule [Fig. 19.4]. [For nerves of smell, see p. 234.]

Arteries of the septum

The nasal septum is supplied by: (1) the sphenopalatine artery, a branch of the maxillary artery; (2) ethmoidal branches of the ophthalmic artery; and (3) branches of the superior labial arteries [Fig. 19.5].

Roof of the nasal cavity

The roof of the nasal cavity is curved and approximately 7–8 cm long. The anterior and posterior parts are sloping, and the middle part is nearly horizontal. The anterior part is formed by the nasal part of the frontal bone, the nasal bone, and the junction of lateral and septal cartilages. The middle part is formed by the cribriform plate of the ethmoid. The posterior part is formed by the anterior and inferior surfaces of the body of the sphenoid [Fig. 19.3].

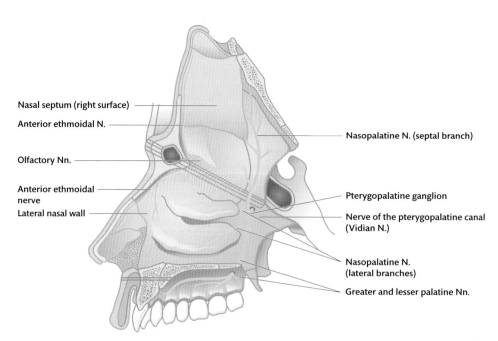

Fig. 19.4 Nerve supply of the nasal septum and lateral wall of the nose.

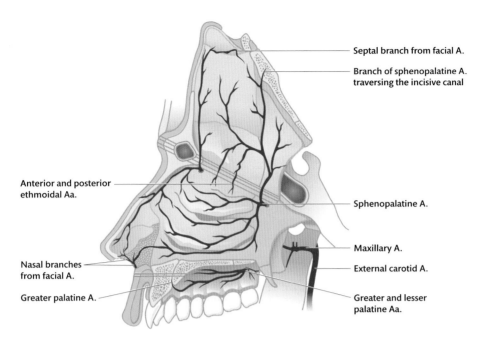

Septal branch from facial A.

Branch of sphenopalatine A. traversing the incisive canal

Anterior and posterior ethmoidal Aa.

Sphenopalatine A.

Maxillary A.

Nasal branches from facial A.

External carotid A.

Greater palatine A.

Greater and lesser palatine Aa.

Fig. 19.5 Arterial supply of the nasal septum and lateral wall of the nose.

Floor of the nasal cavity

The floor is about 5 cm long and 1–1.5 cm wide. It is formed by the palatine process of the maxilla and the horizontal process of the palatine bone. It is concave transversely and is slightly higher anteriorly than posteriorly [Figs. 19.2, 19.3].

Lateral wall

The lateral wall of the nasal cavity is irregular due to the presence of three projecting **conchae** or turbinates—the superior, middle, and inferior conchae. The meatuses are the spaces inferior to the conchae—the superior, middle, and inferior meatuses. Identify the bones that form the lateral wall of the nose—maxilla, ethmoid, palatine—on a dry skull. Adjoining the lateral wall are the air sinuses (air-filled spaces in the bones) which communicate with the nasal cavity. The **ethmoidal sinus** lies between the upper part of the nasal cavity and the orbit. It consists of anterior, middle, and posterior **ethmoidal air cells**. Inferior to this is the **maxillary sinus** which lies below the orbit [Fig. 19.2].

There are three distinct regions in the lateral wall of the nose [Fig. 19.3].

1. The **vestibule of the nose** lies immediately above the nostril.
2. The **atrium of the middle meatus** is above and slightly behind the vestibule. It lies immediately anterior to the middle meatus. The lateral wall of the atrium is concave, except close to the nasal bone where there is a small elevation—the agger nasi.
3. **Nasal conchae and meatuses** [Figs. 19.2, 19.3]. The conchae are three bony plates, which project from the lateral wall of the nose and curve inferiorly. They are covered with a thick, highly vascular mucoperiosteum. The upper two conchae are processes of the ethmoid bone. The inferior concha is a separate bone.

The **superior concha** lies in the posterosuperior part of the nasal cavity and is very short. Its free anterior border begins a little inferior to the middle of the cribriform plate, and it passes postero-inferiorly to end immediately anterior to the lower part of the body of the sphenoid. The **middle concha** is much larger than the superior concha and extends from the atrium to the level of the choanae.

The **inferior concha** is slightly longer than the middle concha and lies about midway between the middle concha and the floor of the nose.

The space posterosuperior to the superior concha is the **spheno-ethmoidal recess**. The sphenoidal air sinus opens into it [Fig. 19.3]. The **superior meatus** is a narrow space between the superior and middle conchae. The posterior ethmoidal cells open into it by one or more orifices. These openings can be exposed by forcing the margin of the superior concha upwards [Fig. 19.6].

The **middle meatus** is much longer and deeper than the superior meatus. To expose it, tilt the middle concha forcibly upwards [Fig. 19.6]. The anterosuperior part of the middle meatus has a funnel-shaped opening—the **infundibulum**—which leads to the frontal air sinus. On the lateral wall of the middle meatus is a deep, curved groove which begins at the infundibulum and runs postero-inferiorly. This is the **hiatus semilunaris**. The anterior ethmoidal and maxillary air sinuses open into it. The upper margin of the hiatus semilunaris is formed by a prominent bulge—the **bulla ethmoidalis**—on which is the opening of the middle ethmoidal air cells. The **opening of the maxillary sinus** [see Fig. 11.3; Figs. 19.2, 19.6] lies in the posterior part of the hiatus semilunaris and leads to the upper medial wall of the sinus. ➲ Infections tend to spread from the frontal to the maxillary sinus, because the position of the openings of the two sinuses favour the flow of material from the frontal into the maxillary sinus.

The **inferior meatus** is the horizontal passage between the inferior concha and the floor of the nose. The nasolacrimal duct opens into the anterior part of the inferior meatus, close to the attached border of the inferior concha [Fig. 19.6].

Using the instructions given in Dissection 19.2, dissect out the nasolacrimal duct.

DISSECTION 19.2 Nasolacrimal duct

Objective

I. To expose the nasolacrimal duct.

Instructions

1. Remove the anterior part of the inferior concha with scissors, and expose the opening of the nasolacrimal duct. Pass a probe upwards along the duct to confirm its continuity with the lacrimal sac [Figs. 19.4, 19.7].

2. Break away the thin plate of bone which separates the duct from the nose, and expose the length of the duct. Expose the lacrimal sac by continuing the bone removal upwards to the level of the eye.

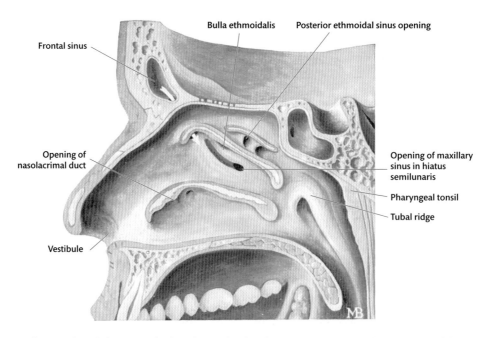

Fig. 19.6 Sagittal section through the nose and palate. The conchae have been cut away to expose the meatuses and the openings into them.

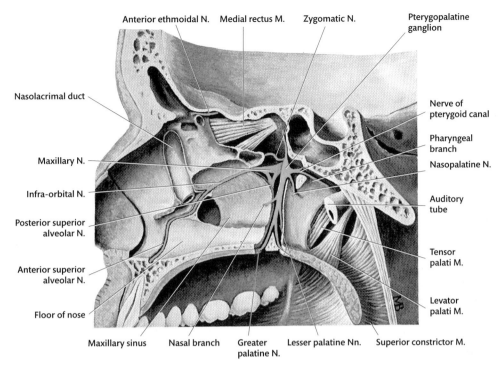

Anterior ethmoidal N. Medial rectus M. Zygomatic N. Pterygopalatine ganglion

Nasolacrimal duct

Maxillary N.

Infra-orbital N.

Posterior superior alveolar N.

Anterior superior alveolar N.

Floor of nose

Nerve of pterygoid canal

Pharyngeal branch

Nasopalatine N.

Auditory tube

Tensor palati M.

Levator palati M.

Maxillary sinus Nasal branch Greater palatine N. Lesser palatine Nn. Superior constrictor M.

Fig. 19.7 The mucous membrane and a large part of the bone of the lateral wall of the nose have been removed to expose the maxillary sinus. The maxillary, infra-orbital, anterior superior alveolar, and palatine nerves have been exposed by removal of the bony wall of their canals. The pterygopalatine fossa and ganglion are also exposed. The ethmoid has been broken into to expose the orbit.

Orifice of the nasolacrimal duct

The opening of the nasolacrimal duct may be wide, patent, and circular, or it may be covered by a fold of membrane. In a few cases, the orifice is so small that it is difficult to find [see Fig. 4.15].

Mucosa of the lateral wall of the nasal cavity

Apart from the vestibule, the lateral wall is covered with mucous membrane which is tightly adherent to the underlying periosteum and forms a **mucoperiosteum**. This mucoperiosteum is continuous: (1) through the nasolacrimal duct, with the ocular conjunctiva; (2) through the openings of the sinuses with the lining of the air sinuses in the frontal, ethmoid, maxilla, and sphenoid bones; and (3) through the choanae with the mucous membrane of the nasopharynx.

The mucoperiosteum on the lateral wall is divisible into the upper yellowish **olfactory region** in the area of the superior concha, and the remainder which comprises the **respiratory region**. These regions cannot be differentiated by the naked eye. In the respiratory region, the mucoperiosteum is

thick and spongy, especially on the free margins and posterior extremities of the middle and inferior conchae, due to the presence of a rich venous plexus in it. The venous channels and rapid blood flow in the mucoperiosteum due to many arteriovenous anastomoses, ensure that the inspired air is warmed and moistened. Dust particles in the inspired air are trapped on the mucus covering the surface and moved posteriorly towards the choanae by the cilia. ➲ The mucoperiosteum on the inferior concha may be swollen by distended venous channels. It may impinge on the nasal septum and effectively reduces the cross-sectional area of the nasal cavity.

Nerves and vessels on the lateral wall of the nasal cavity

General sensation from the lateral wall of the nasal cavity is carried by branches of the maxillary nerve, and the anterior ethmoidal nerve. The **anterior ethmoidal nerve** is a branch of the nasociliary nerve in the orbit. It reaches the anterosuperior part of the lateral wall of the nose through the anterior ethmoidal foramen and the cribriform plate of the ethmoid [Fig. 11.3]. Fibres of the **maxillary**

DISSECTION 19.3   Vessels and nerves of the nasal cavity

Objective

I. To expose the vessels and nerves of the nasal cavity.

Instructions

1. Trace the **nasopalatine nerve** from the nasal septum across the roof of the nasal cavity to the sphenopalatine foramen in the lateral wall.

2. By careful dissection, attempt to display one or more of the nasal branches of the pterygopalatine ganglion and the sphenopalatine artery running with the nasopalatine nerve.

3. Carefully reflect the mucous membrane on the medial pterygoid lamina anteriorly.

4. Attempt to find the **posterior nasal branches of the pterygopalatine ganglion**. These are minute twigs which pass through the sphenopalatine foramen and supply the mucous membrane on the posterior part of the septum, the superior and middle conchae, some ethmoidal cells, and

the lateral wall of the nasal part of the pharynx [Fig. 19.4].

5. Two **nasal branches of the greater palatine nerve** pierce the perpendicular plate of the palatine bone. They supply the mucous membrane on the posterior parts of the conchae and meatuses.

6. The **anterior ethmoidal nerve** [Fig. 19.4] descends in a groove on the deep surface of the nasal bone. Its branches supply the anterosuperior parts of the septum, roof, and lateral wall of the nose.

7. The **sphenopalatine branch of the maxillary artery** is the main arterial supply to the mucous membrane. It enters the nasal cavity through the sphenopalatine foramen and is distributed with the various nerves [Fig. 19.5].

8. The anterior and posterior **ethmoidal arteries** also supply the anterosuperior region, the anterior reaching as far inferiorly as the anterior end of the inferior concha.

nerve reach the walls of the nasal cavity through branches of the pterygopalatine ganglion and the anterior superior alveolar nerve [Fig. 19.4]. The maxillary nerve also carries post-ganglionic sympathetic fibres from the carotid plexus (via the deep petrosal nerve) and post-ganglionic parasympathetic nerve fibres from the pterygopalatine ganglion to the glands in the lateral wall.

The **olfactory nerves** are the nerves of smell. They are the central processes of the olfactory cells in the epithelium of the olfactory area. These fine, non-myelinated nerve fibres run in shallow grooves and small canals in the bone deep to the mucous membrane. They unite to form 12–20 olfactory nerves which pass through the cribriform plate of the ethmoid and pierce the meninges to enter the olfactory bulb [Fig. 19.4].

Dissection 19.3 provides instructions on dissecting the nerves and vessels of the nasal cavity.

Important structures related to the lateral wall of the nose

The **pterygopalatine ganglion**, a short segment of the **maxillary nerve**, and the terminal part of the **maxillary artery** lie adjacent to the lateral wall of the nose [Fig. 19.7]. The pterygopalatine ganglion lies in the pterygopalatine fossa, lateral to the sphenopalatine foramen and the perpendicular plate of the palatine bone.

The greater and lesser palatine branches of the pterygopalatine ganglion will be dissected following the instructions provided in Dissection 19.4.

DISSECTION 19.4   Greater and lesser palatine nerves

Objective

I. To expose the greater and lesser palatine nerves.

Instructions

1. The mucoperiosteum has already been stripped from the perpendicular plate of the palatine bone.

Find the greater palatine nerve which is seen shining through this very thin plate of bone, as it descends on the lateral side of the bone to reach the palate. It runs with the **descending palatine branch** from the maxillary artery.

2. Break through the perpendicular plate of the palatine bone, and expose part of the greater palatine nerve. Then open up the whole length of the canal by levering off the remainder of the lamina lying medial to the nerve. Superiorly, the **greater palatine nerve** joins the pterygopalatine ganglion at the level of the sphenopalatine foramen.

3. Inferiorly, where the canal reaches the hard palate, cut out a narrow, transverse strip of the hard palate to open into the palatine foramen, through which the greater palatine nerve reaches the hard palate.

4. Remove the fibrous sheath covering the greater palatine nerve, and expose the **lesser palatine nerves** which run with it in the upper part of their course. Inferiorly, the lesser palatine nerves pass through separate bony canals.

5. Turn to the inferior surface of the palate, and follow the greater palatine nerve and artery in it.

Greater palatine nerve

The greater palatine nerve is the largest branch of the pterygopalatine ganglion [Fig. 19.7]. It descends vertically through the greater palatine canal and foramen with the **descending palatine branch** of the maxillary artery and enters the inferior surface of the hard palate at its postero-lateral corner. It runs forwards in a groove on the inferior surface of the bony palate, close to its lateral margin. At the incisive fossa, it communicates with the terminal branches of the nasopalatine nerve. It supplies the gum and the mucous membrane of the hard palate, including the palatine mucous glands which indent the inferior surface of the bone.

The greater palatine nerve gives: (1) two **posterior nasal** branches through the perpendicular plate of the palatine bone to the mucous membrane of the nose; and (2) the **lesser palatine nerves** which descend through the lesser palatine canals. The more medial of the lesser palatine nerve emerges immediately posterior to the palatine crest and enters the soft palate to supply its mucous membrane and glands. The more lateral nerve, when present, supplies the mucous membrane of the soft palate near the palatine tonsil.

Using the instructions given in Dissection 19.5, dissect the pterygopalatine ganglion and maxillary nerve.

DISSECTION 19.5 Pterygopalatine ganglion and maxillary nerve

Objectives

I. To remove the lateral wall of the nasal cavity. **II.** To expose the ethmoidal air cells. **III.** To expose the maxillary nerve and its branches. **IV.** To identify the pterygopalatine ganglion.

Instructions

1. Remove the three nasal conchae.

2. Beginning just posterior to the infundibulum, strip away the thin medial wall of the ethmoidal air cells, noting their continuity with the nasal mucous membrane through the apertures already described.

3. Remove the mucous membrane lining the individual cells and the bony walls between them, and expose the medial surface of the orbital lamina of the ethmoid.

4. Break away the medial wall of the maxillary sinus between the nasolacrimal duct and the greater palatine canal, and examine the interior of the maxillary sinus [see Fig. 15.4].

5. Expose the maxillary nerve in the pterygopalatine fossa by removing the intervening bone through the maxillary sinus. This also exposes the anterior surface of the pterygopalatine ganglion and the terminal parts of the maxillary artery.

6. Chip away the sphenoid medial to the ganglion, taking care to preserve the pharyngeal branch of the ganglion and the nerve of the pterygoid canal which enters the posterior surface of the ganglion.

7. Follow the infra-orbital nerve anteriorly by chipping away the floor of the infra-orbital groove and canal.

8. Find the **anterior superior alveolar branch** of the infra-orbital nerve, and trace it forwards. Attempt to find its branches to the upper teeth, gums, and mucous membrane of the maxillary sinus.

Pterygopalatine ganglion

The pterygopalatine ganglion is one of the four parasympathetic ganglia of the head. It is small, triangular in shape and lies in the superior part of the pterygopalatine fossa near the sphenopalatine foramen. It is surrounded by the terminal branches of the maxillary artery [see Fig. 15.4; Fig. 19.7].

Roots of the pterygopalatine ganglion

The pterygopalatine ganglion is suspended from the inferior aspect of the maxillary nerve by two stout **ganglionic roots**, which are nerves entering the ganglia. The sensory trigeminal fibres in these roots pass directly through the ganglion into its branches.

Sympathetic and parasympathetic nerve fibres enter the ganglion in the **nerve of the pterygoid canal**. This nerve is formed by the union of the greater petrosal nerve and deep petrosal nerve. The greater petrosal nerve is a branch of the facial nerve carrying preganglionic parasympathetic fibres to the ganglion. The deep petrosal nerve is a branch of the internal carotid plexus carrying post-ganglionic sympathetic fibres [see Fig. 13.8]. The preganglionic parasympathetic fibres synapse in the ganglion.

Branches of the pterygopalatine ganglion

Branches of the pterygopalatine ganglion contain post-ganglionic parasympathetic, sympathetic, and sensory nerves. They supply the lacrimal gland and glands in the nose, palate, and pharynx. The named branches are: (1) the palatine branches—the greater and lesser palatine nerves; (2) the **orbital branches**—2–3 thin filaments which enter the orbit through the inferior orbital fissure to supply the orbital periosteum (sensory) and the lacrimal gland (secretory); (3) the **nasopalatine** and **posterior nasal branches** passing through the sphenopalatine foramen to the mucous membrane of the nose; and (4) the **pharyngeal branch** which passes posteriorly through the palatovaginal canal to the mucous membrane of the sphenoidal air sinus and the roof of the pharynx.

Termination of the maxillary artery

The third part of the maxillary artery enters the pterygopalatine fossa through the pterygomaxillary fissure [see Fig. 15.3]. It breaks up into branches which accompany the nerves in the pterygopalatine fossa (infra-orbital, posterior superior alveolar, greater palatine, nasopalatine, pharyngeal, and nerve of the pterygoid canal) and carry the same names.

Maxillary air sinus

The maxillary air sinus is the largest of the paranasal air sinuses. It occupies the whole of the body of the maxilla and has the shape of an irregular three-sided pyramid. The **apex** is directed laterally and extends into the zygomatic process of the maxilla. The **base** is the lower part of the lateral wall of the nose. The sides are the different surfaces of the maxilla—the orbital, anterior, and infratemporal sides. The sinus lies superior to the molar and premolar teeth. The lowest part of this sinus is opposite the second premolar and first molar tooth, and is approximately 1 cm below the level of the floor of the nose [see Figs. 11.3, 13.11, 17.7, 17.10; Figs. 19.2, 19.7].

Nasal opening

The maxillary air sinus opens into the middle meatus of the nasal cavity through an aperture in the superior part of its base. The high position of the aperture makes it difficult for fluid in the sinus to drain into the nose when the head is in an erect position, until the sinus is nearly filled [see Fig. 11.3; Fig. 19.2].

The infra-orbital groove and canal run forwards in the bone of the roof of the sinus. The canal bends inferiorly towards the infra-orbital foramen and produces a marked ridge in the angle between the orbital and anterior surfaces of the sinus. The posterior superior alveolar nerve and vessels run in the lower part of the infratemporal and anterior walls of the sinus. The anterior superior alveolar nerve and vessels are in the orbital and anterior surfaces [see Fig. 15.4; Fig. 19.7]. The **mucous membrane** of the sinus is supplied by branches of these nerves and by branches of the greater palatine nerve. The sinus is lined with ciliated columnar epithelium which moves mucus on its surface towards the opening into the nose. ⊃ In some situations, the bone which separates the nerves from the mucous membrane of the sinus may be absent, and this, combined with the fact that the alveolar nerves supply both the teeth and the mucous lining of the sinus, may be responsible for the sensation of toothache which frequently accompanies inflammation in the sinus.

Sphenoidal air sinuses

Using the instructions given in Dissection 19.6, dissect the sphenoidal air sinus.

The paired sphenoidal air sinuses occupy a variable extent of the body of the sphenoid bone. They may extend into the wings and pterygoid processes, and even into the basilar part of the occipital bone. Each opens by a small, round hole into the spheno-ethmoidal recess [see Fig. 8.12; Fig. 19.3].

Position

Each sinus lies posterior to the nasal cavity and superior to the nasopharynx. Posteriorly, a thick layer of bone usually separates it from the cranial cavity, the basilar artery, and the pons. Above the sphenoidal sinus lie the pituitary gland, intercavernous sinuses, and the cavernous sinuses further laterally [see Figs. 3.4B, 8.12, 8.13A; Fig. 19.3].

DISSECTION 19.6 Sphenoidal air sinus

Objective

I. To study the sphenoidal air sinus.

Instructions

1. Examine these sinuses on the two halves of the bisected skull [Fig. 19.3]. As the septum between them is not median, it may be necessary to break down the septum to open the sinus which is not exposed by the cut through the skull.

2. Find the nasal openings into the sinuses in their anterior walls.

See Clinical Applications 19.1 and 19.2 for the practical implications of the anatomy discussed in this chapter.

CLINICAL APPLICATION 19.1 Sinusitis

Infections commonly spread from the nasal cavity into the paranasal air sinuses. Inflammation and swelling of the mucous lining of the paranasal sinuses is known as sinusitis. The opening of the maxillary sinus into the nasal cavity is situated high on the medial wall. It is also small and easily blocked by swelling of the mucosa. These factors lead to an accumulation of secretions within the sinus, associated with pain and heaviness of the head. The proximity of the floor of the sinus to the upper molars [Fig. 19.2A], and the common sensory nerves to both, often makes it difficult to locate the primary pathology.

Fluid in the maxillary sinus may drain at night when the patient lies on one side. (The position of the ostia is such that the right sinus will drain when the patient lies on the left, and vice versa.) In contrast, the frontal air sinus drains best when the head is erect and is often painful and heavy early in the morning.

The relation of the ostia of the frontal sinus to that of the maxillary sinus in the middle meatus is such that infection from the frontal sinus often tracks into the maxillary sinus.

CLINICAL APPLICATION 19.2 Pollen allergy

An 8-year-old girl returned from a school outing, looking tired and feverish. By evening, she complained of a headache, itching of her nose and eyes, and a sore throat. She also started coughing and had watering of her eyes and a running nose. She told her parents that it all started when she was playing in a field and had begun with a bout of repeated sneezing. The family physician examined her and treated her for pollen allergy.

Study question 1: which part of the nervous system supplies the glands in the nasal cavity? (Answer: the parasympathetic system.)

Study question 2: what nerves are responsible for secretions of the glands in the nasal cavity? Trace the entire secretomotor pathway. (Answer: preganglionic para-

sympathetic fibres runs in the facial nerve. They leave the facial nerve in the greater petrosal nerve, run in the nerve of the pterygoid canal, reach the pterygopalatine ganglion, and synapse with cells in the ganglion. Post-ganglionic fibres from the ganglion reach the walls of the nasal cavity through branches of the maxillary nerve and medial posterior superior nasal branches of the ganglion.) The lacrimal glands are supplied by parasympathetic nerves from the pterygopalatine ganglion, which run through the zygomatic and lacrimal nerves.

Pollen allergy also causes conjunctivitis and sinusitis which could account for the itching of the eyes and headache in this patient.

CHAPTER 20
The larynx

Introduction to the larynx

The larynx is the upper expanded part of the airway which is modified for sound production. Its walls are supported by a number of cartilages [Figs. 20.1, 20.2, 20.3, 20.4, 20.5, 20.6]: (1) the ring-like cricoid cartilage inferiorly; (2) the V-shaped thyroid cartilage at a higher level than the cricoid; the thyroid cartilage consists of two laminae set at an angle to each other; (3) the unpaired leaf-shaped epiglottis in the midline; and (4) the paired arytenoid cartilages on the superior margin of the cricoid. In addition, two small paired nodules of cartilage—the corniculate and cuneiform cartilages—are seen on the inlet of the larynx. Familiarize yourself with the location and inter-relations of these cartilages using the figures.

The lower part of the larynx is vertical and parallel to the laryngeal part of the pharynx which lies posterior to it. The upper part (within the concavity of the thyroid cartilage) curves [see Fig. 17.3]

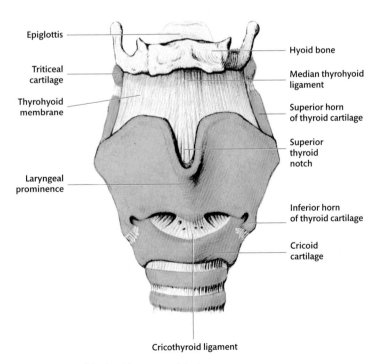

Epiglottis

Triticeal cartilage

Thyrohyoid membrane

Laryngeal prominence

Hyoid bone

Median thyrohyoid ligament

Superior horn of thyroid cartilage

Superior thyroid notch

Inferior horn of thyroid cartilage

Cricoid cartilage

Cricothyroid ligament

Fig. 20.1 Anterior aspect of the cartilages (blue) and ligaments of the larynx.

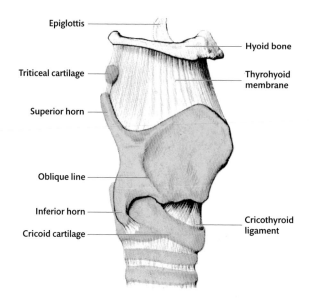

Fig. 20.2 Lateral view of the cartilages (blue) and ligaments of the larynx.

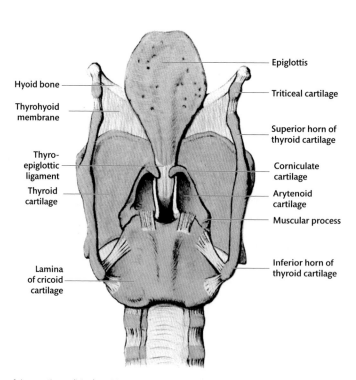

Fig. 20.3 Posterior aspect of the cartilages (blue) and ligaments of the larynx.

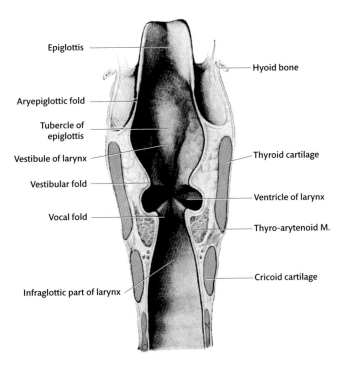

Epiglottis

Hyoid bone

Aryepiglottic fold

Tubercle of
epiglottis

Vestibule of larynx

Thyroid cartilage

Vestibular fold

Ventricle of larynx

Vocal fold

Thyro-arytenoid M.

Cricoid cartilage

Infraglottic part of larynx

Fig. 20.4 Coronal section through the larynx to show its parts. Cartilage = blue.

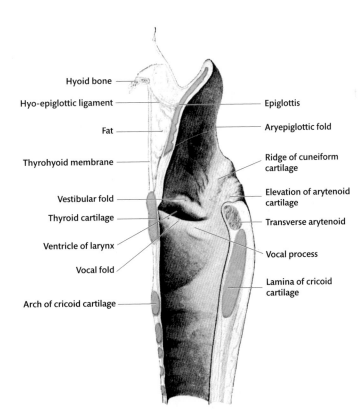

Hyoid bone

Hyo-epiglottic ligament

Epiglottis

Fat

Aryepiglottic fold

Thyrohyoid membrane

Ridge of cuneiform
cartilage

Elevation of arytenoid
cartilage

Vestibular fold

Thyroid cartilage

Transverse arytenoid

Ventricle of larynx

Vocal fold

Vocal process

Lamina of cricoid
cartilage

Arch of cricoid cartilage

Fig. 20.5 Median section through the larynx to show the lateral wall of its right half. Cartilage = blue.

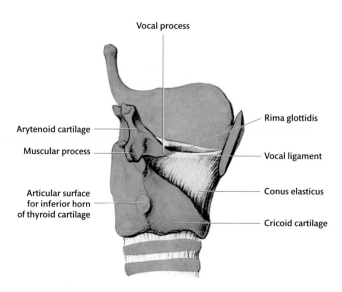

Vocal process

Arytenoid cartilage

Muscular process

Articular surface
for inferior horn
of thyroid cartilage

Rima glottidis

Vocal ligament

Conus elasticus

Cricoid cartilage

Fig. 20.6 Dissection to show the conus elasticus and vocal ligament. The right lamina of the thyroid cartilage has been removed. Cartilage = blue.

back to open into the pharynx through a vertical orifice—the **inlet of the larynx**. On either side of the inlet, part of the pharyngeal cavity projects forwards as the **piriform recess** [see Fig. 17.7].

Cartilages, ligaments, and joints of the larynx

Thyroid cartilage

The thyroid cartilage is the largest of the laryngeal cartilages and consists of two laminae or plates of hyaline cartilage. In the midline anteriorly, the inferior parts of the two laminae are fused together. The superior parts of the laminae are separated from each other by the deep **superior thyroid notch** [Fig. 20.1] and project anteriorly to form the **laryngeal prominence**. The angle at which the laminae meet varies (from 90 to 120 degrees). It is more acute in the male, making it more prominent than in the female.

The thyroid laminae diverge posteriorly and end in the posterior margins, which are lateral to the **piriform recesses** of the pharynx. Each posterior margin extends superiorly and inferiorly as slender horns (**cornua**) of the thyroid cartilage [Figs. 20.2, 20.3]. The **superior horns** are attached to the corresponding greater horns

of the hyoid bone by the thyrohyoid ligaments. The **inferior horns** articulate with the cricoid cartilage.

The lateral surfaces of the thyroid cartilage are relatively flat, except for a raised, oblique line on each lamina [Fig. 20.2]. The inferior constrictor of the pharynx, the pre-tracheal fascia, and the sternothyroid and thyrohyoid muscles are attached to the oblique line.

Thyrohyoid membrane and ligaments

The thyrohyoid membrane ascends up from the superior border of the thyroid cartilage, passes deep to the concavity of the hyoid bone, and is attached to the upper margin of the hyoid bone. Anteriorly, the membrane is thickened to form the **median thyrohyoid ligament**. This ligament is separated from the posterior surface of the body of the hyoid bone by a bursa, which lessens the friction between them when the upper border of the thyroid cartilage is drawn up behind the hyoid bone in swallowing. The lateral thyrohyoid ligaments are thickened posterior margins of the thyrohyoid membrane. Each contains a small cartilaginous nodule—the **triticeal cartilage** [Figs. 20.1, 20.2, 20.3]. The thyrohyoid ligament is pierced by the internal laryngeal branch of the superior laryngeal nerve and the superior laryngeal vessels.

DISSECTION 20.1 Thyrohyoid membrane

DISSECTION 20.1 Thyrohyoid membrane

Objective

I. To expose the thyrohyoid membrane and study its attachments.

Instructions

1. Cut through the thyrohyoid muscle to expose the thyrohyoid membrane and the vessels and nerve piercing it.

2. Define the attachments of the membrane.

Using the instructions given in Dissection 20.1, study the thyrohyoid membrane.

Cricoid cartilage

The cricoid cartilage is shaped like a signet ring. The horizontal inferior margin is at the level of the sixth cervical vertebra. The narrow **arch of the cricoid** lies anteriorly [Fig. 20.1]. Traced laterally from the arch, the upper margin of the cricoid cartilage [Fig. 20.6] slopes upwards, deep to the thyroid cartilage, to form the **lamina of the cricoid cartilage** [Fig. 20.3]. The cricothyroid membrane extends upwards from the upper margin of the cricoid cartilage to the thyroid cartilage. It is thickened in the midline anteriorly to form the **cricothyroid ligament**. The cricoid is attached to the trachea by the membranous, elastic **cricotracheal ligament** [Fig. 20.1].

Arytenoid cartilages

Each of the paired arytenoid cartilages is shaped like a three-sided pyramid [Fig. 20.3]. It rests on the superior surface of the cricoid lamina and forms a synovial joint with it [Figs. 20.3, 20.6].

Each arytenoid cartilage has a **muscular process** which projects laterally and gives attachment to the crico-arytenoid muscles, and a **vocal process** which projects anteriorly and gives attachment to the vocal ligament [Fig. 20.6]. The apex of the arytenoid cartilage extends upwards, curves posteromedially, and has the corniculate cartilage resting on it. The transverse arytenoid muscle is attached to the posterior surface of each arytenoid cartilage [see Fig. 20.10]. The thyro-arytenoid and vocalis muscles are attached to the anterolateral surfaces [Fig. 20.4; see also Fig. 20.11].

Clean and define the cricothyroid muscle and cricothyroid membrane by following the instructions provided in Dissection 20.2.

Cricothyroid joint

The inferior horns of the thyroid cartilage articulate with the lamina of the cricoid cartilage by a synovial joint—the cricothyroid joint [Fig. 20.3]. The two cricothyroid joints allow the cricoid cartilage to rock around a horizontal axis passing through both of them. This movement swings the superior margin of the lamina of the cricoid cartilage and the attached arytenoid cartilages either towards or away from the anterior part of the thyroid **cartilage** and slackens or tightens

DISSECTION 20.2 Cricothyroid muscle and cricothyroid membrane

Objectives

I. To expose the cricothyroid muscle. **II.** To expose the cricothyroid membrane. **III.** To identify the cricothyroid joint.

Instructions

1. Turn the sternothyroid muscle upwards, and define its attachment to the thyroid cartilage.

2. Identify the attachments of the inferior constrictor to the thyroid and cricoid cartilages and to the fascia covering the cricothyroid muscle.

3. Expose the cricothyroid muscle by removing the fascia over it and reflecting the divided parts of the inferior constrictor [see Fig. 17.5].

4. Trace the inferior horn of the thyroid cartilage to its articulation with the cricoid cartilage.

5. Expose the cricothyroid ligament at the anterior border of the cricothyroid muscle.

6. Note that the cricothyroid membrane passes deep to the cricothyroid muscle.

the elastic vocal ligament which is attached to it [p. 246] [Fig. 20.6].

Epiglottis

The epiglottis is a thin, leaf-shaped cartilage. It forms the upper part of the anterior wall of the larynx, and the superior margin of the inlet of the larynx [Fig. 20.3]. It is posterior to the base of the tongue, hyoid bone, and median thyrohyoid ligament. The epiglottis tapers inferiorly and is attached to the posterior surface of the thyroid cartilage in the midline by the strong **thyro-epiglottic ligament**. It is convex anteriorly in its superior part, and convex posteriorly in the lower part. The lower part bulges into the larynx as the **epiglottic tubercle** [Fig. 20.4]. Numerous mucous and serous glands lie on the surface of the epiglottis.

Ligaments of the epiglottis

The thyro-epiglottic ligament has been described earlier. In addition, the anterior surface of the epiglottis is also attached to the upper surface of the hyoid bone by the loose, fibro-elastic **hyo-epiglottic ligament** [Fig. 20.5]. This is separated from the thyro-epiglottic and median thyrohyoid ligaments by fat, which is displaced when the thyroid cartilage is drawn up inside the hyoid bone. The epiglottis is also attached to the tongue by the median and lateral **glosso-epiglottic folds** of mucous membrane [see Figs. 17.7, 18.1] and to the arytenoid cartilages by the **aryepiglottic folds** [see Fig. 17.7].

Dissection 20.3 provides instructions on dissection of the ligaments of the epiglottis.

Crico-arytenoid joints

The crico-arytenoid joints are synovial joints between the base of the arytenoid cartilage and the

lamina of the cricoid cartilage. At these joints, the arytenoid cartilages: (1) slide transversely to come closer together or move apart on the lamina of the cricoid; and (2) rotate around a vertical axis [Figs. 20.7, 20.8], so as to approximate or separate the vocal processes (and hence the vocal ligaments). The arytenoid cartilages are prevented from slipping anteriorly on the cricoid lamina by the strong posterior capsule of the joint [Fig. 20.3].

Structure of laryngeal cartilages

The thyroid, cricoid, and basal parts of the arytenoid cartilages are composed of hyaline cartilage and tend to ossify, even in early adult life. In old age, they may be completely ossified. The apex and vocal process of the arytenoid cartilage and the other cartilages are made up of elastic fibrocartilage and do not ossify.

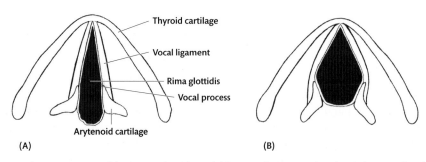

Fig. 20.7 Diagrams to show movements of the arytenoid cartilages. (A) Position during quiet breathing—the rima glottidis is partially open. (B) Position during forced respiration—the rima glottidis is wide open.

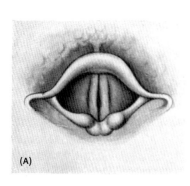
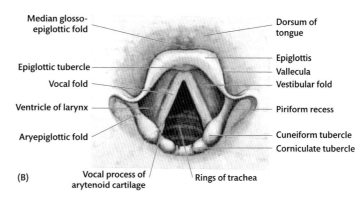

Median glosso-epiglottic fold

Dorsum of tongue

Epiglottic tubercle

Epiglottis

Vocal fold

Vallecula

Vestibular fold

Ventricle of larynx

Piriform recess

Aryepiglottic fold

Cuneiform tubercle

Corniculate tubercle

Vocal process of arytenoid cartilage

Rings of trachea

(A)

(B)

Fig. 20.8 Laryngoscopic view of the cavity of the larynx. (A) During phonation. The rima glottidis is closed by approximation of the vocal folds. (B) During moderate respiration. The rima glottidis is widely open.

Exterior of the larynx

The inlet of the larynx is an almost vertically placed opening. It is bound anterosuperiorly by the epiglottis, on each side by the aryepiglottic fold of mucous membrane, and inferiorly by the interarytenoid fold of mucous membrane. The vertical posterior wall of the larynx below the inlet is made up of the lamina of the cricoid cartilage, surmounted by the two arytenoid cartilages, covered by mucous membrane [see Fig. 17.7]. The anterior wall of the larynx is made up of: (1) the epiglottis which curves upwards and backwards from its attachment to the internal surface of the thyroid cartilage; (2) the thyroid cartilage; and (3) the arch of the cricoid cartilage [Fig. 20.1]. The lateral wall of the upper part is formed by the **aryepiglottic fold**. Each fold has two small nodules of cartilage—the **corniculate** and **cuneiform cartilages**—embedded in its margin near the arytenoid cartilage [see Fig. 17.7].

Interior of the larynx

The interior of the larynx is divided into superior and inferior parts by anteroposterior folds projecting from the lateral walls—the **vocal folds**. Above each vocal fold is a subsidiary **vestibular fold** which is separated from the vocal fold by a narrow, horizontal groove—the **ventricle of the larynx** [Fig. 20.4]. The two pairs of folds narrow the middle part of the laryngeal cavity. The part of the laryngeal cavity above the vestibular folds is the **vestibule of the larynx**. The part below is the **infraglottic part of the larynx**.

Vestibule of the larynx

The superior part, or vestibule of the larynx extends from the inlet of the larynx to the vestibular folds. It has a long **anterosuperior wall** consisting of the mucous membrane covering the epiglottis and thyro-epiglottic ligament, and a short **posterior wall** formed by the mucous membrane covering the apex of the arytenoid and corniculate cartilages. The lateral walls are the aryepiglottic folds which slope inwards towards the vestibular folds and separate the vestibule of the larynx from the piriform recess of the pharynx [Figs. 20.4, 20.5].

Vestibular folds

Vestibular folds are soft, flaccid folds of mucous membrane which extend from the thyroid to the arytenoid cartilages. They contain: (1) numerous mucous glands; (2) a thin band of fibro-elastic tissue; and (3) a few muscle fibres. They lie further apart than the vocal folds and play little or no part in sound production [Fig. 20.5]. The space between the two vestibular folds is the **rima vestibuli**.

Ventricle and saccule of the larynx

The ventricle of the larynx is the narrow groove between the vestibular and vocal folds [Figs. 20.4, 20.5]. The saccule of the larynx is a narrow, blind diverticulum which passes posterosuperiorly between the vestibular fold and the thyroid cartilage. It may reach up to the upper border of the thyroid cartilage.

Dissection 20.4 provides instructions on dissection of the ventricle and saccule of the larynx.

Vocal folds

Each vocal fold is wedge-shaped in the coronal section [Fig. 20.4]. The apex projects medially into the laryngeal cavity. The base lies against the lamina of the thyroid cartilage. The superior surface is nearly horizontal and forms the inferior wall of the ventricle. The inferior surface slopes inferolaterally to the superior border of the cricoid cartilage. Each fold contains the conus elasticus, vocal ligament, and muscle fibres covered with mucous membrane.

Conus elasticus and vocal ligament

The conus elasticus is a thin layer of fibro-elastic tissue on the inferomedial surface of each vocal fold, immediately deep to the mucous membrane. It is an elastic membrane which is attached inferiorly to the arch of the cricoid cartilage. It slopes superomedially to end in a free margin which stretches from the back of the thyroid cartilage (close to the midline) to the vocal process of the corresponding arytenoid cartilage [Fig. 20.6]. The free edge of each membrane is a thickened elastic band known as the **vocal ligament**. The membranes on the right and left sides together form the **conus elasticus**. Anteriorly, the conus elasticus is continuous with the cricothyroid ligament. The mucous membrane covering the vocal ligament is tightly bound to it.

The muscle fibres in the vocal fold lie between the conus elasticus and the lamina of the thyroid cartilage. They arise from the thyroid cartilage and vocal ligament anteriorly. Most of them pass horizontally backwards to the arytenoid cartilage (**thyro-arytenoideus**). The most medial fibres arise from the vocal ligament and form the **vocalis muscle**. The most lateral fibres sweep superiorly to the epiglottis—the **thyro-epiglotticus** [see Fig. 20.11].

Using the instructions given in Dissection 20.5, expose the vocal fold and conus elasticus.

Rima glottidis

The rima glottidis is a midline fissure between the free margins of the vocal folds and the vocal processes of the arytenoid cartilages. The anterior part of the rima lies between the two vocal folds, and the posterior part between the two arytenoid cartilages [Figs. 20.7, 20.8]. It is the narrowest part of the laryngeal cavity and lies behind the thyroid cartilage. The shape of the rima glottidis is continually changing [Fig. 20.8] due to movements of the arytenoid cartilages on the cricoid and of the cricoid relative to the thyroid cartilage. The posterior part of the rima is progressively widened when: (1) the arytenoid cartilages are displaced laterally on the cricoid; and (2) the arytenoids are rotated such that their vocal processes turn laterally [Figs. 20.7B, 20.8B]. If the lamina of the cricoid is tilted forwards with the arytenoids in this position, the vocal ligaments are slackened and the opening can be widened further to allow the free passage of air in forced respiration.

The rima glottidis is narrowed or closed when the arytenoid cartilages are: (1) drawn together; and (2) rotated so that their vocal processes come into apposition [Figs. 20.7A, 20.8A]. The additional tightening of the vocal ligaments by tilting of the cricoid lamina backwards effectively prevents the passage of air. This tightly closed position is taken up prior to the explosive discharge of air in coughing and sneezing. During these actions, the intrathoracic pressure is raised by contraction of the expiratory muscles, following which the tension in the vocal folds is released suddenly.

When the rima glottidis is closed, attempts to draw air into the thorax push the sloping vocal folds more firmly together and prevent inspiration, a situation which arises in laryngeal spasm.

Delicate variations in the following factors are responsible for changes in the pitch and volume of the voice: (1) the tension and length of the vocal cords; (2) the width of the rima glottidis; and (3) the intensity of expiratory effort. The lower pitch of the male voice is due to the greater length of the vocal folds in them (approximately 2.5 cm), as compared with those in the female (approximately 1.7 cm).

Infraglottic part of the larynx

Superiorly, the infraglottic part of the larynx is narrowed by the vocal folds. Inferiorly, the cavity of the larynx is circular at the level of the arch of the cricoid cartilage where it is continuous with the trachea [Fig. 20.9].

Muscles of the larynx

The small muscles of the larynx move the parts of the larynx on each other. They are concerned with alterations in the length and tension of the vocal folds and in changing the size of the rima glottidis.

Cricothyroid

The cricothyroid is seen on the external surface of the larynx anteriorly. It passes posterosuperiorly from the anterolateral part of the cricoid cartilage to the inferior horn, inferior margin, and lower part of the deep surface of the lamina of the thyroid cartilage [Fig. 20.9]. **Nerve supply**: external branch of the superior laryngeal nerve. **Action**: it draws the arch of the cricoid posterosuperiorly, rotating the entire cartilage around the cricothyroid joints, so that the lamina is tilted posteriorly. This movement causes stretching and tightening of the vocal ligaments and raises the pitch of the voice.

Using the instructions given in Dissection 20.6, identify the muscles of the larynx.

Posterior crico-arytenoid

The posterior crico-arytenoid arises from the posterior surface of the lamina of the cricoid cartilage,

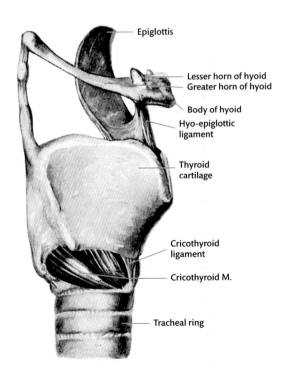

Fig. 20.9 The right cricothyroid muscle.

Epiglottis

Lesser horn of hyoid
Greater horn of hyoid

Body of hyoid
Hyo-epiglottic ligament

Thyroid cartilage

Cricothyroid ligament

Cricothyroid M.

Tracheal ring

DISSECTION 20.6 Muscles of the larynx

Objectives

I. To identify and study the posterior crico-arytenoid, thyro-arytenoid, and oblique arytenoid muscles.
II. To identify and trace the recurrent laryngeal nerve.

Instructions

1. Identify the recurrent laryngeal nerve entering the larynx, deep to the inferior constrictor muscle.

2. Strip the mucous membrane from the posterior surface of the arytenoid and cricoid cartilage. Note the attachment of the longitudinal oesophageal muscle fibres to the median part of the cricoid lamina.

3. Identify the posterior crico-arytenoid, transverse arytenoid, and oblique arytenoid muscles [Fig. 20.10]. The transverse arytenoid and oblique arytenoid have been divided in the midline, but the oblique arytenoid can be followed into continuity with the aryepiglottic muscle by stripping the mucous membrane from the margin of the aryepiglottic fold.

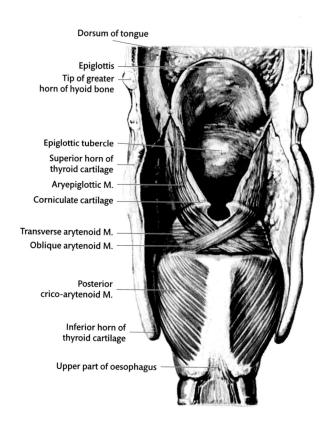

Dorsum of tongue

Epiglottis

Tip of greater horn of hyoid bone

Epiglottic tubercle

Superior horn of thyroid cartilage

Aryepiglottic M.

Corniculate cartilage

Transverse arytenoid M.

Oblique arytenoid M.

Posterior crico-arytenoid M.

Inferior horn of thyroid cartilage

Upper part of oesophagus

Fig. 20.10 Muscles on the posterior surface of the larynx.

runs laterally, and converges on the laterally directed muscular process of the arytenoid cartilage [Fig. 20.10]. **Nerve supply**: recurrent laryngeal branch of the vagus. (All intrinsic muscles of the larynx, except the cricothyroid, are supplied by the recurrent laryngeal nerve.) **Action**: the upper, more horizontal fibres rotate the arytenoid, so that its vocal process is directed laterally and the rima glottidis is opened. The lower, more vertical fibres pull the arytenoid laterally, further increasing the size of the rima. It is the sole abductor of the vocal folds.

Transverse and oblique arytenoid muscles

The transverse and oblique arytenoids extend between the two arytenoid cartilages and draw them together, closing the rima glottidis. The continuity of the oblique arytenoid and aryepiglottic muscles ensures that the arytenoid cartilages are drawn together, closing the rima, while the epiglottis is pulled down over the laryngeal inlet, during passage of food or fluid into the pharynx [Fig. 20.10].

Using the instructions given in Dissection 20.7, study the cricothyroid joint.

DISSECTION 20.7 Cricothyroid joint

Objectives

I. To open the cricothyroid joint.   **II.** To examine the thyro-arytenoid and lateral crico-arytenoid muscles.

Instructions

1. On one side, remove the cricothyroid muscle, the lower part of the lamina, and the inferior horn of the thyroid cartilage, thus opening the cricothyroid joint. Take care not to cut the recurrent laryngeal nerve (the inferior laryngeal nerve) which is deep to the posterior part of the thyroid cartilage.

2. Examine the thyro-arytenoid muscle in the vocal fold which is now exposed [Fig. 20.11], with the lateral crico-arytenoid muscle inferior to it.

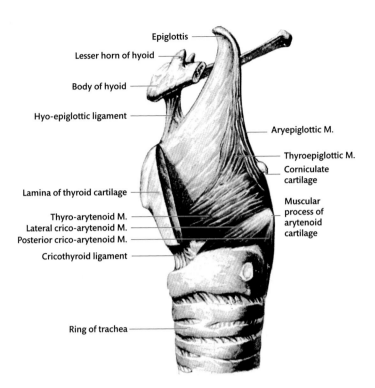

Epiglottis

Lesser horn of hyoid

Body of hyoid

Hyo-epiglottic ligament

Aryepiglottic M.

Thyroepiglottic M.

Corniculate cartilage

Lamina of thyroid cartilage

Thyro-arytenoid M.
Lateral crico-arytenoid M.
Posterior crico-arytenoid M.

Muscular process of arytenoid cartilage

Cricothyroid ligament

Ring of trachea

Fig. 20.11 Muscles in the lateral wall of the larynx.

Lateral crico-arytenoid muscle

The lateral crico-arytenoid muscle takes origin from the superior border of the posterior part of the arch of the cricoid cartilage and is inserted into the muscular process of the arytenoid cartilage [Figs. 20.11, 20.12]. **Action**: it pulls the muscular process anteriorly, rotating the arytenoid so that its vocal process swings medially and closes the rima glottidis.

Thyro-arytenoid and vocalis

The thyro-arytenoid takes origin from the posterior surface of the thyroid cartilage, close to the midline, and is inserted into the anterolateral surface of the arytenoid cartilage. The upper lateral fibres sweep superiorly to the epiglottis—the **thyro-epiglottic** muscle. Some of the deeper fibres arise from the vocal ligament and pass to the vocal process of the arytenoid cartilage. These fibres constitute the **vocalis** muscle [Figs. 20.11, 20.12]. **Action**: the main mass of the muscle pulls the arytenoid anteriorly and slackens the vocal ligament.

The vocalis tends to tighten the anterior part of the ligament, while simultaneously slackening the posterior part—a position taken up by the vocal cords in whispering. The thyro-epiglottic and aryepiglottic muscles play a minor role in closing the laryngeal inlet.

Extrinsic muscles

The extrinsic muscles of the larynx raise and lower the larynx during swallowing. The **thyrohyoid**, acting from a fixed hyoid bone and assisted by the **stylopharyngeus** and **palatopharyngeus**, raises the larynx inside the hyoid bone. The elevated epiglottis is tipped backwards by the bulging posterior surface of the tongue (assisted by the aryepiglotticus and thyro-epiglotticus). It comes into contact with the elevated arytenoid cartilages, closes the laryngeal orifice, and allows the tip of the epiglottis to direct the bolus away from the larynx. The **sternothyroid** returns the larynx to its original position and opens the laryngeal orifice.

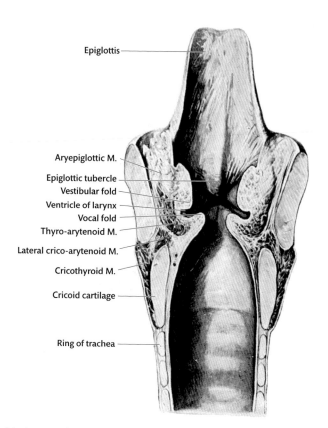

Epiglottis

Aryepiglottic M.
Epiglottic tubercle
Vestibular fold
Ventricle of larynx
Vocal fold
Thyro-arytenoid M.
Lateral crico-arytenoid M.
Cricothyroid M.
Cricoid cartilage
Ring of trachea

Fig. 20.12 Coronal section of the larynx to show the position of the muscles.

Nerves and vessels of the larynx

Superior laryngeal nerve

The **superior laryngeal** branch of the vagus divides into internal and external nerves [see Fig. 17.5]. The **internal laryngeal nerve** pierces the thyrohyoid membrane with the superior laryngeal artery and supplies the lateral wall of the piriform recess, through a number of small branches. Some branches pass in the aryepiglottic fold to the base of the tongue and epiglottis. Others descend to supply the mucous membrane on the internal surface of the larynx, as far as the vocal folds, and the mucous membrane covering the posterior surfaces of the arytenoid and cricoid cartilages. One branch descends deep to the thyroid cartilage to join a similar branch from the recurrent laryngeal nerve. It contains sensory and autonomic fibres.

The **external laryngeal nerve** supplies the cricothyroid muscle.

Recurrent laryngeal nerve

The recurrent laryngeal branch of the vagus ascends in the groove between the trachea and oesophagus. It enters the larynx by passing deep to the lower border of the inferior constrictor, posterior to the cricothyroid joint [see Fig. 17.5]. It supplies all the intrinsic muscles of the larynx, except the cricothyroid, and the mucous membrane below the rima glottidis. It communicates with the internal laryngeal branch of the superior laryngeal nerve and is accompanied by the inferior laryngeal branch of the inferior thyroid artery.

Fig. 20.13A and B show the vocal cords, cartilages, and relations of the larynx in a cross-sectional view.

See Clinical Applications 20.1 and 20.2 for the practical implications of the anatomy discussed in this chapter.

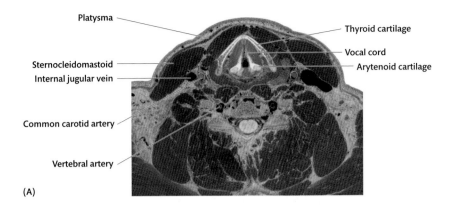

Platysma
Thyroid cartilage
Vocal cord
Sternocleidomastoid
Arytenoid cartilage
Internal jugular vein
Common carotid artery
Vertebral artery

(A)

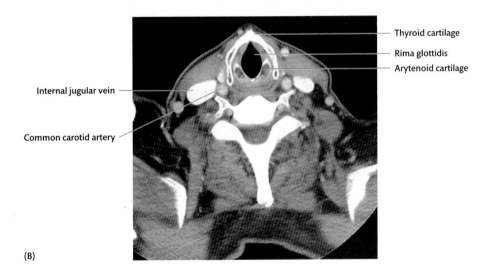

Thyroid cartilage
Rima glottidis
Arytenoid cartilage
Internal jugular vein
Common carotid artery

(B)

Fig. 20.13 (A) Horizontal section through the neck at the level of the vocal cords. (B) Contrast enhanced axial CT section at the level of the vocal cords.

Image A courtesy of the Visible Human Project of the US National Library of Medicine.

CLINICAL APPLICATION 20.1 Injury to the recurrent and superior laryngeal nerves

Injury to the recurrent laryngeal nerve on one side leads to hoarseness of voice, due to paralysis of the vocal cord on that side. The paralysed vocal cord cannot adduct to close the rima. Some degree of compensatory movement of the vocal cord of the other side will occur with time. In bilateral paralysis of the cords, the voice is almost totally lost. In such cases, abduction of the cords is also lost (paralysis of the posterior crico-arytenoids), and the patient will not be able to take a deep breath. Attempt to do so will result in stridor—a loud, high-pitched sound—and a sense of anxiety.

Injury to the superior laryngeal nerve will result in loss of sensation in the vestibule. Accidental aspiration of food particles during swallowing will not be detected, and the aspirate will enter the larynx. In addition, paralysis of the cricothyroid muscle will make it hard to raise the pitch of the voice.

CLINICAL APPLICATION 20.2 Laryngoscopy

The larynx can be visualized in the living by a procedure known as laryngoscopy. In direct laryngoscopy, an instrument—the laryngoscope—is inserted into the mouth, past the tongue and epiglottis, towards the inlet of the larynx. The laryngoscope allows the doctor to visualize the vestibule of the larynx, the vestibular fold, and the vocal folds. When the rima glottidis is open, the infraglottic part of the larynx can also be seen through the laryngoscope [Fig. 20.8].

In indirect laryngoscopy, a small hand-held mirror is held at the back of the throat, and a light is shone into the patient's mouth. The mirror is angulated, so as to get a reflection of the larynx on the mirror. The piriform recess of the pharynx can also be examined in this way.

Table 20.1 provides an overview of the movements of the larynx.

Table 20.2 provides an overview of movements taking place during sneezing and coughing.

Table 20.1 Movements of the larynx

Movement	Muscles	Nerve supply
As a whole		
Elevation (this closes the laryngeal orifice)	Thyrohyoid (hyoid fixed)	C. 1 ventral ramus
	Stylopharyngeus	Glossopharyngeal
	Palatopharyngeus	Pharyngeal plexus
Depression (this opens the laryngeal orifice)	Sternothyroid	Ansa cervicalis
Of vocal cords		
Abduction	Posterior crico-arytenoid	Recurrent laryngeal
Adduction	Lateral crico-arytenoid	Recurrent laryngeal
	Oblique and transverse arytenoid	Recurrent laryngeal
Tightening	Cricothyroid	External laryngeal
	Vocalis	Recurrent laryngeal
Slackening	Thyro-arytenoid	Recurrent laryngeal
	Vocalis	Recurrent laryngeal

Table 20.2 Sneezing and coughing

Movement	Muscles	Nerve supply
1. A breath is taken in:		
Inspiration	See Vol. 2	
2. Intrathoracic pressure is raised by:		
(a) Tensing and adducting vocal cords	Cricothyroid	External laryngeal
	Oblique and transverse arytenoids, lateral crico-arytenoid	Recurrent laryngeal
(b) Contracting expiratory muscles	Oblique and transverse abdominals	Intercostal and subcostal
	Internal intercostal, transversus thoracis	Intercostal
	Levator ani and sphincter urethrae	Pudendal
3(a) Sneezing Palate depressed against posterior part of tongue to separate mouth from pharynx	Palatopharyngeus	Pharyngeal plexus
	Palatoglossus	Pharyngeal plexus
3(b) Coughing Palate raised, tensed, and pulled against posterior pharyngeal wall to separate oral and nasal parts of pharynx	Levator palati	Pharyngeal plexus
	Tensor palati	Mandibular
	Superior constrictor	Pharyngeal plexus
	Palatopharyngeus (horizontal part)	Pharyngeal plexus
4. Vocal cords suddenly abducted to release intrathoracic air pressure through nose or mouth	Posterior crico-arytenoid	Recurrent laryngeal

The parts numbered 1, 2, and 4 of the sequence are the same in both activities.

CHAPTER 21
The contents of the vertebral canal

Introduction

The vertebral canal lies behind the vertebral bodies and intervertebral discs, and in front of the spines and laminae of the vertebrae [Fig. 21.1]. The main content of the vertebral canal is the spinal cord, the meninges surrounding the spinal cord, the blood vessels supplying the cord, and the spinal nerves. The external features of the spinal cord and its coverings and blood supply are described in this chapter. The internal features are described later in the section on the brain and spinal cord.

255

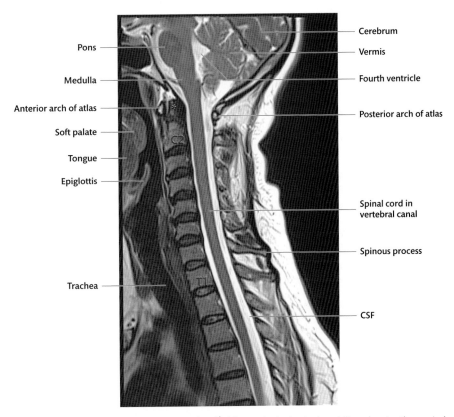

Pons
Medulla
Anterior arch of atlas
Soft palate
Tongue
Epiglottis
Trachea

Cerebrum
Vermis
Fourth ventricle
Posterior arch of atlas
Spinal cord in vertebral canal
Spinous process
CSF

Fig. 21.1 T2-weighted sagittal magnetic resonance imaging (MRI) of the cervical spine in the midline, showing the cervical and upper thoracic vertebrae (C. 2–T. 4). The spinal cord is seen within the vertebral canal, surrounded by the hyperintense (bright) cerebrospinal fluid.

DISSECTION 21.1 Opening of the vertebral canal

Objectives

I. The lower lumbar and sacral parts of the vertebral canal may have been opened already. In this session, you will: (1) open the remainder of the vertebral canal to see the entire length of the spinal cord; and (2) see the course of the spinal nerves within the vertebral canal.

Instructions

1. Remove all the remaining muscles of the back to expose the laminae and spines of the vertebrae and the dorsum of the sacrum.

2. Follow the dorsal rami of the spinal nerves towards the intervertebral foramina, noting their course relative to the vertebrae and especially the articular processes.

3. Remove the posterior wall of the vertebral canal by sawing through the lateral parts of the laminae and dividing the ligamenta flava in a coronal plane. Do not saw completely through the laminae, but complete the division with a chisel or bone forceps to avoid cutting the spinal cord and its coverings (meninges). (It is often possible to cut the cervical laminae entirely with bone forceps by starting at the upper end where the right half of the skull has been removed.)

4. When a length of spines, laminae, and ligamenta flava has been removed, test the elasticity of these ligaments by stretching the specimen.

5. Note the extensive venous plexus which surrounds the spinal dura mater. It is very obvious when filled with blood.

Using the instructions given in Dissection 21.1, remove the vertebral spines and laminae to open into the vertebral canal.

Epidural

The epidural space lies between the periosteum of the vertebral canal and the spinal dura mater. The space is filled with loose areolar tissue, semi-liquid fat, a network of veins—the internal vertebral venous plexus—and the small arteries which supply the structures in the vertebral canal [Fig. 21.2]. The veins correspond to the dural venous sinuses in the cranium and are continuous with them through the foramen magnum.

Spinal arteries in the epidural space

Small spinal arteries arise from arteries in the cervical, thoracic, lumbar, and sacral regions from the ascending cervical, vertebral [see Fig. 9.8], posterior intercostal [Vol. 2, Fig. 4.14], lumbar [Vol. 2, Fig. 13.1], and lateral sacral arteries. They enter the vertebral canal through the intervertebral foramina and join the anterior and posterior spinal arteries [p. 262] to supply the spinal cord, its nerve roots and meninges, and the surrounding bone and ligaments.

Internal vertebral venous plexus

The internal vertebral venous plexus extends throughout the length of the vertebral canal and may be divided into four subordinate longitudinal channels: two anterior and two posterior venous channels [Fig. 21.2].

The posterior plexuses lie on the deep surfaces of the laminae and ligamenta flava. The anterior plexuses are on the posterior aspect of the vertebral bodies near the edges of the posterior longitudinal ligament. The four plexuses are united to each other by dense transverse plexuses opposite the laminae and receive the veins from the bones and contents of the vertebral canal. The **basivertebral veins** from the back of each vertebral body are especially large [Vol. 2, Fig. 1.7]. The internal vertebral venous plexus communicates through the intervertebral foramina with the body wall veins—the vertebral, posterior intercostal, lumbar, and lateral sacral veins. The plexus contains no valves and is capable of considerable distension. It may drain into, or receive, blood from any of the body wall veins, transmitting blood from areas of high venous pressure to areas of lower venous pressure. For example, the internal vertebral venous plexus may transmit blood from tributaries of the inferior vena cava (lateral sacral and lumbar veins) to tributaries of the superior vena cava (posterior intercostal and vertebral veins) when there is a pressure difference between the two. ⊃ Because of its multiple communications, the internal vertebral venous plexus is implicated in the spread of some pelvic tumours, e.g. spread of cancer of the prostate to the vertebral bodies, and even to the skull.

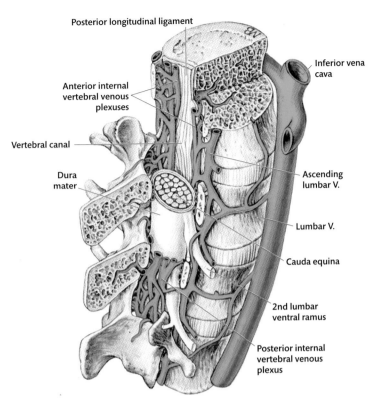

Posterior longitudinal ligament

Anterior internal
vertebral venous
plexuses

Vertebral canal

Dura
mater

Inferior vena
cava

Ascending
lumbar V.

Lumbar V.

Cauda equina

2nd lumbar
ventral ramus

Posterior internal
vertebral venous
plexus

Fig. 21.2 Dissection of the upper four lumbar vertebrae to show the internal vertebral venous plexuses and their communications with the inferior vena cava.

Meninges of the spinal cord

The spinal cord is covered by the same three layers of meninges as the brain—the pia mater, arachnoid mater, and dura mater. The meninges extend from the foramen magnum down the vertebral canal as three separate tubular sheaths around the spinal cord. The sheaths terminate at different levels, as described below.

Using the instructions given in Dissection 21.2, identify the spinal meninges and the spinal nerve roots.

Spinal dura mater

The tough fibrous sleeve of the dura extends from the margin of the foramen magnum to the second sacral vertebra. At the foramen magnum, it is fused with the meningeal layer of the cranial dura, and at the second sacral vertebra, it closes onto the arachnoid and filum terminale [Fig. 21.4]. (The filum terminale is an extension of the pia mater beyond the caudal end of the spinal cord. It is attached inferiorly to the coccyx.) The dura is separated from the walls of the vertebral canal by the epidural space, except at certain locations. It is attached: (1) to the posterior longitudinal ligament on the bodies of the second and third cervical vertebrae; and (2) to the intervertebral foramina by the extensions around the roots of the spinal nerves. These attachments hold the dural sheath close to the vertebral bodies, so that the spinal cord is as close to the axis of movement between the vertebrae as possible, and is not greatly affected by these movements [Fig. 21.3].

The dura mater forms a separate sheath for each dorsal and ventral root. The adjacent surfaces of these sheaths fuse at the medial surface of the spinal ganglion [Figs. 21.3, 21.5]. But the dura on the posterior surface of the dorsal root remains as a separate layer until it fuses with the distal part of the ganglion and becomes continuous with the **epineurium** of the nerve [Fig. 21.5].

Spinal arachnoid

The thin, transparent arachnoid membrane lines the dural sac throughout its length, but is separated

DISSECTION 21.2 Spinal meninges and spinal nerve roots

Objectives

I. To study the spinal meninges in the vertebral canal.
II. To identify and trace the dorsal and ventral nerve roots.

Instructions

1. Remove the veins and fat from the external surface of the **dura mater**.

2. Follow one of the prolongations of the dura over a spinal nerve into an intervertebral foramen by cutting away the articular processes.

3. Make a small incision in the dura mater in the midline. This allows the **arachnoid** to fall away from it. Introduce the blade of scissors into the incision, and split the dura mater longitudinally, taking care not to damage the underlying transparent arachnoid.

4. If the arachnoid is not damaged, the subarachnoid space should be inflated by injecting water or air beneath the arachnoid.

5. Split the arachnoid longitudinally, and pull its edges apart. Note the trabeculae attaching it to the pia mater on the surface of the spinal cord.

6. Below the first lumbar vertebra, note a collection of the lower lumbar and sacral spinal nerve roots. This is the **cauda equina** [Fig. 21.2]. The cauda

equina descends in the subarachnoid space, and individual nerve roots of the cauda exit the vertebral canal at each vertebral level.

7. Gently pull the spinal cord to one side to expose the projection of the pia mater from its lateral aspect—the **ligamentum denticulatum**. The ligamentum denticulatum sends pointed teeth-like extensions through the arachnoid to the dura between the points of emergence of the spinal nerves [Fig. 21.3]. These extensions are more easily seen if the dorsal rootlets of one or two spinal nerves are cut away from the spinal cord and reflected laterally.

8. Fold the cut edges of the dura mater and arachnoid laterally to expose the emergence of one or more spinal nerves through them. Note that each spinal nerve makes two separate openings in the dura and arachnoid—one for the dorsal root, and one for the ventral root.

9. Follow the dorsal root to the spinal cord, and note how the rootlets enter it.

10. Follow one or more ventral roots in a similar manner, dividing one or more teeth of the ligamentum denticulatum so that the spinal cord may be rotated to expose the exit of the rootlets which make up the ventral root.

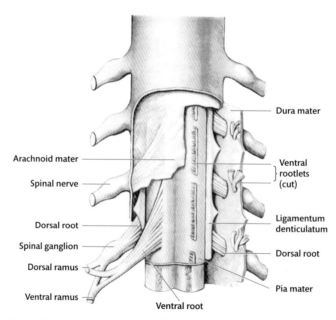

Fig. 21.3 Meninges of the spinal cord and mode of origin of spinal nerves. The contribution of each root to both rami is shown diagrammatically in the lowest spinal nerve on the left.

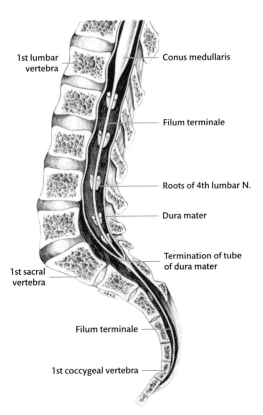

1st lumbar vertebra

Conus medullaris

Filum terminale

Roots of 4th lumbar N.

Dura mater

Termination of tube of dura mater

1st sacral vertebra

Filum terminale

1st coccygeal vertebra

Fig. 21.4 Sagittal section through the lower part of the vertebral canal.

from it by the **subdural space**. The dura and arachnoid mater fuse with each other: (1) at the intervertebral foramen around the spinal nerves; (2) on the filum terminale at S. 2 level; and (3) where the teeth of the ligamentum denticulatum pass through the arachnoid to the dura mater. The arachnoid mater extends along each spinal nerve root and usually fuses with the medial part of the spinal ganglion [Fig. 21.5].

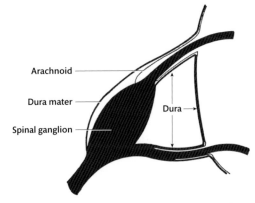

Arachnoid

Dura mater

Spinal ganglion

Dura

Fig. 21.5 Diagram to represent the meningeal relation of a spinal nerve.

Deep to the arachnoid lies a relatively wide **subarachnoid space** containing **cerebrospinal fluid**. Only a few strands of connective tissue pass from the deep surface of the arachnoid to the pia mater around the spinal cord, and these are mainly on the posterior aspect of the cord. The space is also crossed by the ligamentum denticulatum.

Spinal pia mater

The pia mater around the spinal cord is a firm vascular membrane closely adherent to the spinal cord. At the lower end of the spinal cord, it continues over the filum terminale. The pia ensheathes each rootlet of the spinal nerve, as it crosses the subarachnoid space and becomes continuous with the **perineurium** of the spinal nerves. The pia mater also extends into the nervous tissue for a short distance over each vessel entering the spinal cord and carries a short sleeve of subarachnoid space around the vessel. This space is the **perivascular space**. The pia extends into the anterior median fissure of the spinal cord and is thickened at the mouth of the fissure to form a median longitudinal, glistening band—the **linea splendens**.

Ligamentum denticulatum

The ligamentum denticulatum is a thin ridge of pia mater on each side of the spinal cord, midway between the attachments of the ventral and dorsal nerve roots. This ligament extends from the foramen magnum to the first lumbar vertebra (the lower limit of the spinal cord). It is made up of 21 pointed projections of pia mater which extend laterally from the surface of the spinal cord. The projections cross the subarachnoid space, pierce the arachnoid mater, cross the subdural space, and get attached to the dura mater, in the interval between two adjacent spinal nerves. The first projection is at the foramen magnum; the last is between the twelfth thoracic and first lumbar nerves. The two ligaments (right and left) together suspend the spinal cord in the subarachnoid space from these points of attachments and allow some movement of the dura mater without corresponding movement of the spinal cord [Fig. 21.3].

Filum terminale

The filum terminale is a thin filament which extends from the narrowed end of the spinal cord (**conus medullaris**) to the coccyx. It lies among the descending roots of the lumbar and sacral nerves (the cauda equina) but is readily differentiated from them by its silvery appearance and attachments [Fig. 21.4].

It is composed chiefly of the pia mater surrounding a continuation of the central canal, and some neural elements which can be traced in it for nearly half its length. At the level of the second sacral vertebra, the spinal arachnoid and dura mater fuse with the filum (and the subdural and subarachnoid spaces end). The filum continues through the sacral canal and fuses with the periosteum on the back of the coccyx or the last piece of the sacrum [Fig. 21.4].

The spinal cord

The spinal cord begins at the foramen magnum as the inferior continuation of the medulla oblongata of the brain. In the adult, it ends opposite the intervertebral disc between the first and second lumbar vertebrae, and approximately one vertebra lower in the newborn. The end of the spinal cord rises when the vertebral column is flexed and descends when it is extended.

The average length of the spinal cord is 45 cm. It is nearly cylindrical in shape. The diameter increases in regions which give rise to the large nerves of the limbs, because of the increased number of nerve cells within the spinal cord at these regions. These enlargements occur in the cervical and lumbar regions and are known as the **cervical** and **lumbar swellings** of the spinal cord. The cervical swelling extends from the fourth cervical vertebra to the first thoracic vertebra (it has a maximum transverse diameter of 14 mm at the sixth cervical vertebra). The lumbar swelling extends from the tenth to twelfth thoracic vertebrae (it has a maximum transverse diameter of 12 mm at the twelfth thoracic vertebra). The end of the spinal cord rapidly tapers to a point, forming the **conus medullaris**.

Spinal nerves

Thirty-one pairs of spinal nerves are attached to the spinal cord: eight cervical, 12 thoracic, five lumbar, five sacral, and one coccygeal nerve [Figs. 21.2, 21.3]. The first seven cervical nerves leave the vertebral canal above the corresponding vertebrae; the eighth emerges between the seventh cervical and first thoracic vertebrae; and the remaining nerves emerge below the corresponding vertebrae.

Spinal nerve roots

Each spinal nerve is formed by the union of the dorsal and ventral roots. The roots are attached to the spinal cord by a series of dorsal and ventral rootlets [Fig. 21.3]. The **dorsal root** is larger than the ventral root (except in the first cervical nerve which frequently has no dorsal root) and has an oval swelling—the **spinal ganglion**—on it where it joins the ventral root. The dorsal root is composed of afferent (sensory) nerve fibres which are processes of the cells in the spinal ganglion. The ventral rootlets arise from cells in the spinal cord and unite to form the **ventral root**. It consists of efferent (motor) nerve fibres. The dorsal and ventral roots unite at the spinal ganglion to form the **spinal nerve**, which contains both sensory and motor fibres [see Fig. 7.7].

The rootlets of the dorsal roots enter the spinal cord on the dorsolateral aspect, on a slight furrow—the **posterolateral sulcus**. The rootlets of the ventral roots emerge from the ventrolateral aspect of the spinal cord over a broader strip [Figs. 21.3, 21.5]. The part of the spinal cord to which any one pair of nerves is attached is called a **spinal segment**. There are 31 spinal segments in the spinal cord.

The size of a root is directly proportional to the amount of tissue it supplies. The roots of nerves contributing to the limb plexuses are large, especially those which innervate the lower limb. The roots of the thoracic and upper cervical segments are small, except the first thoracic nerve which innervates part of the upper limb.

The roots of the spinal nerve vary in length because the spinal cord is shorter than the vertebral canal. (The spinal cord is shorter than the vertebral canal due to differential growth between the two during intrauterine life) By birth, the lower end of the spinal cord has moved from its original position in the coccyx to the third lumbar vertebra; and by adulthood, it has ascended to the level of the lower border of the first lumbar vertebra. Despite the shortening of the spinal cord, the spinal nerves continue to exit the vertebral canal at the intervertebral foramen below the numerically

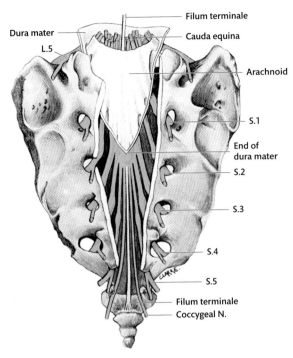

Fig. 21.6 Posterior view of the meninges and spinal nerves in the sacral canal.

Labels on figure:
Filum terminale
Dura mater
Cauda equina
L.5
Arachnoid
S.1
End of dura mater
S.2
S.3
S.4
S.5
Filum terminale
Coccygeal N.

Table 21.1 Vertebral levels of spinal segments

Vertebral levels (spines)	Spinal segments
Foramen magnum—sixth cervical	Cervical 1–8
Sixth cervical—fourth thoracic	Thoracic 1–6
Fourth thoracic—ninth thoracic	Thoracic 7–12
Tenth thoracic—first lumbar	Lumbar and sacral

corresponding vertebra. As the upper part of the spinal cord is relatively fixed during development, the upper spinal roots are short (1.5–2 cm) and horizontal. The nerve roots of the lower spinal nerves run obliquely downwards and laterally to the intervertebral foramen and are progressively elongated (27 cm in S. 5). The **cauda equina** is made up of dorsal and ventral roots of the lumbar, sacral, and coccygeal nerves. These nerves descend as a leash around the filum terminale in the subarachnoid space, inferior to the termination of the spinal cord [Figs. 21.2, 21.6].

Vertebral levels of spinal segments

Shortening of the spinal cord results in individual spinal segments lying at a higher level than the corresponding vertebra, as shown in Table 21.1.

⊃ In patients with spinal cord injury following a vertebral fracture, the level of the spinal injury can be predicted from the level of vertebral injury using information given in Table 21.1. For example, a fracture of T. 9 vertebra is likely to affect T. 12 segment of the spinal cord (T. 9 spinal segment will be unaffected).

Exit of spinal nerves

Almost all the spinal nerves emerge through an intervertebral foramen. The first cervical nerve emerges between the posterior arch of the atlas and the occiput, the second between the posterior arch of the atlas and the vertebral arch of the axis, and the fifth sacral and coccygeal nerves emerge through the lower end of the sacral canal. The other sacral nerves additionally have a separate sacral foramen (ventral and dorsal sacral foraminae) for the ventral and dorsal rami.

Meningeal branch of the spinal nerve

A slender meningeal branch is formed at each level from the spinal nerve and the sympathetic trunk. It runs back into the vertebral canal through the intervertebral foramen. It is sensory to the walls and contents of the vertebral canal and its blood vessels [see Fig. 7.7].

Spinal ganglia

The spinal ganglion is also known as the dorsal root ganglion or sensory ganglion. It is made up of a collection of nerve cell bodies on the dorsal root [Figs. 21.3, 21.5]. It lies in the intervertebral foramina, except for the sacral and coccygeal ganglia which lie in the sacral canal [Fig. 21.6]. The first two cervical ganglia lie above and below the atlas, behind the articular facets. Each ganglion gives rise to a peripheral process to the peripheral nerve, and a central process to the dorsal root on which the ganglion lies. There are no synapses in the ganglia.

Spinal nerve

Each spinal nerve is formed by the union of a dorsal and a ventral root, lateral to the spinal ganglion. It divides almost immediately into a **dorsal** and a **ventral ramus** [see Fig. 7.7].

Using the instructions given in Dissection 21.3, study the spinal cord.

DISSECTION 21.3 Spinal cord

Objectives

I. To remove the spinal cord and its meninges. **II.** To identify and trace the spinal accessory nerve. **III.** To identify and trace the branches of the anterior spinal artery.

Instructions

1. Cut across the spinal nerves in the intervertebral foramina, leaving as long a piece attached to the dura as possible.

2. Pull on the dura, and divide its attachments to the posterior longitudinal ligament.

3. Remove the spinal cord and meninges in one piece.

4. Split the dura mater along the middle anteriorly to expose the arachnoid and pia mater, and the ligamenta denticulata.

5. Find the rootlets of the **spinal part of the accessory nerve**, posterior to the ligamentum denticulatum in the upper cervical region. Follow them to the nerve, and trace the nerve cranially in front of the dorsal roots [see Fig. 8.9].

6. Remove the linea splendens from the ventral surface of the anterior median fissure, and expose the anterior spinal artery.

7. Follow the artery cranially and caudally, and try to expose the arteries joining it on the ventral roots.

8. With a hand lens, examine the small branches of the artery on the surface of the spinal cord, and the perforating branches passing into the anterior median sulcus when the artery is lifted gently away from the spinal cord.

Arteries of the spinal cord

The spinal cord is supplied by a single median anterior spinal artery and paired posterior spinal arteries. Throughout its length, many thin-walled arteries reach the anterior and posterior spinal arteries on the roots of the spinal nerves. These arteries arise from the vertebral arteries, ascending cervical arteries (in the cervical region), posterior intercostal arteries (in the thoracic region), lumbar arteries (in the lumbar region), and lateral sacral arteries (in the sacral region). They are smaller and more numerous on the dorsal than on the ventral roots.

The anterior spinal artery is formed on the anterior surface of the medulla oblongata of the brain by the union of two roots, one from each vertebral artery [see Fig. 26.3]. It descends on the anterior surface of the spinal cord, through the length of the spinal cord, dorsal to the linea splendens. It receives 3–10 spinal arteries from the vessels on the ventral roots. The largest of these supplies the lumbar swelling and usually enters from the left, frequently on the tenth thoracic ventral root.

The anterior spinal artery gives rise to many small perforating vessels which enter the spinal cord at the anteromedian fissure. They branch to supply the central parts of the spinal cord, including most of the grey matter (nerve cell bodies) and the deeper parts of the surrounding white matter (nerve fibres). Small vessels also pass backwards on the surface of the spinal cord to anastomose with the **posterior spinal arteries** which course longitudinally beside the entry point of the dorsal rootlets. The **posterior spinal arteries** arise as branches of the posterior inferior cerebellar or vertebral arteries on the medulla oblongata [see Fig. 26.3]. They run down along the entry points of the dorsal rootlets. They are fed by numerous small arteries on the dorsal roots and are much smaller than the anterior spinal artery. The posterior spinal arteries send branches onto the posterior surface of the spinal cord to complete an irregular, circular anastomosis, from which branches pass radially into the white matter. All the arteries which enter the spinal cord are end-arteries. This pattern of surface anastomosis with perforating end-arteries is present throughout the central nervous system.

The veins of the spinal cord, though small, numerous, and tortuous, are larger than the arteries. They anastomose freely on the surface of the spinal cord and form six more or less perfectly longitudinal channels—one anteromedian, one posteromedian, two close to the attachment of the dorsal rootlets, and two close to the attachment of the ventral rootlets. They are continuous above with the veins of the medulla oblongata and drain laterally along the spinal nerve roots to the internal vertebral venous plexus.

The structure of the spinal cord is described in Chapter 27 in the section on the brain and spinal cord.

See Clinical Applications 21.1, 21.2, and 21.3 for the practical implications of the anatomy discussed in this chapter.

CLINICAL APPLICATION 21.1 Significance of high termination of the spinal cord

The high termination of the spinal cord and the presence of only a leash of roots in the subarachnoid space inferior to it have a number of clinical significances: (1) injuries to the vertebral column below the second lumbar vertebra can damage only spinal nerve roots (and not the spinal cord itself), though the roots of many nerves may be damaged by an injury at one level; and (2) samples of cerebrospinal fluid can be obtained for diagnostic purposes from the subarachnoid space below L. 1 level without fear of injuring the spinal cord. This procedure is a lumbar puncture and is done by introducing a hollow needle into the subarachnoid space between the laminae of the lower lumbar vertebrae.

CLINICAL APPLICATION 21.2 Radiculopathy

Neuropathy is a general term for nerve disorders. Radiculopathy is sensory or motor disturbance caused by pathology of a nerve root. The most common cause of radiculopathy is intervertebral disc herniation. Fig. 21.7 shows herniation of the intervertebral discs between C. 3/C. 4, C. 4/C. 5, and C. 5/C. 6. [See also Vol. 2, Fig. 1.10 for disc herniation between L. 4/L. 5 and L. 5/S. 1.]

Other causes of radiculopathy are presence of osteophytes, spinal stenosis, and trauma.

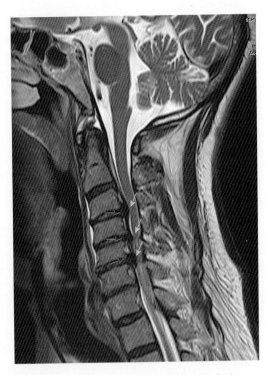

Fig. 21.7 T2-weighted sagittal MRI of the cervical spine, showing intervertebral disc prolapse between C. 3/C. 4, C. 4/C. 5, and C. 5/C. 6 (red arrows) and compression of the dural sac (yellow arrows).

CLINICAL APPLICATION 21.3 Cauda equina syndrome

A 45-year-old man was lifting a heavy load when he coughed and immediately experienced sharp pain in both gluteal regions. Over the next few days, he continued to have pain and developed loss of sensation over his buttock and genitalia. He also developed constipation and urinary retention.

On examination, his motor function was normal. He had decreased sensation (touch, pain, and temperature) over the buttock, genitalia, anal region, and back of the upper thigh (saddle anaesthesia). Sensation in all other areas was normal. Superficial abdominal reflexes and the cremasteric reflex were normal.

Study question 1: what spinal segments receive sensation from the skin of the gluteal region, perineum, and back of the upper thigh? [Refer to Vol. 1, Fig. 20.2.] (Answer: S. 2 to S. 5/Co.)

Study question 2: what can you deduce about spinal cord function from the finding that the abdominal and cremasteric reflexes are intact? [Refer to Vol. 2, Clinical Application 8.2.] (Answer: spinal segments T. 7–L. 2 are normal.)

A spinal computerized tomogram/myelogram done on the patient revealed a L. 5–S. 1 central disc prolapse compressing the nerves of the cauda equina. (Herniation of the disc posteriorly into the vertebral canal is a central disc herniation. Rootlets of lower segments are located more medially in the cauda equina and are more likely to be affected by a central disc herniation. A posterolateral disc prolapse affects upper segment rootlets, as they lie closer to the intervertebral foramen.) The mass was removed surgically, the dural sac decompressed, and the patient made a good recovery.

CHAPTER 22
The joints of the neck

Cervical joints

Begin the study of this region by reviewing the cervical joints exposed earlier and exposing the remaining joints.

Dissection 22.1 provides instructions on reviewing the atlanto-occipital joint and dissecting the remaining cervical joints.

Each cervical vertebra articulates with the adjacent vertebrae by joints between the bodies and the articular processes. The first cervical vertebra (atlas) articulates with the skull at the atlanto-occipital joint.

The joints between the second to fifth cervical vertebrae are similar to those in the other parts of the vertebral column and allow flexion, extension, lateral flexion, and some rotation. The joints between the first and second cervical vertebrae

DISSECTION 22.1 Cervical joints

Objectives

I. To review the joints already opened. **II.** To expose the remaining cervical joints.

Instructions

1. The joints of the neck have already been partly dissected when the right half of the head was removed. The right atlanto-occipital joint has been opened, and the right alar ligament and the longitudinal fibres of the cruciate ligament have been cut [Fig. 22.1].

2. Expose the ligaments uniting the cervical vertebrae by removing the remnants of muscle from the cervical articular processes and from the laminae and spines which have been removed in one piece.

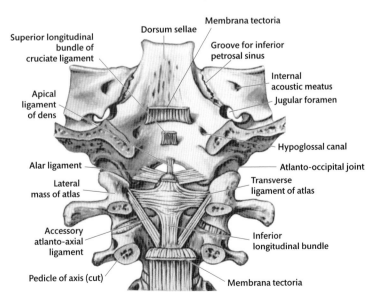

Superior longitudinal bundle of cruciate ligament
Dorsum sellae
Membrana tectoria
Groove for inferior petrosal sinus
Internal acoustic meatus
Jugular foramen
Apical ligament of dens
Hypoglossal canal
Alar ligament
Atlanto-occipital joint
Lateral mass of atlas
Transverse ligament of atlas
Accessory atlanto-axial ligament
Inferior longitudinal bundle
Pedicle of axis (cut)
Membrana tectoria

Fig. 22.1 Diagram showing the main ligaments that connect the occipital bone, atlas, and axis.

are designed to allow rotation of the head from side to side (as in turning the face to the right and left). The joints between the first cervical vertebra (atlas) and the skull allow nodding movements of the skull on the vertebral column (as in flexing and extending the head).

Typical cervical joints

The joints between the lower six cervical vertebrae are typical cervical joints [Fig. 22.2]. The **bodies** of these vertebrae are firmly bound to each other by a flexible intervertebral disc. The disc consists of the **annulus fibrosus** and **nucleus pulposus** and allows a moderate degree of movement between the vertebrae. The intervertebral discs are strengthened anteriorly and posteriorly by the anterior and posterior **longitudinal ligaments**, which are attached principally to the discs and the adjacent parts of the bodies [see Fig. 22.4]. The discs do not cover the entire surface of the vertebral bodies but are replaced laterally by small **synovial joints** where the margins of the inferior vertebra overlap the vertebral body above [Fig. 22.2].

The **vertebral arches** are united by the synovial joints between the superior and inferior articular processes and by a number of ligaments [Fig. 22.2]. The cervical articular facets lie in an oblique coronal plane, which passes anterosuperiorly, and the facets on the two sides are parallel to each other [Fig. 2.3]. The capsules of these joints are lax and permit a considerable range of movement.

Ligaments of vertebral arches

Ligamenta flava

The **ligamenta flava** are wide, flat bands of yellow elastic tissue that run between the anterior surfaces of adjacent laminae. They help to maintain the position of the vertebral column and restore it to that position after they have been stretched by flexion [Fig. 22.3].

Interspinous ligaments

The interspinous ligaments are weak in the cervical region. They pass between adjacent spines and are directly continuous with the supraspinous ligaments and the ligamentum nuchae [see Fig. 7.6].

Joints of the atlas, axis, and occipital bone

The atlas is a ring of bone with a lateral mass on each side. The lateral masses articulate superiorly with the occipital condyles, and inferiorly with the superior articular facets of the axis. The articular surfaces of the atlas for the occiput and for the axis are of different configuration. Those with the occiput permit flexion and extension, and those with the axis permit side-to-side rotation. The occipital bone and the axis are firmly bound to each other by strong ligaments, so that the atlas is held between them like a washer.

Anterior longitudinal ligament

The **anterior longitudinal ligament** [Vol. 2, p. 6] narrows superiorly to be attached to the

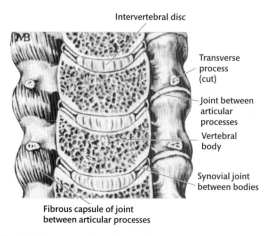

Intervertebral disc

Transverse process (cut)

Joint between articular processes

Vertebral body

Synovial joint between bodies

Fibrous capsule of joint between articular processes

Fig. 22.2 Coronal section through the joints between the bodies of the cervical vertebrae.

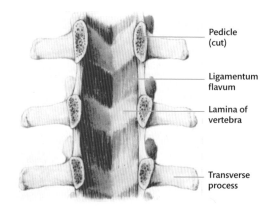

Pedicle (cut)

Ligamentum flavum

Lamina of vertebra

Transverse process

Fig. 22.3 Ligamentum flavum seen from the front after removal of the bodies of the vertebrae in the lumbar region.

anterior tubercle of the atlas. Above this, it continues as a narrow band to the base of the skull and strengthens the median part of the **anterior atlanto-occipital membrane**. (The anterior atlanto-occipital membrane passes from the superior margin of the anterior arch of the atlas to the base of the skull, anterior to the foramen magnum [Fig. 22.4].)

Ligamentum flavum

The **ligamentum flavum** between the atlas and axis is delicate. Between the posterior arch of the atlas and the occipital bone, the ligamentum flavum is known as the **posterior atlanto-occipital membrane** [Fig. 22.4]. It passes from the part of the posterior arch of the atlas between the grooves for the vertebral arteries, to the margin of the foramen magnum and the atlanto-occipital joints [see Fig. 7.4]. The lateral edges arch over the corresponding vertebral artery to reach the posterior surface of the lateral mass of the atlas. These edges may be ossified.

The membrana tectoria, cruciate, and atlanto-axial ligaments are exposed, following the instructions in Dissection 22.2.

Membrana tectoria

The membrana tectoria is a broad ligamentous sheet. It is the superior continuation of the posterior longitudinal ligament. It passes from the posterior surface of the body of the axis to the cranial

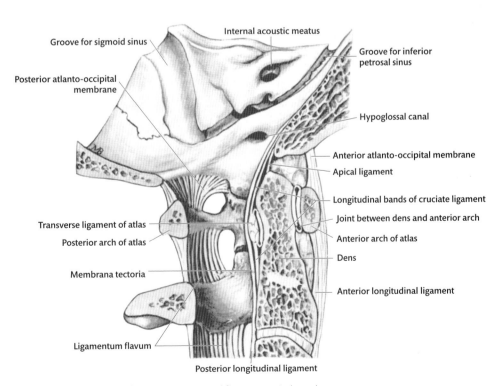

Groove for sigmoid sinus
Internal acoustic meatus
Groove for inferior petrosal sinus
Posterior atlanto-occipital membrane
Hypoglossal canal
Anterior atlanto-occipital membrane
Apical ligament
Longitudinal bands of cruciate ligament
Joint between dens and anterior arch
Transverse ligament of atlas
Anterior arch of atlas
Posterior arch of atlas
Dens
Membrana tectoria
Anterior longitudinal ligament
Ligamentum flavum
Posterior longitudinal ligament

Fig. 22.4 Median section through the foramen magnum and first two cervical vertebrae.

surface of the occipital bone [Figs. 22.2, 22.4]. It holds the axis to the skull and covers the posterior surface of the dens and its ligaments, and the anterior margin of the foramen magnum.

Accessory atlanto-axial ligaments

The **accessory atlanto-axial ligaments** [Fig. 22.1] pass from the posterior surface of the body of the axis to the corresponding lateral mass of the atlas. These strong ligaments help to limit the rotation of the atlas on the axis.

Transverse ligament of the atlas

The **transverse ligament of the atlas** stretches between two tubercles on the medial side of the lateral masses of the atlas [Fig. 2.5]. It extends across the posterior surface of the dens and holds it firmly against the posterior surface of the anterior arch of the atlas. There is a synovial joint between the dens and the ligament, and another between the dens and the anterior arch of the atlas [Fig. 22.4]. As such, the atlas is capable of rotating round the dens but cannot be displaced anteroposteriorly on it.

Cruciate ligament

The cruciate ligament is formed by the transverse ligament of the atlas and the **superior** and **inferior longitudinal bands** which pass from the transverse ligament to the cranial surface of the occipital bone (superior longitudinal band) and the body of the axis (inferior longitudinal band) below [Figs. 22.1, 22.4].

Using the instructions given in Dissection 22.3, expose the apical and alar ligaments of the dens.

DISSECTION 22.3 Ligaments of the dens— apical and alar ligaments

Objective

I. To expose the apical and alar ligaments of the dens.

Instructions

1. If the division of the skull was to the right of the midline, the apical ligament of the dens [Figs. 22.1, 22.4] should still be present with the left half. It may be exposed by removing the superior band of the cruciate ligament.

2. Identify the divided right alar ligament, and expose the left alar ligament passing from the side of the apex of the dens to the occipital condyle.

Apical ligament of the dens

The apical ligament of the dens is a weak, cord-like ligament which stretches from the apex of the dens to the cranial surface of the occipital bone, immediately above the margin of the foramen magnum. It lies anterior to the superior band of the cruciate ligament but does not play a significant part in strengthening the joints [Fig. 22.1]. (It develops around a part of the notochord.)

Alar ligaments

The alar ligaments are very powerful ligaments which arise from the sloping sides of the top of the dens. They pass laterally and slightly upwards to the medial sides of the occipital condyles. They hold the skull to the axis and tighten when the atlas, carrying the skull, rotates round the dens. They are the main factor in limiting rotation at the atlanto-axial joints. The alar ligaments are attached to the skull on the axis of the nodding movements which the skull makes on the atlas, and so do not hinder these movements [Fig. 22.1].

Atlanto-occipital joint

The occipital condyles are kidney-shaped and lie on the anterolateral aspects of the foramen magnum. The articular surfaces are directed laterally and downwards [see Fig. 3.6]. They fit into the superior articular facets of the atlas which are also kidney-shaped. The atlanto-occipital joints allow flexion, extension, and slight side-to-side rocking of the head, but no rotation. The stability of these joints depends on the alar ligaments, the membrana tectoria, and the longitudinal bands of the cruciate ligament, all of which bind the skull to the axis.

Atlanto-axial joints

The **atlanto-axial** joints are formed between the large, nearly circular, slightly curved facets on the inferior surface of the lateral mass of the atlas and superior articular facet of the axis. These facets slope downwards and laterally [Fig. 22.1]. In addition, the dens articulates with the anterior arch of the atlas and the transverse ligament of the atlas. The atlas, carrying the skull with it, rotates around

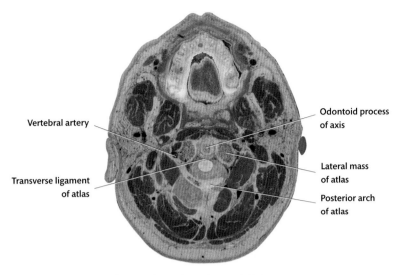

Vertebral artery

Transverse ligament
of atlas

Odontoid process
of axis

Lateral mass
of atlas

Posterior arch
of atlas

Fig. 22.5 Horizontal section through the dens showing the median atlanto-axial joint.

Image courtesy of the Visible Human Project of the US National Library of Medicine.

the dens of the axis [Fig. 22.5]. The lateral atlanto-axial joints are stabilized by the ligaments which bind the axis and the skull together, so that the atlas is held firmly between them.

See Clinical Application 22.1 for the practical implications of the anatomy discussed in this chapter.

CLINICAL APPLICATION 22.1 Fracture of the dens versus rupture of the transverse ligament of the atlas

Fracture of the dens commonly occurs at its base where the dens is united to the body. In an isolated fracture of the dens, the transverse ligament of the atlas is intact. It holds the fractured dens against the anterior arch of the atlas and prevents the fractured segment from impinging on the spinal cord. The most common complication in a fracture of the dens is avascular necrosis of the fractured segment.

Rupture of the transverse ligament of the atlas is a result of pathological softening of the ligament. It results in the dens being free to move posteriorly and impinge on the spinal cord. Spinal cord compression between the posterior arch of the atlas and the dens could result in quadriplegia (paralysis of all four limbs).

CHAPTER 23
MCQs for part 1: Head and neck

Each of the following questions have four options. Please choose the most correct answer.

1. **The sensory innervation to the lower part of the medial surface of the auricle is by the**

   A. Facial nerve

   B. Auriculotemporal nerve

   C. Greater auricular nerve

   D. Lesser occipital nerve

2. **The three cutaneous nerves that pierce the deep fascia at the middle of the posterior border of the sternocleidomastoid include all the following, EXCEPT the**

   A. Supraclavicular nerve

   B. Lesser occipital nerve

   C. Great auricular nerve

   D. Transverse nerve of the neck

3. **The nerve that accompanies the submental artery is the**

   A. Cervical branch of the facial nerve

   B. Mylohoid nerve

   C. Transverse cervical nerve

   D. Great auricular nerve

4. **All of the following statements are true concerning the middle meningeal artery, EXCEPT**

   A. It enters the cranial cavity through the foramen ovale

   B. It has no role in supplying the pia and arachnoid mater

   C. It grooves the inner table of the skull

   D. Rupture of it results in extradural haematoma

5. **The straight sinus is formed by the union of the**

   A. Superior sagittal sinus and inferior sagittal sinus

   B. Superior sagittal sinus and transverse sinus

   C. Superior sagittal sinus and great cerebral vein

   D. Inferior sagittal sinus and great cerebral vein

6. **The emissary vein that traverses through the foramen ovale connects the cavernous sinus with the**

   A. Superior ophthalmic vein
   B. Inferior ophthalmic vein
   C. Pterygoid plexus of veins
   D. Pharyngeal plexus of veins

7. **The following are branches of the hypoglossal nerve, EXCEPT the**

   A. Superior root of the ansa cervicalis
   B. Nerve to the geniohyoid
   C. Nerve to the genioglossus
   D. Nerve to the palatoglossus

8. **In Horner's syndrome, ptosis is due to paralysis of the**

   A. Orbital part of the orbicularis oculi
   B. Palpebral part of the orbicularis oculis
   C. Striated part of the levator palpebrae superioris
   D. Smooth muscle component of the levator palpebrae superioris

9. **The otic ganglion receives preganglionic fibres from the**

   A. Oculomotor nerve
   B. Facial nerve
   C. Glossopharyngeal nerve
   D. Vagus nerve

10. **The muscle that retracts the mandible is the**

    A. Masseter
    B. Temporalis
    C. Medial pterygoid
    D. Lateral pterygoid

11. **The nerve that pierces the sphenomandibular ligament is the**

    A. Auriculotemporal nerve
    B. Lingual nerve
    C. Chorda tympani
    D. Mylohyoid nerve

12. **The muscle that hooks round the pterygoid hamulus is the**

    A. Medial pterygoid
    B. Lateral pterygoid
    C. Tensor palati
    D. Levator palati

13. **The sinuses that open into the hiatus semilunaris are the**
    A. Frontal and anterior ethmoidal
    B. Anterior and middle ethmoidal
    C. Anterior ethmoidal and maxillary
    D. Middle and posterior ethmoidal

14. **The muscle that is responsible for raising the pitch of the voice is the**
    A. Cricothyroid
    B. Posterior crico-arytenoid
    C. Lateral crico-arytenoid
    D. Vocalis

15. **Which one of the following is the remnant of the notochord?**
    A. Alar ligament
    B. Apical ligament
    C. Cruciate ligament
    D. Transverse ligament of the atlas

Please go to the back of the book for the answers.

PART 2

The brain and spinal cord

CHAPTER 24

Introduction to the brain and spinal cord

Introduction

The nervous system consists of two main parts—the central nervous system (CNS) made up of the brain and spinal cord, and the peripheral nervous system (PNS) made up of the spinal nerves, cranial nerves, and the peripheral part of the autonomic nervous system. The brain and spinal cord are discussed in this section.

Structure of the nervous tissue

The CNS contains two types of cells: (1) the **nerve cells** proper; and (2) the connective tissue of the CNS—the **neuroglia**.

Nerve cells or neurons

Nerve cells are variable in size and shape. They have cytoplasmic processes, some of which extend for considerable distances from the cell body. These processes are of two types—axons and dendrites. The **dendrites** are the processes which receive stimuli. They vary greatly from cell to cell but are commonly branched in a complicated fashion and restricted to the vicinity of the cell body. The **axons** are usually thinner than the dendrites and transmit impulses from the cell body either to other nerve cells or to peripheral tissues through the peripheral nerves. Some axons are of considerable length (up to 1 m), and all axons are capable of branching. Most of the axons in the CNS are covered with a fatty **myelin sheath**.

The brain and spinal cord are largely made up of nerve cells. The nerve cell bodies are grouped together and make up the **grey matter**. A collection of nerve cell bodies within the CNS, often having shared functions and connections, are referred to as **nuclei**. Axons of nerve cells are grouped together to form the **white matter**. Groups of axons coming from the same origin, or going to the same destination, often run together in definite pathways and are called **tracts** or **fasciculi**. Dendrites and nerve synapses are usually confined to the grey matter.

In the spinal cord and most of the brainstem, the grey matter lies internally and is covered by a layer of white matter, which consists of longitudinally running axons. In the cerebellum and cerebrum, there is an additional layer of nerve cells on the external surface. This covering of grey matter, or **cortex**, greatly increases the number of nerve cells and the complexity of their interactions.

Neuroglia

The **neuroglia** has three types of cells—the astrocytes, oligodendroglia, and microglia. The astrocytes and oligodendroglia are derived from the ectoderm in common with most of the nervous system. The microglia are derived from the mesoderm, as are the blood vessels. In addition, the ependymal cells lining the cavities of the brain are also part of the neuroglia.

Astrocytes are star-shaped cells with cell processes radiating from them. They pervade the CNS, forming a surface layer throughout it. One or more of the processes extend to cover a segment of an adjacent capillary, so that together the processes of astrocytes cover the capillaries of the CNS. There are two main types of astrocytes: (1) the **protoplasmic astrocytes** which have processes branching repeatedly to form a dense bush—they are found in areas where nerve cells (grey matter) predominate; (2) the **fibrillary astrocytes** found predominantly among the bundles of nerve fibres (white matter). Their long, thin processes branch infrequently.

Oligodendroglia are small cells with few short processes. They form myelin sheaths in the CNS. **Microglia** are small rod-shaped cells. During nerve fibre injury, they ingest particles of degenerating myelin and develop a foam-like cytoplasm. The **ependyma** forms the epithelial lining for the cavities of the brain and spinal cord. It also covers the vascular pia mater which invaginates the ventricles to form the choroid plexuses.

Functionally, the CNS is concerned with the receipt and integration of sensory information (sensory system), production of movement (motor system), memory, emotions, and many other complex higher functions. These complex activities are achieved by passage of impulses through the interconnected networks of cells in the CNS. Each cellular unit is linked into the system by cell junctions, or **synapses**, where nerve cells come together and neuronal impulse from one cell is transferred to another. Passage of impulses can be facilitated or inhibited at the synapse.

It is not possible to give a detailed account of this complex system in this book. But a knowledge of the arrangement of the parts of the CNS and of the major tracts by which they are interconnected is provided. The external features, meninges, and gross structure of the spinal cord have been discussed in Chapter 21. The internal features of the spinal cord are described in Chapter 27.

The brain

The **brain** lies within the cranial cavity. Like the spinal cord, it is surrounded by the **meninges**—dura mater, arachnoid mater, and pia mater. The meninges are continuous with their spinal counterparts at the foramen magnum. As you saw when you removed the brain, the cranial dura mater remains fused with the skull, the arachnoid is separated from the dura by the subdural space, and the pia and arachnoid mater come away with the brain [Chapter 8].

The main **blood vessels** of the brain and spinal cord and their principal branches lie in the subarachnoid space between the arachnoid and pia mater. The smaller vessels ramify on the pia mater before sinking into the substance of the brain.

Before examining the arachnoid, pia mater, and blood vessels which lie between them, you must have some knowledge of the main parts of the brain. With the help of Figs. 24.1 and 24.2, identify the major parts of the brain. Having a brain from which the meninges and blood vessels have been removed will be helpful. If such a specimen is not available, study the brain which was removed in Chapter 8, but avoid damage to the meninges during this preliminary examination. Confirm the relations of the parts of the brain to the skull by using a dry skull.

Parts of the brain

The brain is made up of the cerebrum, cerebellum, diencephalon, midbrain, pons, and medulla oblongata [Figs. 24.1, 24.2]. The midbrain, pons, and medulla together constitute the brainstem.

External features of the cerebrum

The **cerebrum** is the largest part of the brain. It is composed of the two **cerebral hemispheres** which are partially separated from each other by the falx cerebri in the midline. The hemispheres cover the other parts of the brain superiorly, so that these parts can only be seen on the inferior surface [Fig. 24.2]. The surface area of each hemisphere is increased by extensive folding and the presence of a number of grooves known as **sulci**, between which are blunt ridges known as **gyri**.

Each hemisphere has three surfaces: (1) the convex **superolateral surface** [Fig. 24.1]; (2) the medial surface, partly in contact with the falx cerebri; and (3) the **inferior surface** [Fig. 24.2]. The superolateral surface is convex. It ends anteriorly at the frontal pole and posteriorly at the occipital pole. The temporal pole is the most anterior part of the temporal lobe [Fig. 24.1]. The medial surface is not seen on the external aspect of the brain. The inferior surface consists of **orbital** and **tentorial** parts. The orbital part lies in the anterior cranial fossa, on the roof of the orbit, and the nasal cavity [see Fig. 3.9]. It is separated from the tentorial part of the inferior surface by a deep horizontal fissure known as the stem of the lateral sulcus, into which the lesser wing of the sphenoid fits. Posteriorly, the tentorial part rests on the tentorium cerebelli and ends in the occipital pole [see Fig. 8.6]. The occipital pole fits

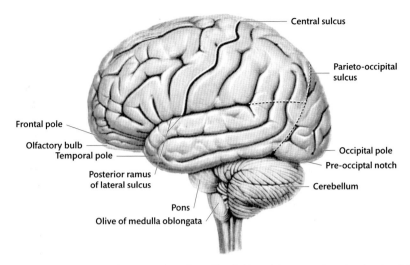

Fig. 24.1 Lateral surface of the brain to show the main sulci and gyri. The division of the supero-lateral surface into lobes by the central sulcus and two arbitrary lines is shown.

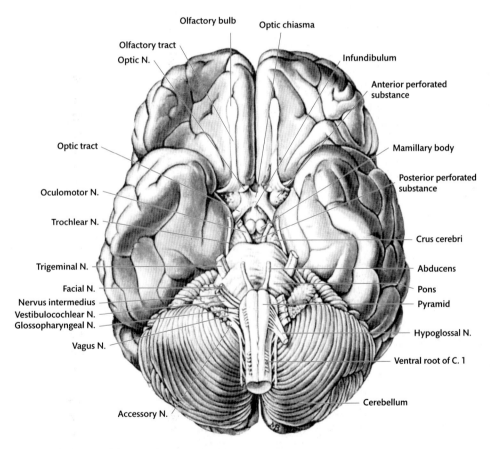

Fig. 24.2 The base of the brain and the cranial nerves.

into the fossa on the occipital bone in the area between the grooves for the superior sagittal and transverse sinuses [see Fig. 8.10]. Anteriorly, the tentorial surface lies on the floor of the middle cranial fossa and extends forwards below the lesser wing of the sphenoid into the anterior extremity of the fossa.

External features of the diencephalon

The **diencephalon** consists of the **epithalamus** and **thalamus** superiorly, and the **hypothalamus** and **subthalamus** inferiorly. It is almost entirely hidden from view by the cerebral hemispheres. The inferior surface of the hypothalamus is visible on the inferior surface of the brain between the optic chiasma anteriorly, the optic tracts anterolaterally, and the crus cerebri posterolateral [Fig. 24.2]. It lies superior to the sella turcica of the sphenoid bone.

External features of the cerebellum

The **cerebellum** is the second largest part of the brain. It lies in the posterior cranial fossa, inferior to the tentorium cerebelli, and overlaps the posterior surfaces of the midbrain, pons, and medulla oblongata [Fig. 24.2]. A large number of closely set transverse **fissures** run across the surface of the cerebellum. The cerebellum consists of two cerebellar hemispheres and a median portion—the **vermis** [Figs. 24.1, 24.2]. On the inferior surface,

the vermis is deeply placed between the cerebellar hemispheres in a median groove called the **vallecula cerebelli**. The vallecula is partly filled by the falx cerebelli.

External features of the midbrain

The **midbrain** is part of the brainstem. It is the narrow segment which passes through the tentorial notch and joins the diencephalon to the pons. The anterior surface of the midbrain can be seen in continuity with the base of brain. It consists of the **crus cerebri** which are two broad bundles of nerve fibres, descending from the cerebral hemispheres and entering the pons inferiorly [Figs. 24.2, 24.3]. The posterior part of the interpeduncular fossa lies between them [p. 282]. The posterior surface of the midbrain is hidden from view in the whole brain. It is known as the **tectum** and consists of four small swellings—the **colliculi**. They are the paired **superior** and **inferior colliculi**. The tectum is deeply buried between the cerebellum and the cerebral hemispheres and will be seen

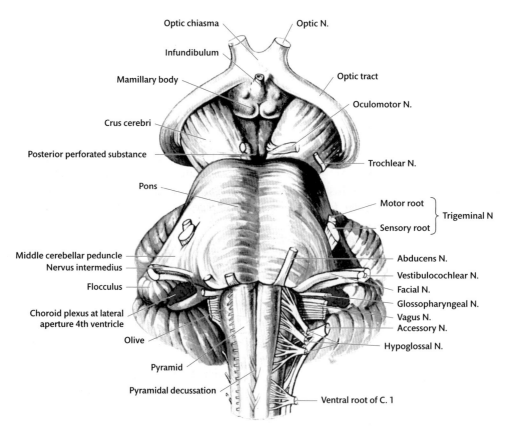

Fig. 24.3 Anterior surface of the brainstem.

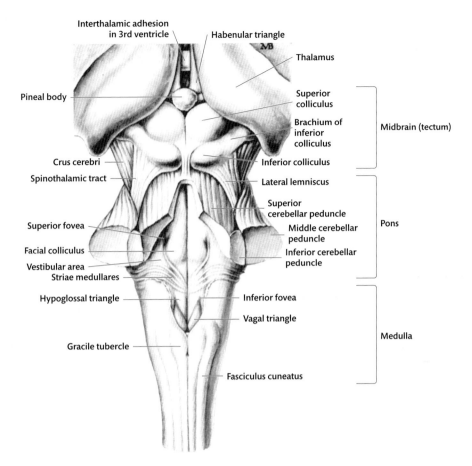

Interthalamic adhesion
in 3rd ventricle — Habenular triangle

Thalamus

Pineal body — Superior
colliculus

Superior
colliculus

Brachium of
inferior
colliculus

Midbrain (tectum)

Crus cerebri — Inferior colliculus

Spinothalamic tract — Lateral lemniscus

Superior
cerebellar peduncle

Superior fovea — Middle cerebellar
peduncle

Facial colliculus — Inferior cerebellar
peduncle

Vestibular area
Striae medullares

Hypoglossal triangle — Inferior fovea

Vagal triangle

Gracile tubercle

Fasciculus cuneatus

Pons

Medulla

Fig. 24.4 Posterior view of the brainstem.

later [Fig. 24.4]. The oculomotor—the third cranial nerve—emerges from the anterior surface of the midbrain, medial to the crus cerebri [Fig. 24.2].

External features of the pons

The **pons** is the part of the brainstem between the midbrain and medulla. Seen from the ventral aspect, it is a broad band of transversely running fibres. On each side, it narrows posteriorly to form the rounded **middle cerebellar peduncle**, which extends posteriorly into the cerebellum. The thick **trigeminal nerve**—the fifth cranial nerve—marks the junction of the pons and middle cerebellar peduncle [Figs. 24.2, 24.3, 24.5]. The dorsal aspect of the pons is not seen on the external surface. It forms the upper part of the floor of the fourth ventricle [Fig. 24.4].

Medulla oblongata

The **medulla oblongata** is the conical, white structure which extends inferiorly from the pons

and joins the spinal cord at the foramen magnum. A **median fissure** divides the ventral surface of the medulla into right and left halves. The **pyramid** is a longitudinal ridge on each side of the fissure. Posterolateral to the pyramid is an oval swelling— the **olive** [Figs. 24.3, 24.5]. The dorsal surface of the medulla is hidden from view. The upper part forms the floor of the fourth ventricle. The lower part is in direct continuation with the dorsal aspect of the spinal cord [Fig. 24.4].

The sixth, seventh, and eighth cranial nerves are attached to the junction of the pons and medulla. The sixth cranial nerve is attached ventrally (in line with the groove between the pyramid and olive), and the seventh and eighth laterally. The ninth, tenth, and eleventh cranial nerves are attached to the lateral surface of the medulla, posterior to the olive, in a linear series of rootlets. The twelfth cranial nerve is attached as a series of rootlets in the groove between the pyramid and olive.

The brain

281

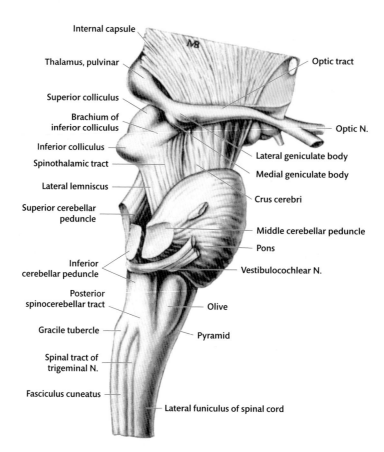

Internal capsule

Thalamus, pulvinar

Superior colliculus

Brachium of
inferior colliculus

Inferior colliculus

Spinothalamic tract

Lateral lemniscus

Superior cerebellar
peduncle

Inferior
cerebellar peduncle

Posterior
spinocerebellar tract

Gracile tubercle

Spinal tract of
trigeminal N.

Fasciculus cuneatus

Optic tract

Optic N.

Lateral geniculate body

Medial geniculate body

Crus cerebri

Middle cerebellar peduncle

Pons

Vestibulocochlear N.

Olive

Pyramid

Lateral funiculus of spinal cord

Fig. 24.5 Lateral view of the brainstem.

Use the instructions given in Dissection 24.1 to identify the parts and salient features of the brain.

Base of the brain

Having identified the parts of the brain and salient surface projections, it is useful to study in further detail the base of the brain.

Interpeduncular fossa

The interpeduncular fossa is a rhomboid-shaped space on the base of the brain, bounded by the pons posteriorly, the crus cerebri (or cerebral peduncles) posterolaterally, the optic tracts anterolaterally and the optic chiasma anteriorly [Fig. 24.3]. The crus cerebri project downwards from the cerebral hemispheres and are crossed laterally by the optic tracts. They converge into the pons.

Structures in the interpeduncular fossa

The following structures are seen in the interpeduncular fossa: (1) the **oculomotor nerves**, which

emerge immediately dorsomedial to the corresponding crura; (2) the **posterior perforated substance**, a layer of grey matter in the angle between the crus cerebri—it is pierced by branches of the posterior cerebral arteries; (3) the **mammillary bodies**, a pair of small, white, spherical bodies which protrude, side by side, from the ventral surface of the hypothalamus, immediately anterior to the posterior perforated substance; and (4) the **tuber cinereum**, a slightly raised area of grey matter between the mammillary bodies and the optic chiasma. The **infundibulum**, a narrow stalk which connects the hypothalamus to the hypophysis (pituitary gland), rises from the tuber cinereum. (The infundibulum was cut when the brain was removed.)

Anterior perforated substance

The anterior perforated substance is a small area of grey matter. It is bound anteriorly by the diverging striae of the olfactory tract, medially by the optic chiasma and tract, and posteriorly by the uncus—a part of the cortex of the temporal lobe [Fig. 24.6].

DISSECTION 24.1 Parts of the brain

Objective

I. To identify the cerebrum, cerebellum, midbrain, pons, and medulla oblongata on the exterior of the brain.

Instructions

1. Identify the superolateral surface of the cerebral hemisphere, and the frontal, occipital, and temporal poles.

2. Identify the inferior surface of the cerebral hemisphere and the temporal pole. The posterior part is hidden from view by the cerebellum. Raise the cerebellum gently to visualize this part.

3. Identify the two cerebellar hemispheres and the vermis.

4. Identify the midbrain, pons, and medulla oblongata [Fig. 24.3].

5. Identify the crus cerebri of the midbrain and the oculomotor nerve.

6. Trace the ventral aspect of the pons laterally, and identify the middle cerebellar peduncle and the cut end of the trigeminal nerve.

7. On the ventral aspect of the medulla, identify the median fissure, pyramid, and olive.

8. Identify the cut ends of the sixth to twelfth cranial nerves.

Optic chiasma

The optic chiasma lies across the midline between the anterior perforated substance of either side. It receives the optic nerves anteriorly and gives rise to the optic tracts posteriorly. It is made up of crossing fibres from the nasal half of each retina [Figs. 24.2, 24.6].

Optic tracts

Each optic tract begins at the posterolateral corner of the optic chiasma. It passes posterolaterally between the anterior perforated substance and the tuber cinereum. It then lies superior to the medial aspect of the temporal lobe on the lateral aspect of the crus cerebri [Figs. 24.2, 24.6].

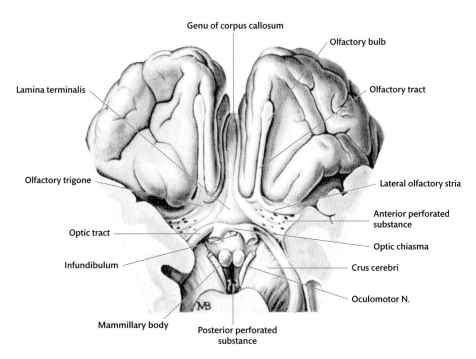

Fig. 24.6 Orbital surfaces of the hemispheres and the interpeduncular fossa. The frontal lobes have been separated slightly to show the genu of the corpus callosum, and the optic chiasma has been turned inferiorly to uncover the lamina terminalis.

Lamina terminalis

The lamina terminalis is a thin, grey membrane which extends superiorly from the optic chiasma and forms the anterior wall of the third ventricle. It can be seen by bending the optic chiasma gently downwards. Confirm the continuity of the lamina terminalis with the anterior perforated substance on both sides [Fig. 24.6].

Superficial attachments of the cranial nerves

Twelve pairs of cranial nerves are attached to the brain. They are: (1) olfactory; (2) optic; (3) oculomotor; (4) trochlear; (5) trigeminal; (6) abducens; (7) facial; (8) vestibulocochlear; (9) glossopharyngeal; (10) vagus; (11) accessory; and (12) hypoglossal.

Each cranial nerve enters or leaves the brain at its superficial attachment. In motor nerves, the fibres in the nerve arise within the brain and leave at the superficial attachment. In sensory nerves, the fibres enter the brain at the superficial attachment and terminate on nuclei within the brain. The first pair of cranial nerves is attached to the cerebrum, the second to the diencephalon, the third and fourth to the midbrain, the fifth to the pons, the sixth to eighth to the junction of the pons and medulla, and the ninth to twelfth to the medulla oblongata. The eleventh is attached to the cervical spinal cord as well. The cranial nerves may be attached to the ventral, lateral, or dorsal surface of the brain. The nerves with ventral and lateral attachments are seen on the base of the brain.

Cranial nerves with ventral attachments

Olfactory nerves

Approximately 20 **olfactory nerves** on each side pass through the cribriform plate of the ethmoid to the olfactory bulb. They are unusual in that they arise from the olfactory cells in the nasal mucous membrane and consist of bundles of minute, non-myelinated nerve fibres [Fig. 24.2].

Optic nerve

The optic nerve is a thick, cylindrical nerve. It is composed of myelinated nerve fibres which arise in the retina. The optic nerve ends by joining the anterolateral angle of the optic chiasma [Fig. 24.2].

Oculomotor nerve

The oculomotor nerve arises as a compact bundle of rootlets at the medial aspect of the cerebral peduncle in the posterior part of the interpeduncular fossa [Fig. 24.3].

Abducens nerve

The abducens nerve emerges at the inferior border of the pons, immediately lateral to the pyramid [Fig. 24.3].

Hypoglossal nerve

The hypoglossal nerve is formed by the union of rootlets which arise from the anterior aspect of the medulla oblongata in the groove between the pyramid and the olive [Fig. 24.3]. They are directly in line with the ventral rootlets of the first cervical nerve.

Cranial nerves with lateral attachments

Trigeminal nerve

The **trigeminal nerve**, the largest of the cranial nerves, is attached to the junction of the pons and the middle cerebellar peduncle. It consists of two roots: a larger posterolateral **sensory root** consisting of loosely packed nerve bundles; and a smaller anterosuperior **motor root** which is compact and closely applied to the sensory root [Fig. 24.3].

Facial and vestibulocochlear nerves

The facial and vestibulocochlear nerves, with the small **nervus intermedius** between them, emerge on the inferior border of the pons, posterior to the olive, and in the same vertical line as the other laterally attached cranial nerves [Fig. 24.3].

The facial nerve is motor. The nervus intermedius [Fig. 24.3] carries sensory and parasympathetic fibres associated with the facial nerve. It lies between the facial and vestibulocochlear nerves. The vestibulocochlear nerve is sensory. It splits at the medulla oblongata into a cochlear part passing posterior to the inferior cerebellar peduncle [Fig. 24.5] and a vestibular part passing anterior to it.

Glossopharyngeal, vagus, and accessory nerves

The glossopharyngeal, vagus, and accessory nerves arise as a series of rootlets from a groove posterior to the olive in the medulla oblongata, and from the lateral aspect of the spinal cord as far inferiorly as the fifth cervical spinal segment. The rootlets which form the glossopharyngeal nerves can only be differentiated from the others because they

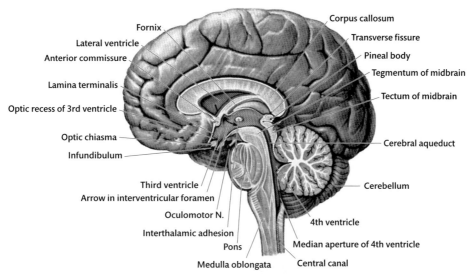

Fig. 24.7 Medial surface of the right half of a bisected brain to show the ventricles. The arrow passes through the interventricular foramen from the lateral to the third ventricle. (The septum pellucidum has been removed to expose the lateral ventricle.) Ependymal lining of ventricles = blue.

pierce the dura mater separately at the jugular foramen. A part of the accessory nerve may still be attached to the brain in the specimen. If a portion of the spinal cord is present, the spinal and cranial roots may be seen [Figs. 24.2, 24.3].

Cranial nerve with dorsal attachment

Trochlear nerve

The thin **trochlear nerve** is the only cranial nerve with a dorsal attachment. It decussates within the midbrain and emerges from the dorsal surface, lateral to the median plane. The proximal part will be seen later when the anterior lobe of the cerebellum is removed. A part of it may be seen here winding around the lateral aspect of the crus cerebri towards the interpeduncular fossa, immediately superior to the pons [Fig. 24.2].

Use the instructions given in Dissection 24.2 to identify the 12 pairs of cranial nerves.

The ventricular system

The ventricular system is a hollow, fluid-filled system derived from the cavities of the primitive brain vesicles. It is lined by ependyma. Each cerebral hemisphere has a **lateral ventricle** which communicates with the single midline third ventricle through the interventricular foramen, or **foramen of Monro** [Fig. 24.7]. The

DISSECTION 24.2 Surface attachment of cranial nerves

Objective

I. To identify the surface attachment of the cranial nerves.

Instructions

1. Identify the surface attachments of the cranial nerves.

2. Remove the small blood vessels and pia mater from the medulla oblongata, leaving the nerve roots in position as far as possible.

third ventricle is a narrow slit-like cavity of the diencephalon. Posteriorly, it continues with the **cerebral aqueduct** of the midbrain, which in turn communicates with the fourth ventricle. The **fourth ventricle** is a wide tent-shaped cavity between the pons and medulla and the cerebellum [see Figs. 32.1, 32.2]. Inferiorly, the cavity of the fourth ventricle is continuous with the central canal in the inferior part of the medulla and the spinal cord.

The ventricles are filled with cerebrospinal fluid (CSF) and contain the choroid plexus which produces it. The roof of the fourth ventricle has one median and two lateral apertures. Through these apertures CSF leaves the ventricle and enters the subarachnoid space around the brain and spinal cord [see Fig. 25.1].

Development of the brain and spinal cord

The brain and spinal cord develop from the neural tube. The cavity of the neural tube persists as the ventricular system in the brain and as the central canal of the spinal cord. The parts of the brain developed from each of the primitive brain vesicles (forebrain, midbrain, and hindbrain vesicles) and the cavity enclosed within them are listed in Table 24.1.

Table 24.1 Developmental origin and ventricular system in parts of the brain

During development	In the adult	Ventricular system
Forebrain	Cerebrum	Lateral ventricle
	Diencephalon	Third ventricle
Midbrain	Midbrain	Cerebral aqueduct
Hindbrain	Medulla oblongata Pons Cerebellum	Fourth ventricle

CHAPTER 25
The meninges of the brain

Introduction

The brain is surrounded by the same three membranes which surround the spinal cord—the dura mater, arachnoid mater, and pia mater [see Fig. 8.1]. The meninges of the brain and spinal cord are continuous with each other at the foramen magnum.

Dura mater

The cranial dura mater has been seen and described during the dissection of the head [Chapter 8], but its parts should be reviewed in relation to the brain.

Arachnoid mater

The arachnoid mater is an exceedingly thin, almost transparent membrane which lines the internal surface of the dura mater and, for the most part, has exactly the same shape as the dural sac. The arachnoid is separated from the dura mater by a capillary space—the **subdural space**—which contains a film of fluid. This arrangement allows movement between the dura mater and the brain (enclosed in the arachnoid and pia mater), except where the arachnoid and dura are fused. Fusion of the arachnoid and dura occurs where both meninges are pierced by structures entering or leaving the brain (e.g. nerves and blood vessels), where the arachnoid granulations pierce the dura mater, and where the ligamentum denticulatum is attached to the dura mater [Chapter 21].

Subarachnoid space

The subarachnoid space, between the arachnoid and pia mater, is filled with **cerebrospinal fluid** (CSF). The fluid acts as a mobile buffer to distribute and equalize pressures within the skull [Fig. 25.1].

Filaments, or **trabeculae**, traverse the subarachnoid space from the arachnoid to the pia mater and are numerous in some situations, e.g. on the surfaces of the cerebral hemispheres. The dense trabeculae form a kind of fluid-filled sponge which helps to protect the surface of the brain from damage against the skull or the dural folds, when it moves within the dura mater. The trabeculae also bind the pia and arachnoid tightly together in these situations. Elsewhere, and especially where the pia mater is widely separated from the arachnoid, the mesh is less dense and the CSF can flow more freely. The larger arteries and veins of the brain lie in the subarachnoid space and send branches into the substance of the brain. A sleeve of pia mater and subarachnoid space, called the **perivascular space**, surround each branch for a short distance within the brain substance.

Subarachnoid cisterns

In certain situations, the brain closely covered by pia mater lies some distance from the arachnoid lining the dura mater. In these situations, the subarachnoid space is large and is known as **subarachnoid cisterns**. Like the subarachnoid space everywhere else, the subarachnoid cisterns are filled with CSF. Cisterns are principally found around the brainstem and cerebellum, on the base

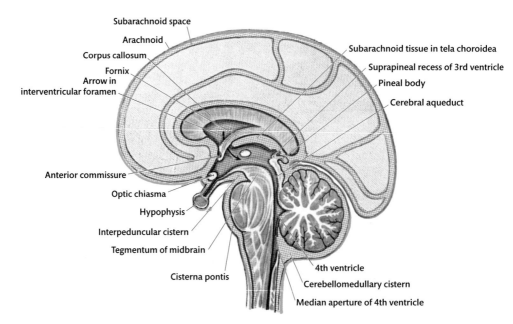

Subarachnoid space
Arachnoid
Corpus callosum
Fornix
Arrow in interventricular foramen
Subarachnoid tissue in tela choroidea
Suprapineal recess of 3rd ventricle
Pineal body
Cerebral aqueduct
Anterior commissure
Optic chiasma
Hypophysis
Interpeduncular cistern
Tegmentum of midbrain
Cisterna pontis
4th ventricle
Cerebellomedullary cistern
Median aperture of 4th ventricle

Fig. 25.1 Diagram of a median section of the brain to show membranes and cisterns. Red = pia mater; blue stipple = subarachnoid space and ventricles; blue = arachnoid; pink = surface view of shallow subarachnoid space. The lines of blue stipple running over the pink area indicate the places where the subarachnoid space is deeper around the branches of the anterior and posterior cerebral arteries.

of the brain, around the free margin of the tentorium cerebelli, and in association with the major blood vessels [Fig. 25.1].

The **cerebellomedullary cistern** lies in the angle between the cerebellum, medulla oblongata, and the occipital bone. It is continuous inferiorly with the posterior part of the spinal subarachnoid space [Fig. 25.1]. ➲ The cerebellomedullary cistern is accessible through a needle introduced anterosuperiorly through the posterior atlanto-occipital membrane, between the posterior arch of the atlas and the posterior margin of the foramen magnum—cisternal puncture.

The **cisterna pontis** lies anterior to the pons and medulla oblongata [Fig. 25.1]. It contains the vertebral and basilar arteries. It is continuous: (1) posteriorly around the medulla oblongata with the cerebellomedullary cistern; (2) inferiorly with the spinal subarachnoid space; and (3) superiorly with the interpeduncular cistern.

The **interpeduncular cistern** fills the interpeduncular fossa [Fig. 25.1]. At the superior border of the pons, the arachnoid turns anteriorly above the sella turcica and is stretched between the temporal lobes of the hemispheres. Here it forms the floor of the interpeduncular cistern. This cistern contains the arterial circle—the circle of Willis [see Fig. 8.9].

Arachnoid villi and granulations

Arachnoid villi are minute protrusions of the arachnoid mater into the dural venous sinuses through apertures in the dura mater. (They are similar to, but smaller and more numerous than, the arachnoid granulations shown in Fig. 25.2.) They are particularly common in the superior sagittal sinus and its lateral lacunae. The arachnoid villi contain subarachnoid tissue, CSF, and a number of thin tubules which pass through the middle of each villus. The tubules and spaces between the arachnoid trabeculae are continuous with the subarachnoid space at the base of the villus. The tubules open into the venous sinus at the apex of the villus. When the pressure of the CSF exceeds that in the venous sinus, the spaces fill with fluid, the villi bulge into the sinus, and the central tubules become patent and allow CSF to flow into the venous sinus. If the venous pressure exceeds that of the subarachnoid space, the villi collapse, effectively closing the central tubules and preventing the reflux of blood into the subarachnoid space. In effect, the arachnoid villi are one-way valves for the passage of CSF into the venous system. With increasing age, the size of

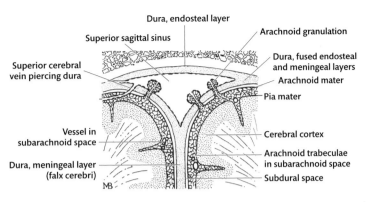

Fig. 25.2 Diagrammatic transverse section through the superior sagittal sinus and surrounding structures. Note the arrangement of the arachnoid granulations.

the villi increases till they form arachnoid granulations which often indent the overlying bone of the skull.

Communications of the subarachnoid space

The subarachnoid space communicates with: (1) the cavity of the dural venous sinus through the arachnoid villi; and (2) the ventricles of the brain through three small openings in the roof of the fourth ventricle.

Using the instructions given in Dissection 25.1, explore the extent and contents of the subarachnoid space.

The pia mater is adherent to the surface of the brain and follows the irregularities of its surface closely.

The blood vessels of the brain lie in the subarachnoid space on the surface of the pia mater. They break up into branches on the pia mater and

---

DISSECTION 25.1 Subarachnoid space

Objectives

I. To study the extent of the subarachnoid space. **II.** To identify and trace the vertebral and basilar arteries. **III.** To identify the choroid plexus in the median and lateral apertures of the fourth ventricle.

Instructions

1. If the arachnoid is complete, divide it along the anterior aspect of the medulla oblongata and pons to expose the vertebral and basilar arteries and their branches [see Fig. 26.3].

2. Note the arachnoid trabeculae.

3. Cut posteriorly through the arachnoid into the cerebellomedullary cistern, and identify the posterior inferior cerebellar branch of the vertebral artery. This branch winds posteriorly on the medulla oblongata, on its way to the cerebellum.

4. Identify the apertures in the roof of the fourth ventricle (the cavity of the hindbrain) by the tuft of

finely granular material (**choroid plexus**) which protrudes through each [see Fig. 24.3]. The **median aperture** can be seen in the depths of the cerebellomedullary cistern by gently depressing the medulla away from the cerebellum [see Fig. 29.4]. The **lateral apertures** face anteriorly and lie immediately posterior to the glossopharyngeal nerve. Pick up the tuft of choroid plexus protruding through the lateral aperture, and pull it gently towards the cerebellum—the aperture will be seen immediately anterior to the choroid plexus at the end of a sleeve-like extension of the thin roof of the fourth ventricle [see Figs. 24.3, 29.4].

5. Extend the median incision in the arachnoid into the interpeduncular fossa which lodges the **interpeduncular cistern**. Note the blood vessels in the cistern and the fact that its floor is perforated posteriorly by the oculomotor nerves and anteriorly by the internal carotid arteries and the infundibulum (stalk of the pituitary).

anastomose there, before passing into the substance of the brain as end-arteries. If a small piece of the pia mater is stripped from the surface of the brain, a number of minute blood vessels are seen entering the brain substance from its deep surface.

Choroid plexus and tela choroidea

In certain situations, the walls of the ventricles are thin and consist only of the lining epithelium—the **ependyma**. In these regions, the overlying pia mater gets invaginated into the cavities as a series of vascular tufts. These tufts carry the ependyma before them and form the **choroid plexuses** of the ventricles [see Fig. 32.3]. The pial element of the choroid plexus is known as the **tela choroidea**. The choroid plexuses are the source of CSF within the ventricles. From the ventricles, the CSF enters the subarachnoid space through the apertures in the roof of the fourth ventricle. The CSF circulates slowly in the subarachnoid space and drains into the dural venous sinuses through the arachnoid granulations and villi.

See Clinical Application 25.1 for the practical implications of the anatomy discussed in this chapter.

CLINICAL APPLICATION 25.1 Subarachnoid haemorrhage

A 54-year-old man complained of sudden onset of severe headache accompanied by vomiting. Soon after, he became unconscious and had a generalized seizure. Clinical examination revealed moderately elevated blood pressure, papilloedema, and focal neurological deficits. Imaging studies showed a bleed in the subarachnoid space—a subarachnoid haemorrhage (SAH).

Study question 1: what are the contents of the subarachnoid space? (Answer: the subarachnoid space contains CSF and the major blood vessels of the brain.)

Study question 2: what are the causes of an SAH? (Answer: the usual causes of an SAH include rupture of an aneurysm [Clinical Application 26.1], localized dilatation of a vessel, arteriovenous malformation [Clinical Application 26.2], or head trauma.)

Study question 3: what is the cause for the headache and vomiting? (Answer: headache and vomiting are typical signs of raised intracranial pressure. In this patient, raised intracranial pressure is due to collection of blood in the subarachnoid space. This pressure is transferred around the optic nerve, and also explains the papilloedema.)

Study question 4: how is this condition managed? (Answer: blood pressure is controlled by antihypertensive medication. Bleeding is controlled by applying surgical clips or an endovascular coil.)

CHAPTER 26
The blood vessels of the brain

The intracranial vessels (with the exception of the dural venous sinuses) [Chapter 8] have much thinner walls than extracranial vessels of comparable size, as they are enclosed in, and supported by, the surrounding cranium. The walls of most of the veins are so thin that they are impossible to see, unless filled with blood.

Veins of the cerebral hemispheres

Most of the cerebral veins lie on the surface of the hemisphere in the subarachnoid space. They drain into the dural venous sinuses by piercing the arachnoid, crossing the subdural space and piercing the dura [see Fig. 8.3].

Veins of the superolateral surface

The **superior cerebral veins** [Fig. 26.1] converge on the superior sagittal sinus, the anterior and posterior veins entering the sinus obliquely from in front and behind. They all pass inferior to the lateral lacunae of the sinus. Most of the **inferior cerebral veins** converge on the superficial middle cerebral vein, but those of the occipital lobe run inferiorly into the transverse sinus [Fig. 26.1].

The **superficial middle cerebral vein** runs anteriorly between the lips of the posterior ramus of the lateral sulcus [see Fig. 24.1] and curves medially into the stem of the lateral sulcus. It ends in the cavernous sinus. Its cut end will be found piercing the arachnoid near the medial end of the stem of the lateral sulcus. Posteriorly, the superficial

middle cerebral vein is frequently connected to the superior sagittal sinus by a wide **superior anastomotic vein**, and to the transverse sinus by the **inferior anastomotic vein** [Fig. 26.1]. ⮡ These anastomotic veins may become important if the cavernous sinus is blocked. The superficial veins also connect with veins in the interior and on the base of the hemisphere by small veins which pierce the hemisphere.

Veins of the inferior surface of the hemisphere

The veins on the inferior surface drain in a number of different directions: (1) anteriorly to the anterior and superficial middle cerebral veins; (2) posteriorly to the basal vein; and (3) directly to the superior petrosal, straight, and transverse sinuses.

Veins of the medial surface of the hemisphere

These veins will be seen later when the hemispheres are separated, but parts of this system can be seen now, so a brief description is given.

The main vein on the medial aspect of the hemisphere is the **great cerebral vein**. It is formed by the union of the two **internal cerebral veins**, inferior to the splenium of the corpus callosum, and ends by uniting with the inferior sagittal sinus to form the straight sinus [see Fig. 8.2A]. (The internal cerebral veins are formed by the union of the thalamostriate vein and the veins draining the choroid plexus of the lateral ventricle at the interventricular foramen [see Fig 32.7].) If the occipital lobes of the hemispheres are gently separated, the cut end of the great cerebral vein

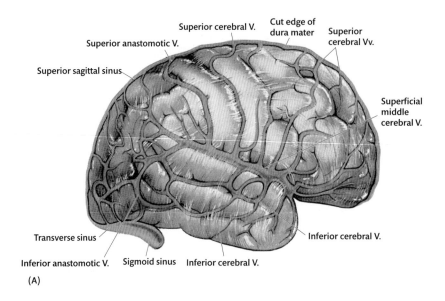

Superior cerebral V.
Cut edge of dura mater
Superior cerebral Vv.
Superior anastomotic V.
Superior sagittal sinus
Superficial middle cerebral V.
Transverse sinus
Inferior anastomotic V.
Sigmoid sinus
Inferior cerebral V.
Inferior cerebral V.

(A)

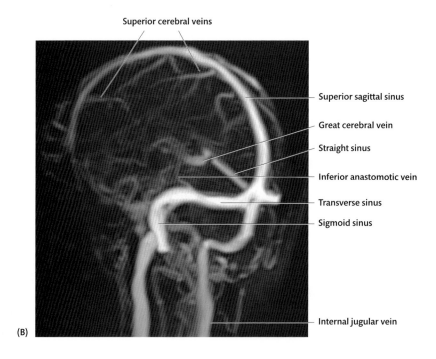

Superior cerebral veins
Superior sagittal sinus
Great cerebral vein
Straight sinus
Inferior anastomotic vein
Transverse sinus
Sigmoid sinus
Internal jugular vein

(B)

Fig. 26.1 (A) Veins of the superolateral surface of the hemisphere, seen through the arachnoid mater. (B) MRI venogram of the brain.

will be seen close to the splenium. The great cerebral vein is joined by a number of symmetrical tributaries from the midbrain and cerebellum, and by the basal veins which curve around the sides of the midbrain to reach it from the inferior surface of the brain.

Each **basal vein** is formed deep in the medial part of the stem of the lateral sulcus by the union of: (1) the **anterior cerebral vein**, which runs with the corresponding artery and enters it from in front; (2) the **deep middle cerebral vein** which lies in the depths of the lateral sulcus on the insula; and (3) the **striate vein** or veins which descend through the substance of the brain and emerge through the anterior perforated substance [see Fig. 24.2].

Using the instructions given in Dissection 26.1, expose the vessels in the lateral sulcus.

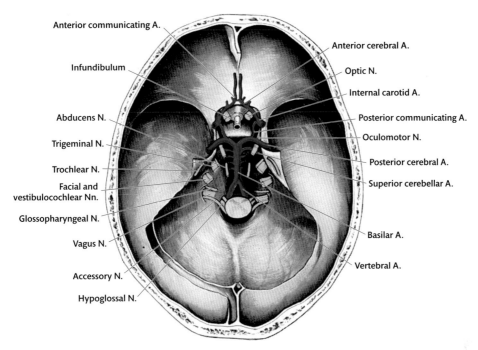

Fig. 26.2 Floor of the cranial cavity after removal of the brain. The arteries at the base of the brain are intact.

DISSECTION 26.1 Exposure of arteries and veins in the lateral sulcus

Objectives

I. To expose the middle cerebral artery and superficial middle cerebral vein in the stem of the lateral sulcus. II. To identify the striate veins and basal veins.

Instructions

1. Divide the arachnoid mater over the stem of the lateral sulcus, and depress the temporal pole to expose the beginning of the middle cerebral artery, the deep middle cerebral vein, the striate veins, and the origin of the basal vein.

2. If the basal vein is filled with blood, it will be seen passing posteriorly close to the optic tract [see Fig. 24.2]. Trace it as far as possible towards the great cerebral vein.

Veins of the cerebellum and brainstem

The veins of the brainstem and cerebellum drain posteriorly to the basal veins, great cerebral veins, and adjacent dural venous sinuses. The veins of the medulla oblongata communicate with those of the spinal cord.

Arteries of the brain

Two internal carotid arteries and two vertebral arteries supply the brain. The vertebral arteries enter the skull through the foramen magnum [Fig. 26.2]. Each internal carotid artery runs through the skull in the carotid canal and the superior part of the foramen lacerum. It then takes a sinuous course through the cavernous sinus and pierces the dural roof of the sinus [see Fig. 8.12; Fig. 26.2]. It ends immediately lateral to the optic chiasma, inferior to the anterior perforated substance, by dividing into its terminal branches—the anterior and middle cerebral arteries [see Fig. 24.2; Figs. 26.3, 26.4].

Vertebral arteries

Each vertebral artery enters the subarachnoid space in the upper part of the vertebral canal by piercing the lateral aspect of the dura and arachnoid mater. It ascends anterosuperiorly through the foramen magnum, curves around the ventrolateral aspect of the medulla oblongata, and unites with the vertebral artery of the other side to form the **basilar artery** at the lower border of the pons. The two vertebral arteries are often of very different calibre [Figs. 26.2, 26.3].

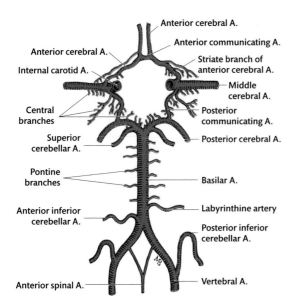

Fig. 26.3 Diagram of the arteries on the base of the brain.

Intracranial branches of the vertebral artery

1. The **posterior spinal artery** is the first intracranial branch. It passes inferiorly on the spinal cord among the dorsal rootlets of the spinal nerves. It commonly arises from the posterior inferior cerebellar artery.

2. The **posterior inferior cerebellar artery** is the largest branch [Fig. 26.3]. It arises from the vertebral artery, soon after it pierces the meninges, and pursues a tortuous course posteriorly on the side of the medulla oblongata, among the rootlets of the hypoglossal, vagus, and glossopharyngeal nerves. It supplies branches to the lateral part of the medulla oblongata, occasionally as far cranially as the inferior border of the pons. It reaches the posterior surface of the medulla oblongata, between the roof of the fourth ventricle and the cerebellum, and supplies the choroid plexus of the fourth ventricle and the inferior surface of the cerebellum. It varies inversely in size with the anterior inferior cerebellar artery but is usually much larger.

3. The **anterior spinal artery** [Fig. 26.3] is formed by the union of a branch from each of the vertebral arteries on the ventral surface of the medulla oblongata, close to the pons. It supplies the median part of the medulla oblongata and continues inferiorly throughout the length of the spinal cord.

Basilar artery

The basilar artery is formed at the inferior border of the pons by the union of the two vertebral arteries. It ends at the superior border of the pons by

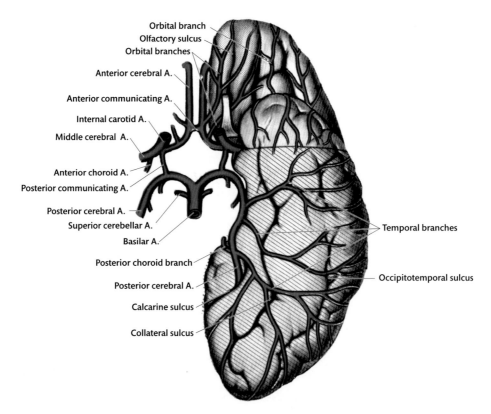

Fig. 26.4 Arteries of the inferior surface of the left hemisphere. The areas supplied by the three cerebral arteries are indicated by: red stipple = anterior cerebral artery; red cross-hatching = posterior cerebral artery; and no colour = middle cerebral artery.

dividing into the two posterior cerebral arteries. It lies in the median groove of the pons in the cisterna pontis, on the basilar part of the occipital bone and the dorsum sellae of the sphenoid [Fig. 26.3].

Branches of the basilar artery

1. The **anterior inferior cerebellar artery** arises at the lower border of the pons and runs laterally, superficial to the sixth, seventh, and eighth cranial nerves. It then loops over the flocculus [see Fig. 24.3] and supplies the antero-inferior part of the cerebellar surface.
2. The **artery of the labyrinth** arises beside, or from, the anterior inferior cerebellar artery [Fig. 26.3]. It accompanies the vestibulocochlear nerve to the internal ear and also supplies the adjacent part of the facial nerve.
3. Numerous slender **pontine branches** pierce the pons, some close to the midline, others further laterally [Fig. 26.3].
4. The large **superior cerebellar artery** arises close to the superior border of the pons. It winds posteriorly along the superior border of the pons and the middle cerebellar peduncle, supplying them and the adjacent part of the midbrain. It also sends many branches to the superior surface of the cerebellum, inferior to the tentorium cerebelli.
5. The two large **posterior cerebral arteries** are the terminal branches of the basilar artery. They diverge at the superior border of the pons [Fig. 26.4]. Each sends a number of fine **central (posteromedial central) branches** into the ventral surface of the midbrain (interpeduncular fossa) and then curves posteriorly around the upper part of the mid-

brain to the inferomedial surface of the corresponding hemisphere. Here it passes towards the occipital pole, giving branches as shown in Figs. 26.4 and 26.5. The posterior cerebral and superior cerebellar arteries run parallel to each other and lie on, and supply, the superior and inferior parts of the midbrain, respectively. The posterior cerebral artery lies above the third and fourth cranial nerves, which arise from the midbrain, and the superior cerebellar artery lies below these nerves [Figs. 26.2, 26.3].

Branches of the posterior cerebral arteries

1. Small **posteromedial central branches** pierce the ventral surface of the midbrain in the interpeduncular fossa. (The passage of these branches creates the **posterior perforated substance**—the perforated tissue in the floor of the interpeduncular fossa.) Similar branches pierce the lateral surface of the midbrain and caudal diencephalon [Fig. 26.3].
2. **Posterior choroid branches** arise on the lateral surface of the midbrain and pass forwards to supply the greater part of the choroid plexus of the lateral and third ventricles [Fig. 26.4].
3. **Cortical branches** supply mainly the inferior surface of the cerebral cortex through named branches, for example the temporal branches [Figs. 26.4, 26.5].

On the anterior surface of the midbrain, each posterior cerebral artery receives a slender **posterior communicating** branch from the corresponding internal carotid artery [p. 296] [Fig. 26.4].

Internal carotid arteries

The cut end of each internal carotid artery can be seen immediately lateral to the optic chiasma. The

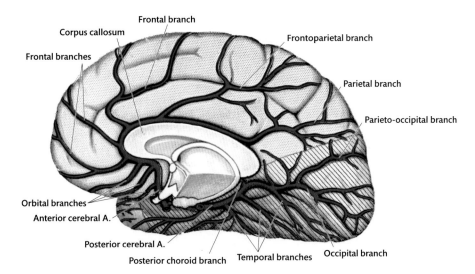

Fig. 26.5 The arteries of the medial and tentorial surfaces of the right hemisphere. Area supplied by the: anterior cerebral artery = red stipple; posterior cerebral artery = red cross-hatching; and middle cerebral artery = no colour.

artery passes into a shallow pit, immediately inferior to the anterior perforated substance [see Fig. 24.2; Fig. 26.2], and gives off the **posterior communicating** and **anterior choroidal** and **ophthalmic arteries**. It ends by dividing into the **middle** and **anterior cerebral** arteries [Figs. 26.3, 26.4].

The **posterior communicating artery** passes posteriorly across the crus cerebri to join the posterior cerebral artery. It completes the arterial circle at the base of the brain [Fig. 26.3]. The posterior communicating artery gives off minute branches to the crus, optic tract, hypophysis, and hypothalamus. The posterior communicating artery is usually a thin vessel, but it may be large on one or both sides and form the major source of blood in the posterior cerebral artery. ⊃ In such cases, occlusion of the internal carotid artery may lead to damage in the territory of the posterior cerebral artery also.

The **anterior choroid artery** arises superior to the posterior communicating artery and passes posterolaterally, close to the optic tract [Fig. 26.4]. It gives branches into the crus cerebri and turns laterally [see Fig. 32.5] to enter the choroid plexus of the inferior horn of the lateral ventricle.

Anterior cerebral artery

Only a small part of this artery can be seen at this stage. (The remainder will be seen when the medial aspect of the hemisphere is exposed.) This initial part of the anterior cerebral artery runs horizontally in an anteromedial direction [Fig. 26.4] to the longitudinal fissure. Here it is joined to the anterior

cerebral artery by the short **anterior communicating artery** [Fig. 26.3], anterosuperior to the optic chiasma. The anterior cerebral artery then bends sharply upwards into the median longitudinal fissure and runs on the medial surface of the cerebral hemisphere [Fig. 26.5].

Branches of the anterior cerebral artery

1. Several thin **central** branches pierce the brain, anterior to the optic chiasma, and enter the anterior hypothalamus.
2. Branches pass to the optic chiasma and the optic nerve.
3. One or more larger recurrent branches arise close to the anterior communicating artery and run to the medial part of the anterior perforated substance. Here they send **medial striate** (**anteromedial central**) branches into the brain substance [Fig. 26.3].
4. Several **cortical branches** are given to the cerebral cortex [Figs. 26.4, 26.5].

Middle cerebral artery

The middle cerebral artery continues in line with the internal carotid artery [Fig. 26.3]. ⊃ As such, particulate matter in the internal carotid artery enters the middle cerebral artery more frequently than the anterior cerebral. The middle cerebral artery runs laterally in the stem of the lateral sulcus and breaks up into a number of branches on the **insula**. These branches emerge through the lateral sulcus and supply most of the superolateral surface of the cerebral hemisphere [Fig. 26.6] and also the

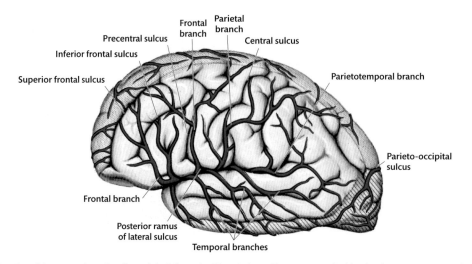

Fig. 26.6 Arteries of the superolateral surface of the left cerebral hemisphere. The areas supplied by the three arteries are indicated by: red stipple = anterior cerebral artery; no colour = middle cerebral artery; and red cross-hatching = posterior cerebral artery.

adjacent parts of the orbital and tentorial surfaces through the cortical branches [Figs. 26.4, 26.5].

The **central branches** of the middle cerebral artery are the numerous small **lateral striate (anterolateral central) arteries** [Fig. 26.3]. They pass superiorly through the anterior perforated substance to the deep nuclei of the hemisphere.

Figs. 26.7A and B are digital subtraction angiograms of the left internal carotid and left vertebral arteries. Fig. 27.6C is a magnetic resonance angiogram of the arterial circle.

The arterial circle—**circle of Willis**—is a communicating channel of arteries made up of the posterior cerebral, posterior communicating, anterior cerebral, and anterior communicating arteries. It extends from the superior border of the pons posteriorly, to the longitudinal fissure anteriorly, and lies principally in the interpeduncular fossa. It forms a route through which blood from the internal carotid artery or the basilar artery may be distributed to all parts of the cerebral hemispheres.

Branches of the cerebral arteries

Two types of branches arise from the cerebral arteries: the cortical and central branches. The **central branches** are numerous and slender, and tend to arise in groups which immediately pierce the surface of the brain to supply the deeper parts. The largest collections of central branches pass through the anterior and posterior perforated

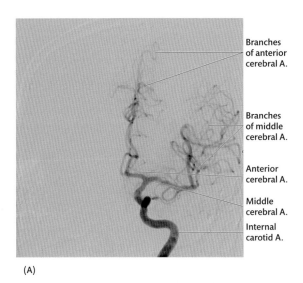

Branches of anterior cerebral A.

Branches of middle cerebral A.

Anterior cerebral A.

Middle cerebral A.

Internal carotid A.

(A)

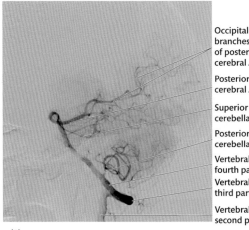

Occipital branches of posterior cerebral A.

Posterior cerebral A.

Superior cerebellar A.

Posterior inferior cerebellar A.

Vertebral A., fourth part

Vertebral A., third part

Vertebral A., second part

(B)

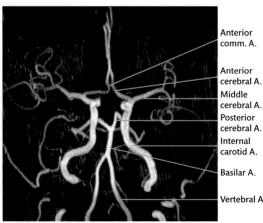

Anterior comm. A.

Anterior cerebral A.

Middle cerebral A.

Posterior cerebral A.

Internal carotid A.

Basilar A.

Vertebral A.

(C)

Fig. 26.7 (A) Digital subtraction angiogram of the left internal carotid artery. (B) Digital subtraction angiogram of the left vertebral artery. (C) Magnetic resonance angiogram of the circle of Willis.

substances [Fig. 26.3]. They do not anastomose to any significant extent within the brain substance. The **cortical branches** ramify over the surface of the cortex and anastomose freely on the pia mater. They give rise to numerous small branches which enter the cortex at right angles and, like the central branches, do not anastomose in it [Figs. 26.4, 26.5, 26.6]. ➔ It follows that blockage of an artery on the pia mater may produce little, if any, damage to the brain, but damage to branches entering the substance of the brain leads to the destruction of brain tissue.

➔ The arteries of the brain are supplied with **sympathetic nerves** which reach them from the carotid and vertebral plexuses. They are extremely sensitive to injury and react by passing into prolonged spasm.

See Clinical Applications 26.1 and 26.2 for the practical implications of the anatomy discussed in this chapter.

CLINICAL APPLICATION 26.1 Aneurysm

An aneurysm of the cavernous part of the right internal carotid artery was noted in a 42-year-old woman who was investigated for double vision [Fig. 26.8]. An aneurysm is a balloon-like swelling in the arterial wall. As it grows, an aneurysm causes pressure symptoms on surrounding structures. A ruptured aneurysm leads to rapid subarachnoid haemorrhage, with high mortality.

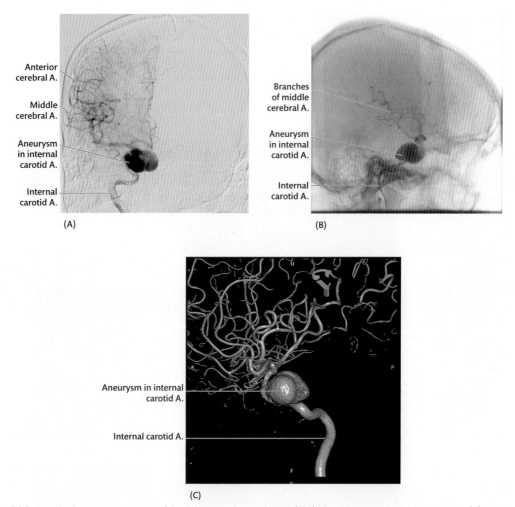

Fig. 26.8 Digital subtraction angiogram of the right internal carotid artery (ICA), showing a cavernous ICA aneurysm. (A) Antero-posterior view. (B) Lateral view. (C) Three-dimensional imaging.

CLINICAL APPLICATION 26.2 Arteriovenous malformations

An arteriovenous malformation (AVM) is a tangled mass of abnormal and poorly formed blood vessels—both arteries and veins. It has a high rate of spontaneous rupture and bleeding. AVMs can occur anywhere in the body, but brain AVMs are of special concern because rupture of them causes subarachnoid haemorrhage [Clinical Application 25.1]. Fig. 26.9 shows an AVM in the middle cerebral artery.

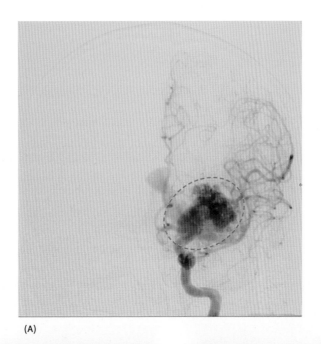

(A)

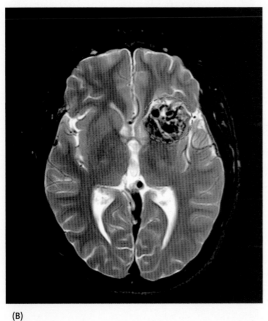

(B)

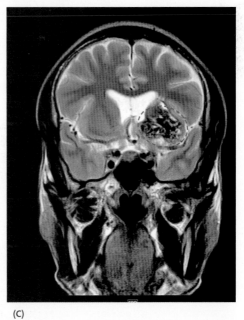

(C)

Fig. 26.9 Arteriovenous malformation in the middle cerebral artery = red circle. (A) Digital subtraction angiogram of the right internal carotid artery. (B) T2-weighted axial magnetic resonance imaging (MRI). (C) T2-weighted coronal MRI.

CHAPTER 27
The spinal cord

The spinal cord extends from just below the fora-men magnum to the intervertebral disc between L. 1 and L. 2. The gross features, coverings, and blood supply of the spinal cord have been described in Chapter 21. The internal arrangement of the grey and white matter of the spinal cord and its connec-tions are described in this chapter.

General arrangement of white and grey matter

In transverse section, the spinal cord is seen to con-sist of an H-shaped core of **grey matter**, consist-ing principally of nerve cell bodies, and an external layer of **white matter**—nerve fibres. (Neuroglia, the cellular connective tissue of the central nerv-ous system, is seen in both the grey and white matter.) The horizontal bar of the H in the grey matter is the **grey commissure**, and it surrounds the central canal. Ventral to the grey commissure, nerve fibres cross the midline, forming the **white commissure**. The two commissures are the only neural continuity between the two halves of the spinal cord, which is otherwise separated into right and left halves [Fig. 27.1].

The **anteromedian fissure** on the spinal cord extends from the midline anteriorly inwards to the white commissure. The **posteromedian septum** extends inwards from the posteromedian sulcus to the grey commissure [Fig. 27.1].

The **central canal** is a narrow tube which runs longitudinally in the grey commissure. It is lined by ependyma and is continuous superiorly with the fourth ventricle of the brain. It ends in the filum terminale. The canal contains cerebrospinal fluid.

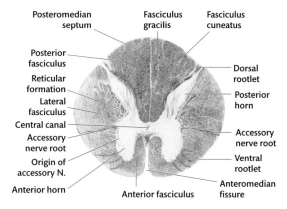

Fig. 27.1 Transverse section through the upper part of the cervi-cal spinal cord.

The anterior and posterior limbs of the H-shaped grey matter are the **anterior** and **posterior horns**. Since the horns extend throughout the length of the spinal cord, they are also known as anterior and posterior **grey columns**. The major-ity of cells in the posterior horn are associated with the sensory system. The cells in the anterior or ven-tral horn give rise to motor nerves. The amount of grey matter at any level is proportional to the amount of tissue supplied by the spinal nerves aris-ing there. As such, the horns are large in the cervi-cal and lumbar swellings (and are mainly responsi-ble for them) [Fig. 27.2].

The **dorsal roots** on each side enter the **postero-lateral sulcus** near the tip of the posterior horn. Here each fibre of the root either enters the poste-rior column and ascends in it or enters the posterior horn. (The fibres may divide into an ascending and a descending branch which run longitudinally in the white matter of the spinal cord, giving off numer-ous collaterals into the grey matter.) The **ventral**

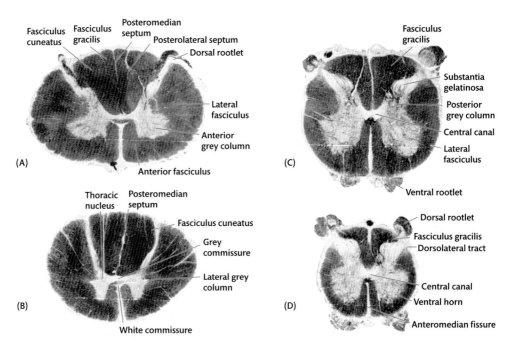

Fig. 27.2 Transverse sections through the cervical (A), thoracic (B), lumbar (C), and sacral (D) regions of the spinal cord.

roots arise mainly from large **motor cells** in the anterior horn.

Grey matter of the spinal cord

Fig. 27.3 summarizes the main terminations of the afferent nerves entering the spinal cord, and the origin of the efferent nerves leaving the spinal cord. The grey matter of the spinal cord is arbitrarily

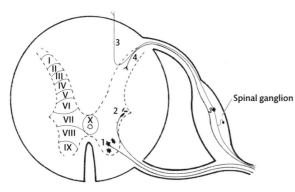

Fig. 27.3 Thoracic spinal segment. On the right is shown the main terminations of the afferent (sensory) nerves entering the spinal cord and the origin of the efferent (motor) nerves leaving the spinal cord. 1 = somatic efferent fibre; 2 = visceral efferent fibre; 3 = afferent fibres entering the posterior column; 4 = afferent fibres ending in the posterior horn. On the left side is shown the position of laminae I–X of Rexed.

divided into ten laminae known as Rexed laminae [Fig. 27.3]. Within the grey matter are a series of discontinuous cell groups which correspond approximately to one or more of these laminae. Laminae I–IV are in the dorsal horn and are the main sites of termination of the sensory fibres entering through the dorsal root. Throughout the spinal cord, the tips of the posterior horns, adjacent to the entry of the posterior roots, are composed of a translucent substance—the **substantia gelatinosa** [Fig. 27.2]. The substantia gelatinosa corresponds to laminae II and III. Laminae V and VI lie at the base of the dorsal horn. The **thoracic nucleus** (also known as Clarke's column) lies in the thoracic and upper lumbar segments at the medial side of the base of the posterior grey column [Fig. 27.2B]. The **lateral grey column**, or **lateral horn**, is a small extension on the lateral aspect of the grey matter, seen in all spinal segments between the first thoracic and second or third lumbar segments [Fig. 27.2B]. It contains the nerve cells which give rise to the preganglionic fibres of the sympathetic system. Neurons in the anterior or ventral horn innervate skeletal muscles. These cells may be grouped into medial, central, and lateral columns. The motor cells innervating the muscles of the limbs lie in the lateral part of the anterior horn. The anterior horn is small in the thoracic and upper cervical regions

[Fig. 27.1]. In the lower cervical and lumbosacral regions, the cells in the lateral group innervate the limb musculature, and the cells in the medial group innervate the axial musculature.

From the above description of nerve cells in the grey matter, it is clear that cells performing the same function lie in the same position at every level of the spinal cord. For example, all cells in the anterior horn will supply skeletal muscle, and cells in the lateral horn will supply smooth muscle and glands. Based on this arrangement, four functional columns are described in the spinal cord: the **general somatic efferent** supplying motor nerves to skeletal muscles; the **general visceral efferent** supplying motor nerves to smooth muscles; the **general visceral afferent**, located in the dorsal horn cells in the thoracic and lumbar regions and receiving sensory input from the viscera; and the **general somatic afferent**, also located in the dorsal horn, but in all segments of the spinal cord, and receiving sensory input from the skin of the body [Fig. 27.2].

The **white matter** of the spinal cord is composed of longitudinally running nerve fibres placed superficial to the grey matter. On each side, the white matter is divided into **posterior**, **lateral**, and **anterior columns**, or **fasciculi**, by the dorsal and ventral roots [Fig. 27.1]. The deepest fibres are short and pass from one segment of the spinal cord to another (**fasciculi proprii**) [Fig. 27.4]. The superficial fibres are long.

Fibres with similar origin and termination are grouped together in the white matter to form **tracts**, or **fasciculi**. Tracts which carry impulses from the brain to the spinal cord are the **descending tracts**. Similarly, tracts which carry sensory impulses from the spinal cord to the brain form the **ascending tracts** [Fig. 27.4]. In each segment of the spinal cord, ascending (sensory) fibres are added to the ascending tracts, and descending (motor) fibres leave the descending tracts to end in the grey matter. As such, both ascending and descending tracts increase in size superiorly, and the volume of white matter increases from below upwards. Note this change in the four sections of the spinal cord depicted in Fig. 27.2.

Descending tracts

The descending tracts originate from the opposite side of the brain and carry motor impulses to the anterior horn cells in the spinal cord. Most of these are crossed tracts, i.e. the fibres cross the midline and terminate on the anterior horn cells of the opposite side. The most important of these—the **lateral**

303

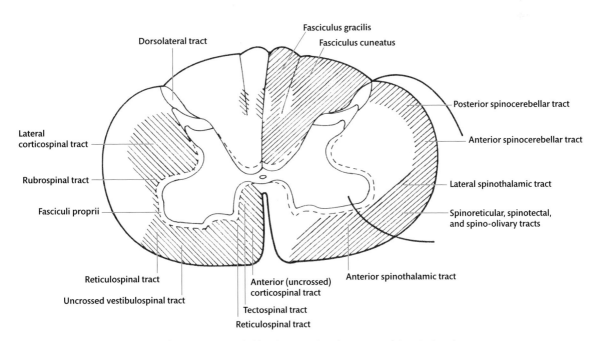

Fig. 27.4 The main ascending (right) and descending (left) pathways in the white matter of the spinal cord.

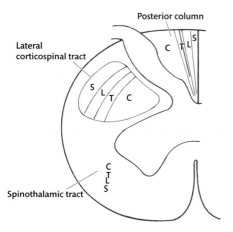

Posterior column

Lateral
corticospinal tract

Spinothalamic tract

Fig. 27.5 Diagrammatic transverse section through half of the cervical spinal cord to show the relative positions of the cervical (C), thoracic (T), lumbar (L), and sacral (S) fibres in the posterior column, spinothalamic tract, and lateral corticospinal tract.

corticospinal tract—originates in the cerebral cortex. The other descending tracts are the rubrospinal (from the red nucleus in the midbrain), reticulospinal (from the reticular formation of the brainstem), vestibulospinal (from the vestibular nuclei in the medulla), and tectospinal (from the tectum of the midbrain) tracts. Note the position of these tracts in Figs. 27.4 and 27.5. In the lateral corticospinal tract, the cervical fibres are the first to leave the tract to end on the anterior horn cells of the cervical spinal cord. They are located most medially. The thoracic, lumbar, and sacral fibres lie sequentially in more lateral positions [Fig. 27.5]. The exact origin of these fibres and the location in different parts of the brainstem will be dealt with in the corresponding sections.

Ascending tracts

The ascending tracts carry sensory impulses from the periphery to various parts of the brain. They are the **dorsal column**, consisting of the **fasciculus gracilis** and **cuneatus** [Figs. 27.2, 27.3, 27.4], **anterior** and **posterior spinocerebellar tracts**, and **anterolateral spinothalamic tracts** [Fig. 27.4]. Sensory information reaches the spinal cord through cells in the spinal or dorsal root ganglion. In the dorsal root, the thicker fibres lie medially and carry sensations of crude touch, pressure, and proprioception. Thinner fibres lie laterally and carry sensations of fine touch, pain, and temperature. The cells of the spinal ganglia are **first-order neurons** [Fig. 27.3]. They end by synapsing with other neurons—**second-order neurons**—in the spinal cord or brainstem.

Posterior column

The **posterior white columns**, or **dorsal columns**, lie between the dorsal roots of the two sides [Fig. 27.2]. They consist of fibres which enter the spinal cord in the dorsal roots and are predominantly concerned with crude touch, vibration, and proprioception. They ascend to the medulla oblongata (fibre marked '3' in Fig. 27.3), giving collaterals for reflex purposes into the posterior horn. New fibres are added at each level and cause the width of the posterior column to increase. The fibres entering through the highest roots, i.e. from the cervical region, lie most laterally [Fig. 27.5]. The fibres in the fasciculus gracilis originate in the lower half of the body; those in the fasciculus cuneatus arise in the upper half. Both groups of fibres give off collaterals to the grey matter throughout their length and ascend without interruption to the nuclei gracilis and cuneatus in the medulla.

In the upper half of the spinal cord, each posterior column is subdivided by a **posterolateral septum** into a slender medial **fasciculus gracilis** (which carries such fibres from the lower half of the body) and a broader lateral **fasciculus cuneatus** which carries fibres from the upper half of the body [Figs. 27.2, 27.4]. The position of this septum is marked on the surface by the **postero-intermediate sulcus**.

Spinothalamic tract

The finer fibres in the dorsal roots (principally concerned with fine touch, pain, and temperature) enter laterally, divide, and ascend or descend for a short distance. Together they form the **dorsolateral tract** overlying the lateral part of the substantia gelatinosa [Fig. 27.3]. These fibres end by synapsing on cells in the posterior horn. Second-order neurons arise from cells in the posterior horn, cross the midline in the anterior white commissure, and ascend to the thalamus in the **spinothalamic tract** [Figs. 27.5, 27.6]. (For further details on the course and termination of the spinothalamic tracts, see Chapters 28 and 30.)

Spinocerebellar tracts

There are two pathways connecting the spinal cord to the cerebellum. (The origin of these tracts is shown in Fig. 27.6.) The **posterior spinocerebellar tract** arises from the cells of the thoracic nucleus (lamina VII of the first thoracic to the second lumbar segments). They receive impulses through branches of the fibres in the fasciculus gracilis and transmit information from the inferior half of the

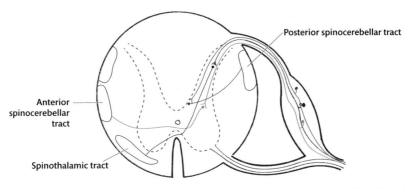

Posterior spinocerebellar tract

Anterior spinocerebellar tract

Spinothalamic tract

Fig. 27.6 Diagrammatic representation of the origin of the spinothalamic (black), posterior spinocerebellar (red), and ventral spinocerebellar (green) tracts.

same side of the body to the cerebellum. This tract ascends in the most posterolateral part of the lateral column of the same side [Figs. 27.4, 27.6].

Fibres of the **anterior** or **ventral spinocerebellar tract** arise from laminae V–VII of the lumbosacral spinal cord [Fig. 27.4]. They cross the midline and ascend in the anterior spinocerebellar tract [Figs. 27.4, 27.6]. They carry information from the lower limb. (For further details on the course and termination of the spinocerebellar tracts, see Chapters 28 and 29.)

See Clinical Applications 27.1 and 27.2 for the practical implications of the anatomy discussed in this chapter.

CLINICAL APPLICATION 27.1 Upper motor neuron and lower motor neuron lesions

The descending motor pathway consists of an **upper motor neuron**, from the motor cortex to the spinal grey matter, and a **lower motor neuron** located in the anterior horn cell. Clinical presentation of lesions affecting the upper motor neurons and lower motor neurons are different.

Signs of upper motor neuron lesions:

1. Hypertonia and exaggerated deep tendon reflexes due to loss of the normal cortical inhibition of the stretch reflex.

2. Absent superficial reflex due to lack of required cortical control.

3. Positive Babinski sign—or upgoing plantar reflex—due to loss of cortical inhibition of primitive reflexes.

Signs of lower motor neuron lesions:

1. Hypotonia and diminished deep tendon reflexes due to damage to the lower motor neurons (efferent limb of reflex).

2. Muscle atrophy resulting from loss of trophic factors normally secreted by the alpha motor neurons.

3. Muscle fasciculations in response to spontaneous action potentials produced by damaged alpha motor neurons.

These clinical findings help to differentiate upper and lower motor neuron lesions, and enable the anatomical localization of a lesion in a patient with paralysis.

CLINICAL APPLICATION 27.2 Hemisection of the spinal cord (Brown-Séquard syndrome)

A man involved in a car accident sustained an injury to the right half of his spinal cord. On examination, he was found to have:

1. Paralysis of the entire right lower limb.

2. Increased muscle tone and exaggerated deep tendon reflexes in the right lower limb, and an upgoing plantar reflex on the right side.

3. Loss of vibration, joint sense, and two-point discrimination on the right side of the body below the level of the umbilicus.

4. Loss of pain and temperature on the left half of the body below the level of the umbilicus.

5. A band of hyperaesthesia and occasional muscle fasciculations on the right side at the level of the umbilicus.

Study questions 1–5: explain the anatomical basis for each of the clinical features seen in this patient.

(Answer 1: paralysis of the right lower limb indicates damage to the corticospinal tract of the right side. The spinal segments involved in motor supply to the lower limb are L. 2 to S. 1. The fact that all movement of the right lower limb is lost means that the corticospinal tract injury is above the level of L. 2. Note: crossing of the corticospinal fibres occurs above the level of the lesion (in the medulla), which explains why the paralysis is on the same side as the lesion.)

(Answer 2: increased muscle tone, exaggerated deep tendon reflexes, and an upgoing plantar reflex on the right lower limb are features of an upper motor neuron lesion and are consistent with damage to the corticospinal tract.)

(Answer 3: loss of vibration, joint sense, and two-point discrimination on the right side of the body below the level of the umbilicus is due to damage to the posterior columns fibres of that side. Fibres carrying these impulses ascend ipsilaterally in the spinal cord. Hence loss of these sensations is on the same side as the lesion.)

(Answer 4: loss of pain and temperature from the left half of the body below the level of the umbilicus is due to damage of the spinothalamic tract on the right side. The origin of these fibres is on the left side [Fig. 27.6], and the second-order neurons cross the midline to ascend on the right. The sensory loss up to the level of the umbilicus localizes the lesion to the T. 10 dermatome.)

(Answer 5: the band of hyperaesthesia at the T. 10 dermatome and muscle fasciculations at this level are most likely due to involvement of the nerve roots and anterior horn cells at the T. 10 level—a lower motor neuron injury. This further indicates that the spinal cord injury occurred at the T. 10 level.)

The combination of neurological lesions discussed above constitutes the Brown-Séquard syndrome. You should know that cases of spinal cord hemisection rarely present this typically.

CHAPTER 28
The brainstem

Introduction

The brainstem consists of the medulla oblongata, pons, and midbrain. Some of the external features of the brainstem have been described and identified in Chapter 24. Review these features using Figs 28.1, 28.2, and 28.3.

External features of the brainstem

Medulla oblongata

The **medulla oblongata** is a conical part of the brainstem which extends from the pons to the spinal cord. It joins the spinal cord approximately at

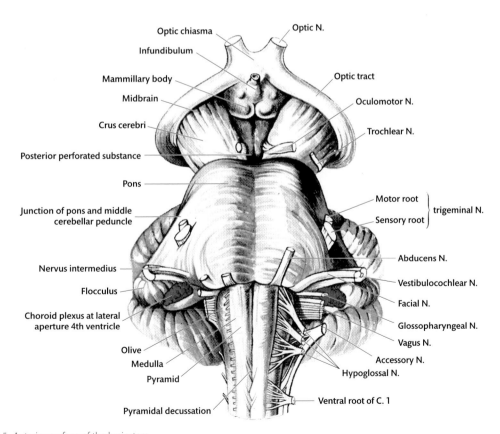

Fig. 28.1 Anterior surface of the brainstem.

Optic chiasma
Optic N.
Infundibulum
Mammillary body
Optic tract
Midbrain
Oculomotor N.
Crus cerebri
Trochlear N.
Posterior perforated substance
Pons
Motor root
Junction of pons and middle cerebellar peduncle
Sensory root
trigeminal N.
Abducens N.
Nervus intermedius
Vestibulocochlear N.
Flocculus
Facial N.
Choroid plexus at lateral aperture 4th ventricle
Glossopharyngeal N.
Olive
Vagus N.
Medulla
Accessory N.
Pyramid
Hypoglossal N.
Pyramidal decussation
Ventral root of C. 1

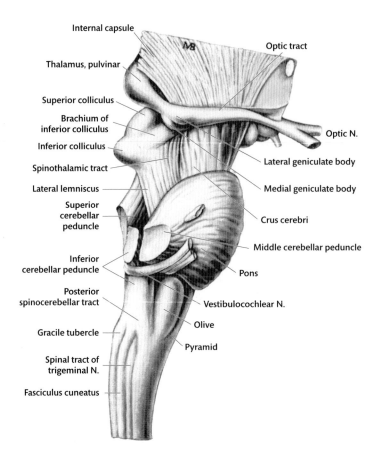

Fig. 28.2 Lateral view of the brainstem.

Internal capsule
Thalamus, pulvinar
Superior colliculus
Brachium of inferior colliculus
Inferior colliculus
Spinothalamic tract
Lateral lemniscus
Superior cerebellar peduncle
Inferior cerebellar peduncle
Posterior spinocerebellar tract
Gracile tubercle
Spinal tract of trigeminal N.
Fasciculus cuneatus

Optic tract
Optic N.
Lateral geniculate body
Medial geniculate body
Crus cerebri
Middle cerebellar peduncle
Pons
Vestibulocochlear N.
Olive
Pyramid

the level of the foramen magnum. (The junction of the medulla and spinal cord is just above the attachment of the first spinal nerve.) It is approximately 2.5 cm long and was once known as the bulb, a term which is still used occasionally, e.g. corticobulbar fibres.

The anterior surface of the medulla oblongata lies against the basilar part of the occipital bone. The posterior surface is lodged in a groove on the anterior surface of the cerebellum—the vallecula cerebelli. A narrow central canal is present in the inferior half of the medulla. This is the continuation of the central canal in the spinal cord. The central canal opens into the fourth ventricle on the posterior surface of the superior half of the medulla oblongata.

Ventral surface of the medulla

Review the description of the ventral surface of the medulla given in Chapter 24. The medulla oblongata has an **anterior median fissure** which is continuous with that of the spinal cord. The **pyramids** are bundles of corticospinal nerve fibres

which originate from cells in the cerebral cortex. In the lower medulla, bundles of fibres from the pyramids cross the midline through the **decussation of the pyramids** [Fig. 28.1]. The **olive** is an oval elevation which lies posterolateral to the pyramid and is separated from it by the rootlets of the hypoglossal nerve [Figs. 28.1, 28.2]. The hypoglossal nerve is attached between the pyramid and the olive. The ninth, tenth, and eleventh cranial nerves are attached to the lateral surface of the medulla, posterior to the olive. The sixth, seventh, and eighth cranial nerves are attached at the upper border of the pons.

Lateral surface of the medulla

The **inferior cerebellar peduncle** lies posterolateral to the olive [Figs. 28.1, 28.2]. It is a thick bundle of fibres on the posterolateral margin of the medulla oblongata. It begins near the middle of the medulla oblongata and passes upwards and slightly laterally to the inferior border of the pons. The inferior cerebellar peduncle is covered by a narrow ridge of grey matter—the **dorsal** and **ventral cochlear**

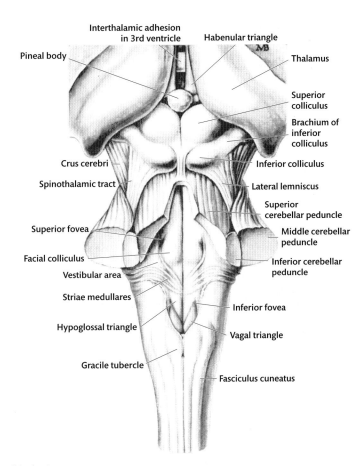

Fig. 28.3 Posterior view of the brainstem.

Labels in figure:
Interthalamic adhesion in 3rd ventricle
Pineal body
Habenular triangle
Thalamus
Superior colliculus
Brachium of inferior colliculus
Inferior colliculus
Crus cerebri
Spinothalamic tract
Lateral lemniscus
Superior cerebellar peduncle
Superior fovea
Middle cerebellar peduncle
Facial colliculus
Inferior cerebellar peduncle
Vestibular area
Striae medullares
Inferior fovea
Hypoglossal triangle
Vagal triangle
Gracile tubercle
Fasciculus cuneatus

nuclei. It then passes medial to the middle cerebellar peduncle and curves posteriorly into the cerebellum. The inferior cerebellar peduncle forms a route of communication between the medulla oblongata and spinal cord and the cerebellum.

The **spinal tract of the trigeminal** nerve is seen as a poorly defined longitudinal ridge, immediately posterior to the inferior cerebellar peduncle.

Posterior surface of the medulla

The inferior part of the posterior surface of the medulla oblongata shows the following features. The **posterior median sulcus** of the spinal cord extends upwards to the inferior angle of the fourth ventricle [Fig. 28.3]. The **fasciculi gracilis** and **fasciculus cuneatus** lie on the posterior surface of the inferior half of the medulla oblongata. The fasciculi gracilis lie one on each side of the posterior median sulcus. They end superiorly in the **gracile tubercle**. The fasciculus cuneatus lies immediately lateral to each fasciculus gracilis. It ends at a slightly higher level in a poorly defined

eminence—the **cuneate tubercle** [see Fig. 27.4; Fig. 28.3].

The upper part of the posterior surface of the medulla forms the lower part of the floor of the fourth ventricle. The floor of the fourth ventricle is diamond-shaped and is formed by the posterior surfaces of the pons and the upper half of the medulla oblongata. It is divided into right and left halves by a **median sulcus**, with a ridge on each side called the **medial eminence**. About the middle of the floor, fine bundles of fibres are seen running laterally towards the inferior cerebellar peduncle. These are the **medullary striae**, and they divide the floor of the ventricle into pontine and medullary parts.

In each half of the medullary part, there is a V-shaped depression (the **inferior fovea**) which divides the floor into three triangular areas. The medial area, part of the medial eminence, overlies the superior part of the hypoglossal nucleus and is known as the **hypoglossal triangle**. The intermediate part overlies the dorsal nucleus of the vagoglossopharyngeal complex and is known as the **vagal triangle**. The lateral part is the inferior part of the **vestibular area**—a poorly defined swelling in the lateral part of the floor of the ventricle, extending superiorly into the inferior part of the pons. It is formed by the **vestibular nuclei** [Fig. 28.3].

Pons

The ventral aspect of the pons forms a prominent bulge on the inferior aspect of the brain, between the medulla and the midbrain. It lies in the posterior cranial fossa, just behind the clivus, and has the basilar artery on it.

Ventral surface of the pons

The ventral aspect of the pons is made up of a bulky ridge composed of transversely running fibre bundles [Fig. 28.1]. This bundle of fibres converges laterally to form the **middle cerebellar peduncle** which enters the cerebellum [Figs. 28.1, 28.2]. The trigeminal nerve is attached to the pons at its junction with the middle cerebellar peduncle. Anterior to the trigeminal nerves, the ridge forms the **ventral part of the pons**. The crus cerebri enter the ventral part at its superior margin, and the pyramids leave it at the inferior margin. Anteriorly, the ventral part of the pons is grooved by the **basilar sulcus** (which lodges the basilar artery), and lies adjacent to the basi-occiput and dorsum sellae of the skull [Fig. 28.1].

Posterior surface of the pons

The posterior aspect of the pons forms the upper part of the floor of the fourth ventricle. A slight swelling in the medial eminence at the inferior part of the pons is the **facial colliculus**. This is produced by the abducens nucleus, with the facial nerve looping round it. Lateral to the facial colliculus a slight groove represents the remains of the sulcus limitans of the developing neural tube and is slightly accentuated at the level of the facial colliculus to form the **superior fovea**. Above the superior fovea, a small area lateral to the medial eminence has a dark colour. This is the **locus coeruleus**. The colour is due to the presence of pigmented cells beneath the ependyma.

Midbrain

The midbrain is the short, thick part of the brainstem which connects the hindbrain, in the posterior cranial fossa, with the cerebrum superior to the tentorium cerebelli. It passes through the tentorial notch. It is about 1.5 cm long and slightly more in width. The narrow tubular part of the ventricular system in the midbrain is the **cerebral aqueduct** [see Fig. 25.1]. It connects the fourth ventricle inferiorly to the third ventricle superiorly.

Ventral surface of the midbrain

The anterior surface of the midbrain can be seen in continuity with the base of the brain. It consists of the **crus cerebri** which descend from the cerebral hemispheres and enters the pons inferiorly [Fig. 28.1]. The posterior part of the interpeduncular fossa lies between them.

Posterior surface of the midbrain

The posterior surface of the midbrain shows four small swellings—the colliculi. They are the paired **superior** and **inferior colliculi** [Fig. 28.3]. This surface is overlapped by the anterior lobe of the cerebellum, pineal body, and splenium of the corpus callosum. The **trochlear nerves** emerge from the dorsal surface of the midbrain, immediately inferior to the inferior colliculi. The **pineal body** lies between, and just above, the two superior colliculi [Fig. 28.3].

Lateral surface of the midbrain

The superior cerebellar peduncles enter the substance of the midbrain, anterior to the inferior colliculi. Each peduncle is crossed obliquely by a ridge of white matter (the **lateral lemniscus** [Fig. 28.2]) which emerges from the superior border of the pons, posterior to the crus cerebri, and passes posterosuperiorly into the inferior colliculus.

On the lateral side of the midbrain, a similar ridge (**brachium of the inferior colliculus** [Fig. 28.2]) passes anterosuperiorly from the inferior colliculus to the **medial geniculate body**—a part of the thalamus.

Internal features of the brainstem

General organization of grey and white matter of the brainstem

The brainstem contains both grey and white matter. The **grey matter** of the brainstem includes the cranial nerve nuclei, as well as other nuclear masses such as the inferior olivary nucleus in the medulla and the red nucleus in the midbrain. The **white matter** of the brainstem includes the ascending and descending tracts of the spinal cord [Chapter 27] and other tracts formed in the brainstem.

The **reticular formation** consists of numerous neurons arranged in ill-defined groups, intermingled with fine bundles of nerve fibres which run mainly in a longitudinal direction.

Cranial nerve nuclei in the brainstem

The nuclei of the third to twelfth cranial nerves lie in the brainstem. The motor nuclei give rise to efferent or motor fibres which leave the brain. The sensory nuclei receive the afferent (sensory) fibres of the cranial nerves. The general arrangement of the cranial nerve nuclei is the same as the arrangement of nuclei in the spinal cord, in that motor and sensory nuclei are grouped together and occupy distinct areas. The nuclei subserving similar functions lie in longitudinal groups or columns which are referred to as **functional columns**. In the upper part of the medulla and pons, where the central canal is replaced by the fourth ventricle, the sensory nuclei (which, in the spinal cord, are dorsal to the motor nuclei) lie lateral to the motor nuclei. Fig. 28.4 shows the comparative positions of the different types of nuclei in the spinal cord and upper medulla.

Position of functional columns

The motor nuclei lie in three columns, based on function: (1) somatic efferent—those supplying skeletal muscles of myotomic origin; (2) special visceral efferent—those supplying skeletal muscles of branchiomeric origin; and (3) general visceral efferent—those supplying smooth muscles and glands (parasympathetic). The somatic efferent column is near the midline; lateral to it is the general visceral efferent column, and more laterally the special visceral efferent column [Fig. 28.5A].

The sensory nuclei lie in four functional columns. Medial to lateral, they are the: (1) general visceral afferent, receiving general sensation from the viscera, including the baroreceptors; (2) special visceral afferent, receiving taste sensation; (3) general somatic afferent, receiving general sensation from the head and neck; and (4) special somatic afferent, receiving impulses from the vestibulo-cochlear system [Fig. 28.5].

A few generalizations about the cranial nerve nuclei should be borne in mind:

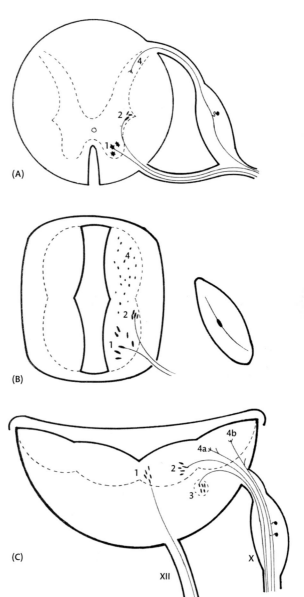

Fig. 28.4 Diagram to illustrate the difference in development between the spinal cord and the medulla. (B) is the basic structure, from which both (A) the thoracic spinal cord and (C) the medulla oblongata arise. Basal lamina: 1 = motor nerves to striated muscles of somite origin (general somatic efferent—or just somatic efferent); 2 = preganglionic autonomic cells (general visceral efferent); 3 = motor nerves to striated muscles of branchial origin. Alar lamina: 4 = sensory terminations: 4a = special visceral afferent (tractus solitarius); 4b = general somatic afferent (trigeminal system).

1. Cells which give rise to motor fibres of a nerve lie at the level of emergence of that nerve. For example, the oculomotor nucleus lies in the midbrain (from which the nerve emerges).
2. Separate nuclei give rise to nerve fibres having different efferent functions within the nerve. For example, the motor nerves to the extraocular mus-

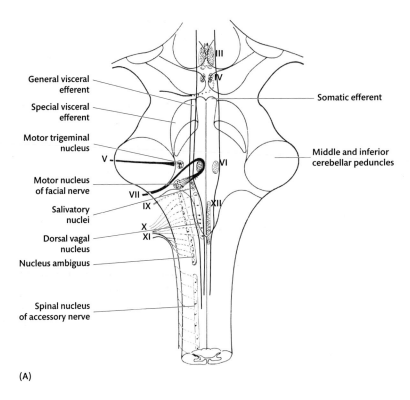

(A)

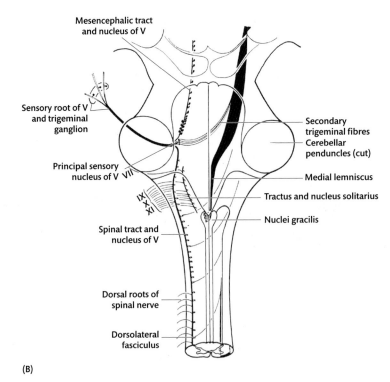

(B)

Fig. 28.5 (A) Posterior view of the brainstem and spinal cord, showing the positions of the cranial nerve motor nuclei—III, IV, V, VI, VII, IX, X, XI, and XII—and the course of the nerves. The nuclei of the somatic efferent column are seen on both sides. The general and special visceral efferents are seen on the left. (B) Posterior view of the brainstem and spinal cord, showing the positions of the cranial nerve sensory nuclei—V, VII, IX, X, and XI. The secondary ascending pathways for the trigeminal are also shown. (The nuclei of cranial nerve VIII are not shown.)

cles of the eyeball and the preganglionic parasympathetic nerve fibres to the iris and ciliary body arise from different oculomotor nuclei within the brain.

3. Where a nerve arises as a series of rootlets, their nuclei of origin will form a continuous column of cells, e.g. hypoglossal nerve.
4. Afferent (sensory) nerve fibres entering through a nerve may run longitudinally in the central nervous system and end in receptive nuclei at a considerable distance from the point of entry.
5. Motor nuclei are under the influence of impulses from the cerebral cortex (motor cortex).
6. Sensory nuclei project to other parts of the brain, mainly the cerebral cortex (sensory cortex) and cerebellum.

Internal features of the medulla

The internal features of the medulla are best studied in a series of transverse sections which show the position of the tracts and nuclei. It is best to have microscopic sections stained with special stains to show the myelin of the nerve fibres. They should be used in conjunction with Figs. 28.6, 28.7, 28.8, and 28.9 which are diagrams based on these sections.

White matter of the medulla

Corticospinal tract

Corticospinal fibres originate in the cerebral cortex and descend through the cerebral hemispheres, the crura cerebri, and the pons to form the pyramid in the medulla oblongata.

In the upper part of the medulla, the pyramidal fibres lie on the ventral aspect and account for the pyramid seen on the external surface [Fig. 28.1]. (See Figs. 28.6, 28.7, 28.8, and 28.9 for the location of the pyramid at different levels.) In the lower medulla, most of the fibres cross in the **motor decussation** to form the **lateral corticospinal tract** [Figs. 28.6, 28.10]. Review the position of the lateral corticospinal tract in the deeper parts of the lateral column of the spinal cord [see Figs. 27.4, 27.5]. The corticospinal fibres which do not cross in the medulla descend either in the anterior fasciculus, as the **anterior corticospinal tract**, or in the lateral fasciculus anterior to the lateral corticospinal tract [Fig. 28.10]. Because the corticospinal fibres pass through the pyramid, the tracts they form are commonly called the **pyramidal tracts**. Each lateral corticospinal tract extends throughout the length of the spinal cord [Fig. 28.10].

Fasciculus gracilus and cuneatus, internal arcuate fibres, and medial lemniscus

Review the formation and position of the fasciculus gracilis and cuneatus in the spinal cord [Chapter 27; see Figs. 27.4, 27.5]. These fasciculi lie on the posterior surface of the inferior half of the medulla oblongata and extend up to the **gracile** and **cuneate tubercle**.

The fibres of the fasciculus gracilis and cuneatus end by synapsing on the **nucleus gracilis** and

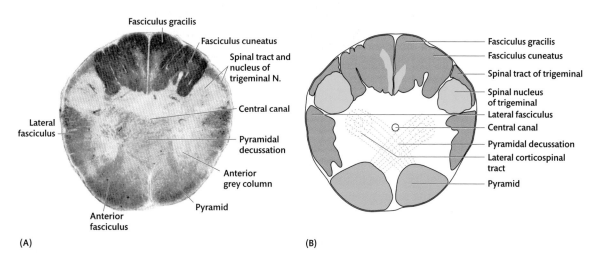

Fig. 28.6 Transverse section through the lowest part of the medulla oblongata. (A) Histology section. Grey matter = white; white matter = grey to black, depending on the density of the myelinated fibres. (B) Structures of interest in (A) are highlighted.

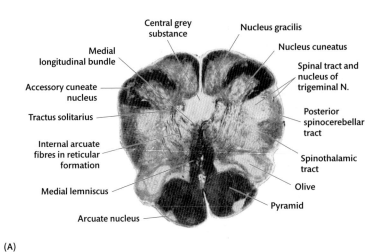

Fig. 28.7 Transverse section of the medulla through the nuclei cuneatus and gracilis. (A) Histology section. Grey matter = white; white matter = grey to black. (B) Structures of interest in (A) are highlighted.

nucleus cuneatus. Second-order neurons arise from the cells of the nucleus gracilis and cuneatus, pass ventrally, and cross the midline anterior to the central canal as the **internal arcuate fibres**. They form the great sensory **decussation** [Fig. 28.7]. After crossing the midline, the fibres form the **medial lemniscus** and ascend [see Fig. 31.28] to the thalamus. In the medulla oblongata, the medial lemnisci are in the form of flat bands, adjacent to the midline and dorsal to the pyramid [Fig. 28.8].

(Note that the fasciculus gracilis and cuneatus in the lower medulla, the internal arcuate fibres in the mid medulla, and the medial lemniscus in the upper medulla are all parts of the same system—the dorsal column–medial lemniscus pathway.)

Spinothalamic tract

The **spinothalamic tract** consists of fibres that arise in the spinal cord from cells in the grey matter [see Figs. 27.4, 27.6]. As in the spinal cord, these fibres retain the lateral position in the medulla. Note the position of the spinothalamic tracts in the medulla at the different level [Figs. 28.6, 28.7, 28.8, 28.9]. They pass through the medulla oblongata, posterior to the olivary nucleus [Fig. 28.8], and give fibres to the reticular formation—the **spinoreticular tract**.

Spinocerebellar tracts

The origin of the fibres in the **posterior spinocerebellar tract** and their position in the spinal cord are described in Chapter 27. They ascend in the posterolateral part of the lateral column of the spinal cord and enter the medulla oblongata, anterior to the spinal tract of the trigeminal nerve. The tract then passes posteriorly over the lateral surface of the spinal tract of the trigeminal and enters the inferior cerebellar peduncle [Figs. 28.2, 28.7].

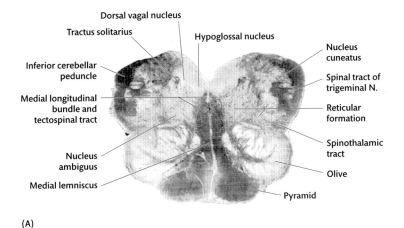

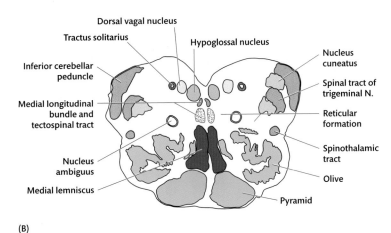

Fig. 28.8 Transverse section through the upper half of the medulla oblongata. (A) Histology section. Grey matter = white; white matter = grey to black. (B) Structures of interest in (A) are highlighted.

The **anterior spinocerebellar tract** passes through the medulla oblongata and pons, anterior to the spinal tract of the trigeminal nerve, and turns posteriorly into the cerebellum over the superior cerebellar peduncle [Fig. 28.2], above the level of entry of the trigeminal nerve.

Grey matter of the medulla

The grey matter of the medulla includes the nuclei of the lower cranial nerves, the nucleus gracilis and cuneatus described earlier, the inferior olivary, accessory olivary, and arcuate nuclei. The cranial nerve nuclei in the medulla include: (1) the spinal nucleus of the trigeminal (cranial nerve (CN) V); (2) nucleus of the tractus solitarius (CN IX); (3) nucleus ambiguus (CN IX, X, XI); (4) hypoglossal nucleus (CN XII); (5) dorsal motor nucleus of the vagus (CN X); (6) cochlear nuclei, and inferior and part of the medial and lateral vestibular nuclei (CN VIII).

Spinal nucleus of the trigeminal

The trigeminal nerve has connections with three sensory, and one motor, nuclei. Of these, only the **nucleus of the spinal tract of the trigeminal** is located in the medulla. Sensory fibres from the area supplied by the trigeminal nerve enter the brainstem at the pons. Some of these fibres descend in the spinal tract of the trigeminal to end in the nucleus of the spinal tract of the trigeminal. The tract and spinal nucleus extend from the level of the lower pons to the upper part of the spinal cord, and are seen throughout the length of the medulla oblongata. The spinal nucleus lies medial to the tract [Figs. 28.5B, 28.6, 28.7, 28.8, 28.9].

The fibres which end in the nucleus caudal to the fourth ventricle are principally concerned with sensations of pain and temperature from the trigeminal area. The spinal tract and nucleus of the trigeminal also receive fibres carrying general

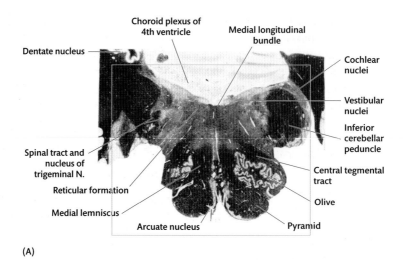

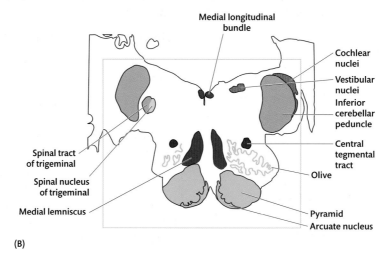

Fig. 28.9 Transverse section through the uppermost part of the medulla oblongata (enclosed in box). (A) Histology section. Grey matter = white; white matter = grey to black. (B) Structures of interest in (A) are highlighted.

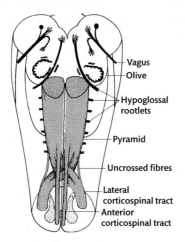

Fig. 28.10 Diagram of the medulla oblongata and spinal cord to show the decussation of the pyramids (corticospinal tracts).

sensation from the territory supplied by the facial, glossopharyngeal, and vagus nerves.

Nucleus of the tractus solitarius

The **nucleus of the tractus solitarius** lies in the upper part of the medulla [Fig. 28.8]. It receives general sensation from the viscera (GVA), and taste sensation from the tongue, epiglottis, and soft palate (SVA) through the facial, glossopharyngeal, and vagus nerves. The sensory fibres from these nerves form the **tractus solitarius** and end in the nucleus [Fig. 28.9].

Cochlear and vestibular nuclei

Sensory fibres from the cochlear nerve end in the **cochlear nuclei** which overlie the superior part of the inferior cerebellar peduncle in the medulla oblongata. The vestibular fibres pass anterior to the same peduncle and spread out into the **vestibular nuclei** in the floor of the fourth ventricle. These nuclei underlie the **vestibular area** [Fig. 28.3] which is partly in the medulla and partly in the pons [Fig. 28.9].

Dorsal motor nucleus of the vagus and inferior salivatory nucleus

Preganglionic parasympathetic fibres in the vagus (GVE) arise in the cells of the **dorsal nucleus of the vagus** [Figs. 28.5A, 28.8]. The superior extremity of this nucleus is the **inferior salivatory nucleus** which gives rise to the preganglionic parasympathetic fibres of the glossopharyngeal nerve.

Nucleus ambiguus

Somatic efferent nerve fibres in the glossopharyngeal, vagus, and accessory nerves arise in the **nucleus ambiguus** and pass into these nerves [Figs. 28.5A, 28.8]. They supply muscles of branchiomeric origin (SVE).

Hypoglossal nucleus

The hypoglossal nerve arises from a single paramedian **hypoglossal** nucleus [Figs. 28.5A, 28.8] which extends throughout the greater part of the medulla oblongata. It supplies the tongue muscles (GSE or simply SE).

Summary of the lower four cranial nerves

The **glossopharyngeal nerve** (CN IX):

1. Supplies the stylopharyngeus (SVE) through fibres which rise in the nucleus ambiguus.
2. Supplies preganglionic parasympathetic fibres to the parotid gland through fibres which arise in the inferior salivatory nucleus (GVE).
3. Carries general sensation from the posterior third of the tongue, pharynx, and external ear to the spinal nucleus of the trigeminal (GSA).
4. Carries sensation from the baroreceptors and chemoreceptors of the carotid body and sinus to the nucleus solitarius (GVA).
5. Carries taste sensation from the posterior third of the tongue to the nucleus solitarius (SVA).

The **vagus nerve** (CN X):

1. Supplies the pharyngeal and laryngeal muscles (SVE) through fibres which arise in the nucleus ambiguus.

2. Supplies preganglionic parasympathetic fibres to the heart, lungs, and much of the gastrointestinal tract through fibres which arise in the dorsal motor nucleus of the vagus (GVE).
3. Carries general sensation from the pharynx and external ear to the spinal nucleus of the trigeminal (GSA).
4. Carries taste sensation from the posterior-most part of the tongue to the nucleus solitarius (SVA).

The **accessory nerve** (CN XI):

1. Supplies the pharyngeal and laryngeal muscles (SVE) through fibres which arise in the nucleus ambiguus—cranial part.
2. Supplies the sternocleidomastoid and trapezius (SVE) through fibres which arise in the cervical spinal cord—spinal part.

The **hypoglossal nerve** (CN XII):

1) Supplies muscles of the tongue (SE) through fibres which arise in the hypoglossal nucleus.

Other nuclei in the medulla

Inferior olivary nucleus

The inferior olivary nucleus lies posterolateral to the pyramid [Figs. 28.8, 28.9]. It has the shape of a crumpled bag of grey matter, with its open mouth facing medially. Its efferent fibres emerge from this mouth and pass to the opposite half of the cerebellum through the inferior cerebellar peduncle [Fig. 28.8].

Arcuate nucleus

The arcuate nucleus lies anterior to the pyramid [Fig. 28.7]. This nucleus and the fibres which arise from it represent an inferior extension of the pontine nuclei and the pontocerebellar fibres. The **anterior external arcuate fibres** and **striae medullares** arise from the arcuate nucleus. The anterior external arcuate fibres pass laterally to the cerebellum in the inferior cerebellar peduncle. Other fibres from the arcuate nucleus [Fig. 28.9] pass posteriorly through the midline of the medulla oblongata and run across the floor of the fourth ventricle to the cerebellum as the striae medullares [Fig. 28.3].

Accessory cuneate nucleus

The accessory cuneate nucleus lies on the lateral aspect of the main cuneate nucleus [Fig. 28.7]. It gives rise to the **posterior external arcuate fibres** which pass superiorly into the inferior cerebellar peduncle. The accessory cuneate nucleus receives collaterals (branches) from the fibres in the fasciculus cuneatus and transmits information carried by the fasciculus cuneatus from the upper half of the body on the same side [Fig. 28.8].

The internal features of the pons are best studied in a series of transverse sections which show the position of the tracts and nuclei [Figs. 28.11, 28.12, 28.13]. The interior of the pons is arbitrarily divided into a ventral and dorsal part. The bulky ridge seen on the ventral aspect of the external surface of the pons lies in the **ventral part of the pons**. The **dorsal part of the pons**, also known as the **tegmentum**, separates the ventral part from the floor of the superior half of the fourth ventricle

[Fig. 28.12; see Fig. 29.1]. It is continuous superiorly with the tegmentum of the midbrain, and inferiorly with the medulla oblongata.

White matter of the pons

The ventral part of the pons contains transverse and longitudinally running fibre bundles. It also contains scattered pontine nuclei. The transverse fibres are the **pontocerebellar fibres** which arise from the **pontine nuclei**, cross the midline, and converge laterally to form the **middle cerebellar peduncle** [Figs. 28.11, 28.12, 28.13]. The bundle of longitudinal fibres are made up of corticospinal, corticonuclear, and corticopontine fibres which descend from the cerebral cortex. As mentioned earlier, the **corticospinal fibres** descend from the cerebral cortex to the spinal cord. Their position in the upper part of the medulla (in the

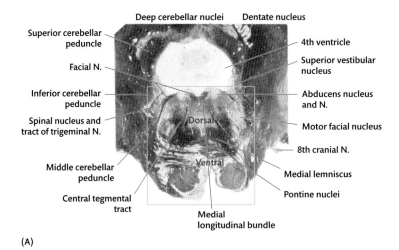

(A)

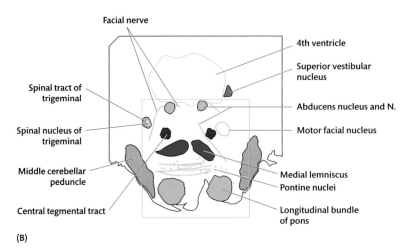

(B)

Fig. 28.11 Transverse section through the inferior part of the pons (enclosed in box). (A) Histology section. Grey matter = white; white matter = grey to black. (B) Structures of interest in (A) are highlighted.

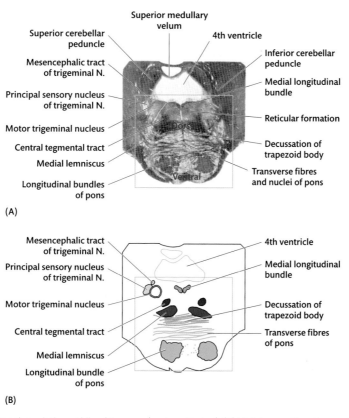

Fig. 28.12 Transverse section through the middle of the pons (enclosed in box). (A) Histology section. Grey matter = white; white matter = grey to black. (B) Structures of interest in (A) are highlighted.

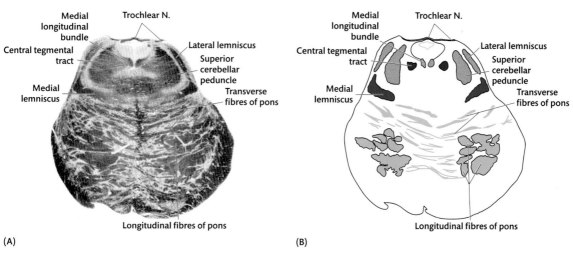

Fig. 28.13 Transverse section through the upper part of the pons. (A) Histology section. Grey matter = white; white matter = grey to black. (B) Structures of interest in (A) are highlighted.

pyramid) and their decussation in the lower part of the medulla have been described. In the pons, these fibres run longitudinally and are continuous with the crura cerebri of the midbrain at the superior margin of the pons, and with the pyramids at its inferior margin. The **corticopontine fibres** run with the corticospinal tract in the midbrain and end in the pontine nuclei. **Corticonuclear fibres** end on the motor cranial nerve nuclei of the pons and the medulla.

The **medial lemniscus** and **spinothalamic tract** enter the pons from the medulla and pass into the dorsal part of the pons. Trace these fibres sequentially through Figs. 28.6, 28.7, 28.8, 28.9, 28.11, and 28.12 to get an idea of the course of these fibres [see also Fig. 31.28]. Note that the medial lemniscus which extended anteroposteriorly in the medulla is now placed transversely.

Another bundle of white matter—the **trapezoid body**—is seen running transversely, just posterior to the ventral part of the pons [Figs. 28.11, 28.12, 28.13]. It consists of auditory fibres which arise in the cochlear nucleus and cross the midline to the opposite side. At the lateral ends of the trapezoid body, these fibres collect to form the **lateral lemniscus** which ascends to the inferior colliculus in the midbrain.

The inferior cerebellar peduncle does not enter the pons but passes dorsally into the cerebellum at the upper border of the medulla [Fig. 28.9]. The dorsal part of the pons also contains the superior extension of the **reticular formation** of the medulla oblongata.

Cranial nerve nuclei in the pons

Motor nucleus of the trigeminal

All four nuclei of the trigeminal nerve—motor, main or chief sensory, mesencephalic, and nucleus of the spinal tract—lie in the pons, but two only partially. The **motor nucleus** lies medially at the level of entry of the trigeminal nerve. It gives rise to the nerves which innervate the muscles of mastication and other muscles derived from the first pharyngeal arch [Fig. 28.5, 28.12].

Main sensory nucleus of the trigeminal

The **main sensory nucleus of the trigeminal nerve** lies lateral to the motor nucleus. It receives tactile information from the trigeminal area.

Spinal nucleus of the trigeminal

The **spinal nucleus of the trigeminal** extends inferiorly from the point of entry of the trigeminal nerve, in the lateral margin of the dorsal part of the inferior pons [Fig. 28.11]. Its continuation in the medulla has been described already.

Mesencephalic nucleus of the trigeminal

A small bundle of fibres—the **mesencephalic nucleus of the trigeminal**—passes dorsally,

between the motor and main sensory nuclei, to the midbrain [Figs. 28.5B, 28.14]. This tract [see Fig. 31.28] contains the proprioceptive fibres from the muscles of mastication and the temporomandibular joint. It differs from all other peripheral sensory neurons in that its cells of origin lie scattered along the tract and are not situated in the trigeminal ganglion.

Abducens nucleus

This small nucleus lies on the floor of the fourth ventricle, in the most inferior part of the pons, close to the midline [Figs. 28.5, 28.11]. It raises a small protuberance on the floor of the ventricle called the **facial colliculus** [Fig. 28.3] because the facial nerve curves around this nucleus [Figs. 28.5A, 28.11].

Facial nucleus

The **motor nucleus of the facial nerve** lies immediately anteromedial to the spinal nucleus of the trigeminal nerve in the most inferior part of the pons [Fig. 28.11]. It supplies the muscles of facial expression and other muscles derived from the second pharyngeal arch. The facial nerve passes posteromedially from the nucleus, curves around the medial and posterior aspects of the abducens nucleus, forming the genu of the facial nerve, and passes anterolaterally to emerge at the inferior border of the pons [Fig. 28.5A].

Superior salivatory nucleus

The preganglionic parasympathetic fibres of the facial nerve arise from the **superior salivatory nucleus**, which lies in the inferior part of the pons, superior to the inferior salivatory nucleus [Fig. 28.5A]. Fibres from this nucleus join the facial nerve as it runs through the pons.

Vestibular nuclei

The vestibular fibres of the vestibulocochlear nerve pass anterior to the inferior cerebellar peduncle and fan out into the **superior, lateral, medial, and inferior vestibular nuclei** in the floor of the fourth ventricle [Figs. 28.3, 28.11]. These nuclei underlie the **vestibular area** which is partly in the medulla [Fig. 28.9].

Cochlear nuclei

Sensory fibres from the cochlear divisions of the vestibulocochlear nerve have already been seen passing into the **cochlear nuclei** which overlie

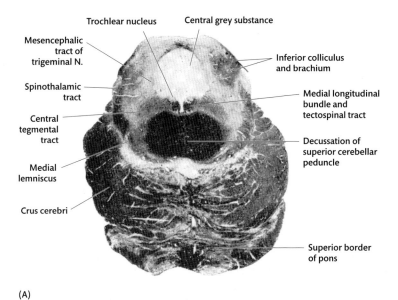

Trochlear nucleus   Central grey substance

Mesencephalic tract of trigeminal N.

Inferior colliculus and brachium

Spinothalamic tract

Medial longitudinal bundle and tectospinal tract

Central tegmental tract

Decussation of superior cerebellar peduncle

Medial lemniscus

Crus cerebri

Superior border of pons

(A)

Trochlear nucleus

Mesencephalic tract of trigeminal N.

Inferior colliculus and brachium

Spinothalamic tract

Medial longitudinal bundle and tectospinal tract

Central tegmental tract

Decussation of superior cerebellar peduncle

Medial lemniscus

Crus cerebri

(B)

Fig. 28.14 Transverse section through the lowest part of the midbrain. (A) Histology section. Grey matter = white; white matter = grey to black. (B) Structures of interest in (A) are highlighted.

the superior part of the inferior cerebellar peduncle in the medulla oblongata [Fig. 28.9].

Summary of cranial nerves V–VIII

The **trigeminal nerve** (CN V):

1. Supplies the muscles of mastication (SVE) through fibres which arise in the motor nucleus of the trigeminal.
2. Carries general sensation from the face, nasal and oral cavities, and meninges to the mesencephalic, main sensory, and spinal nucleus of the trigeminal (GSA).

The **abducens nerve** (CN VI):

1. Supplies the lateral rectus (GSE) through fibres which arise in the abducens nucleus.

The **facial nerve** (CN VII):

1. Supplies the muscles of facial expression (SVE) through fibres which arise in the motor nucleus of the facial nerve.
2. Supplies preganglionic parasympathetic fibres to the submandibular, sublingual, lacrimal, nasal, and oral mucosal glands through fibres which arise in the superior salivatory nucleus (GVE).

3. Carries taste sensation from the anterior two-thirds of the tongue to the nucleus solitarius (SVA).
4. Carries general sensation from a small area on the external ear to the spinal nucleus of the trigeminal (GSA).

The **vestibulocochlear nerve** (CN VII):

1. Carries vestibular and cochlear stimuli to the vestibular and cochlear nuclei (SSA).

The reticular formation in the brainstem

The **reticular formation** consists of numerous neurons arranged in ill-defined groups, mingled with fine bundles of nerve fibres which run mainly in the longitudinal direction. Fibres arising in the reticular formation of the pons and medulla oblongata descend in the spinal cord as the **reticulospinal tract**. Other fibres ascend into the diencephalon—the thalamus and hypothalamus.

The reticular formation receives collaterals of ascending pathways, e.g. spinothalamic tracts, and sensory information from some cranial nerves. It has extensive reciprocal connections with the cerebellum and other parts of the central nervous system.

The midbrain consists of a dorsal part, posterior to the cerebral aqueduct—the **tectum**—and a ventral part—the **cerebral peduncle**. The tectum consists of the two superior and two inferior colliculi. Each cerebral peduncle consists of: (1) the crus cerebri, anteriorly; (2) the tegmentum, posteriorly; and (3) a layer of pigmented cells—**the substantia nigra**—between the two [Figs. 28.15, 28.16].

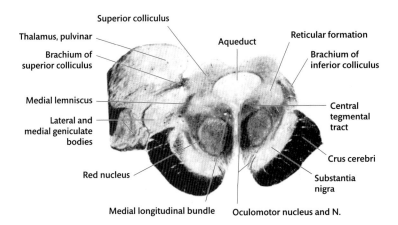

(A)

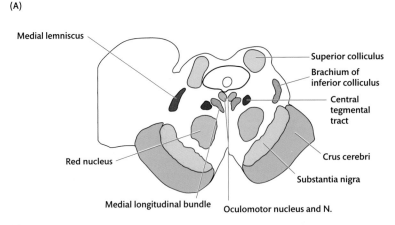

(B)

Fig. 28.15 Transverse section through the upper part of the midbrain. (A) Histology section. Grey matter = white; white matter = grey to black. (B) Structures of interest in (A) are highlighted.

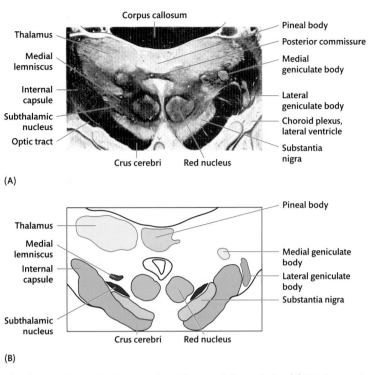

Fig. 28.16 Transverse section through the junction between the midbrain and diencephalon. (A) Histology section. Grey matter = white; white matter = grey to black. (B) Structures of interest in (A) are highlighted.

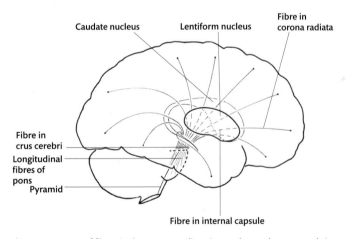

Fig. 28.17 Diagram to show the arrangement of fibres in the corona radiata, internal capsule, crus cerebri, pons, and pyramid.

Crus cerebri

The nerve fibres in the crus are the corticospinal, corticonuclear, and corticopontine fibres. They arise in the cerebral cortex and converge radially on the crus [Fig. 28.17]. Corticopontine fibres from the frontal cortex (frontopontine fibres) lie in its medial part, and corticopontine fibres from the other parts of the cortex (parietopontine, temporopontine, and occipitopontine) lie in its lateral part. The corticospinal and corticonuclear fibres which

arise in the posterior part of the frontal lobe, i.e. near the middle of the hemisphere, lie in the intermediate part of the crus. Of these, the corticonuclear fibres are the most medial, and corticospinal fibres to the lower limb are the most lateral [see Fig. 27.5].

Substantia nigra

The substantia nigra is a curved plate of grey matter which lies between the crus cerebri and the tegmentum. It contains large nerve cells with a considerable amount of melanin in their cytoplasm. These cells have connections with the tegmentum of the midbrain and with the corpus striatum (part of the deep nuclei in the cerebrum) in the ipsilateral hemisphere. They play an important part in the control of muscle tone and activity, and produce dopamine which is passed along their axons to the corpus striatum. The substantia nigra extends from the superior border of the pons into the inferolateral part of the subthalamus, superior to the midbrain [Figs. 28.15, 28.16].

Tegmentum

The tegmentum of the midbrain consists of a thick column of grey and white matter. It is continuous inferiorly with the dorsal part of the pons, and superiorly with the hypothalamus and subthalamus. Posteriorly, it is continuous with the tectum around the cerebral aqueduct. The cerebral aqueduct is surrounded by a thick layer of grey matter (the **central grey substance**), in which lie the nuclei of the oculomotor and trochlear nerves and the mesencephalic nucleus of the trigeminal nerve [Figs. 28.14, 28.15, 28.16]. In addition, the tegmentum contains a number of important nuclei and tracts which are discussed later.

Tectum

The two superior and two inferior colliculi are rounded elevations of grey matter on the posterior surface of the tectum [Fig. 28.3].

Nucleus of the superior colliculus

In the superior colliculi, the grey matter is on the surface and consists of many layers. It receives a bundle of visual fibres from the optic tract through the **brachium of the superior colliculus** [see Fig. 30.5]. The brachium runs over the postero-inferior surface of the thalamus to the colliculus and the region immediately anterior to it (the **pretectal region**). The nucleus of the superior colliculus and the pretectal region are concerned with visual reflexes. The nucleus of the superior colliculus is connected to the cranial nerve nuclei and to the motor cells of the spinal cord through the **tectospinal tract** [see Fig. 27.3, 31.35; Figs. 28.8, 28.14] and is responsible for the reflex turning of the head and eyes towards a source of light.

Nucleus of the inferior colliculus

The nucleus of the inferior colliculus is oval. It receives the lateral lemniscus which transmits impulses from the cochlear nuclei. On the side of the midbrain, a ridge—the **brachium of the inferior colliculus** [Figs. 28.2, 28.15]—passes anterosuperiorly from the inferior colliculus to the **medial geniculate body** of the thalamus [Fig. 28.2]. It transmits auditory impulses to the medial geniculate body for relay to the cerebral cortex.

Cranial nerve nuclei in the midbrain

Trochlear nucleus

The **trochlear nucleus** is the motor nucleus of the trochlear nerve. It lies on the ventral aspect of the peri-aqueductal grey matter at the level of the inferior colliculus, close to the midline [Fig. 28.14]. The nerve emerges from the dorsal surface of the brainstem, immediately inferior to the inferior colliculi. It supplies the superior oblique muscle.

Oculomotor nucleus

The oculomotor nucleus lies at the level of the superior colliculus, on the ventral aspect of the central grey matter [Fig. 28.15]. It gives motor fibres to the extraocular muscles of the eyeball (SE) and preganglionic parasympathetic fibres to the ciliary ganglion (GVE).

Mesencephalic nucleus of the trigeminal

The **mesencephalic tract of the trigeminal nerve** [see Fig. 31.26] ascends from the pons. It contains the proprioceptive sensory fibres from the muscles of mastication. It differs from all other peripheral sensory neurons in that its cells of origin lie scattered along the tract and are not situated in the trigeminal ganglion.

Summary of cranial nerves III–IV

The **oculomotor nerve** (CN III):

1. Supplies the levator palpebrae superioris, inferior oblique, and superior, medial, and inferior rectus muscles in the orbit (GSE) through fibres which arise in the oculomotor nucleus.
2. Supplies preganglionic parasympathetic fibres to the sphincter pupillae and ciliaris muscle through fibres which arise in the Edinger–Westphal component of the oculomotor nucleus (GVE).

The **trochlear nerve** (CN IV):

1. Supplies the superior oblique (GSE) through fibres which arise in the trochlear nucleus.

Other nuclei in the midbrain

Red nucleus

The **red nucleus** is a cylindrical, rod-shaped collection of reddish grey matter in the medial part of the tegmentum at the superior colliculus level. It extends cranially into the subthalamus [Fig. 28.16]. The fibres of the oculomotor nerve run through it, as they run ventrally to emerge between the crus cerebri [Figs. 28.15, 28.16]. The majority of the cells of the red nucleus send their axons to the thalamus. Other small neurons in the caudal part of the red nucleus give origin to the **rubroreticular** and **rubrospinal tracts**.

Reticular formation in the midbrain

The **reticular formation** of the midbrain occupies the lateral parts of the tegmentum between the central grey substance and the medial lemniscus and spinothalamic tract. It is continuous with the reticular formation of the dorsal part of the pons and with the lateral part of the hypothalamus. It is probably intimately concerned with the genesis of complicated reflexes of the righting variety, which may be stimulated by afferent impulses from the vestibular apparatus or from the proprioceptors of the body, or even by visual impulses from the tectum.

White matter of the midbrain

Corticospinal, corticopontine, and corticonuclear fibres

The majority of fibres end in the nuclei of the ventral part of the pons and constitute the **corticopontine fibres**. A smaller number of fibres—the **corticospinal fibres**—run longitudinally through the pons and form the pyramid on the medulla oblongata. A still smaller number end in the motor cranial nerve nuclei in the brainstem—the **corticonuclear fibres**. The majority of corticospinal and corticonuclear fibres cross to the opposite side before they end [Fig. 28.17].

Medial lemniscus and spinothalamic tracts

The **medial lemniscus** and **spinothalamic tracts** [Figs. 28.14, 28.15, 28.16] ascend through the tegmentum from the dorsal part of the pons.

They pass further laterally, as they ascend (the spinothalamic tract intermingling with the medial lemniscus) and lie deep to the brachium of the inferior colliculus in the upper midbrain. At this level, the spinothalamic tract gives off fibres to the superior colliculus—the **spinotectal tract**. In addition to the fibres which these tracts contain in the medulla oblongata, fibres from the sensory nucleus of the trigeminal nerve—the **trigeminothalamic tract**—come to lie medial to them at the midbrain level [Fig. 28.5].

Superior cerebellar peduncle

The superior cerebellar peduncle connects the cerebellum to the midbrain. The fibres cross the midline at the level of the inferior colliculus in the **decussation of the superior cerebellar peduncle** [Fig. 28.14]. Most of the fibres in this peduncle originate in the dentate nucleus of the cerebellum. A large number of these dentato-rubral fibres end in the red nucleus of the midbrain. Some fibres pass directly on to the thalamus (dentato-thalamic tract).

Rubrospinal tract

The **rubroreticular and rubrospinal tracts** arise in the red nucleus. The rubrospinal tracts decussate in the ventral part of the tegmentum (**ventral tegmental decussation**) and descend through the dorsal part of the pons to the lateral part of the medulla oblongata and upper spinal cord.

Medial longitudinal fasciculus

The **medial longitudinal fasciculus** is a small, compact bundle which extends from the upper part of the midbrain to the spinal cord. It lies adjacent to the midline and the nuclei of the oculomotor and trochlear nerves, and maintains this position throughout the brainstem. It is an intersegmental bundle which connects various levels of the brainstem and receives its major single contribution from the vestibular nuclei. In the spinal cord, it is continuous with the anterior intersegmental tract or medial vestibulospinal tract [Figs. 28.6, 28.7, 28.8, 28.9, 28.11, 28.12, 28.13, 28.14, 28.15, 28.16].

Dorsal longitudinal fasciculus

The **dorsal longitudinal fasciculus** lies posterior to the nuclei of the third and fourth cranial nerves in the central grey matter. It connects the hypothalamus with the reticular formations of the midbrain and pons.

Tectospinal tract

The **tectospinal tract** consists of fibres which arise in the deeper layer of the superior colliculus. They curve around the margin of the central grey substance, decussate anterior to the medial longitudinal fasciculus in the **dorsal tegmental decussation**, and descend through the dorsal part of the pons, medulla oblongata, and spinal cord. Fibres of the tectospinal tract end in the reticular formation of the brainstem and spinal cord, and produce reflex movements in response to visual stimuli reaching the superior colliculus, e.g. turning of the head and eyes towards a sudden flash of light [see Fig. 31.35].

Central tegmental tract

The **central tegmental tract** is a large diffuse bundle of fibres, dorsolateral to the red nucleus. It can be traced from the upper midbrain, through the dorsal part of the pons to end in the capsule of the olivary nucleus [Figs. 28.9, 28.11, 28.12, 28.13, 28.14, 28.15, 28.16; see also Fig. 29.8]. It probably transmits a number of different fibres in both directions and forms a pathway uniting the parts of the reticular formation with each other and with the thalamus, subthalamus, and olivary nucleus. It is one of the pathways for the brainstem ascending activating system to reach the intralaminar thalamic nuclei. It also carries cerebello-olivary fibres and may form a link between the corpus striatum and the cerebellum via the reticular formation and olivary nucleus.

Lateral lemniscus

The lateral lemniscus is formed in the pons by fibres which arise in the cochlear nucleus [Fig. 28.13]. It contains fibres from the ipsilateral cochlear nucleus (uncrossed fibres) and from the contralateral nucleus (fibres which have crossed in the trapezoid body [Fig. 28.12]). It ends by synapsing in cells of the inferior colliculus.

See Clinical Applications 28.1 and 28.2 for the practical implications of the anatomy discussed in this chapter.

CLINICAL APPLICATION 28.1 Lateral medullary syndrome (Wallenberg's syndrome)

A 64-year-old man presented in the Neurology clinic with the following signs and symptoms:

1. Gait and limb ataxia on the left side.

2. Vertigo, nausea, and nystagmus.

3. Loss of pain and temperature sensation on the left side of the face.

4. Loss of pain and temperature sensation on the right side of the body.

5. Hoarseness of voice and difficulty in swallowing.

6. Ptosis, miosis, and anhidrosis of the head and neck on the left side.

Based on the clinical findings, a diagnosis of **lateral medullary syndrome** on the left side was made. This syndrome results from ischaemic injury to the posterior inferior cerebellar artery.

Study questions 1–6: explain the anatomical basis for each of the clinical features seen in this patient.

(Answer 1: interruption of the posterior spinocerebellar tracts in the inferior cerebellar peduncle leads to ataxia in the ipsilateral limb.)

(Answer 2: vertigo, nausea, and nystagmus are due to ischaemia of the vestibular nuclei.)

(Answer 3: damage to the spinal nucleus and tract of the trigeminal nerve causes loss of pain and temperature sensation on the same side of the face.)

(Answer 4: damage to the spinothalamic tracts causes loss of pain and temperature sensation from the opposite side of the body. The fibres in the left spinothalamic tract had their origin in the right half of the spinal cord [see Fig. 27.6 for crossing of the spinothalamic fibres].)

(Answer 5: hoarseness of voice and difficulty in swallowing are due to damage to the left nucleus ambiguus. The nucleus ambiguus gives origin to the motor fibres of the glossopharyngeal, vagus, and cranial accessory nerves. Together, these nerves innervate most muscles of the palate, pharynx, and larynx. The gag reflex is also lost on the left side, as the glossopharyngeal nerve forms the efferent limb of the reflex [refer to Clinical Application 18.1].)

(Answer 6: disruption of the central sympathetic pathway in the reticular system interrupts descending fibres from the diencephalon to the thoracolumbar sympathetic outflow. This results in Horner's syndrome on the left.)

In cases of lateral medullary syndrome, the clinical picture is based on the extent to which the related nuclei and pathways are damaged. Note the proximity of the damaged structures in the upper part of the medulla [Fig. 28.8].

CLINICAL APPLICATION 28.2 Herpes zoster ophthalmicus

A 58-year-old male on immunosuppressive therapy developed painful vesicular eruptions on the right side of the face, involving the tip and side of the nose, the forehead, and the upper eyelid. This was preceded with fever and malaise for a few days. The vesicles initially contained clear fluid, later became cloudy, and ruptured to form dry plaques. The pain over the above region persisted for several weeks.

Study question 1: what is the likely diagnosis? (Answer: the clinical presentation is typical of herpes zoster ophthalmicus. The varicella-zoster virus causes overt or subclinical chickenpox infection in childhood and remains latent in some of the trigeminal ganglion cells. The latent virus can be reactivated in elderly, poorly nourished, or immunosuppressed individuals. The virus damages the nerves by causing severe perineural and intraneural inflammation.)

Study question 2: what is the nerve supply to the affected region? (Answer: the nose, upper eyelid, and forehead are supplied by the ophthalmic division of the trigeminal nerve. Herpes zoster characteristically affects the skin supplied by the ophthalmic division of the trigeminal nerve.)

Other complications of this condition include conjunctivitis, keratitis, and uveitis.

Herpes zoster can affect the maxillary and mandibular dermatomes of the trigeminal nerve, and dermatomes of the trunk and other cranial nerves. It is treated with antiviral drugs and topical steroids.

Ramsay Hunt syndrome is herpes zoster infection involving the facial nerve, causing vesicular eruptions of the skin of the external ear, ipsilateral anterior two-thirds of the tongue, severe ear pain, and facial nerve neuropathy. The prognosis is worse than that of Bell's palsy.

CHAPTER 29
The cerebellum

External features of the cerebellum

The cerebellum consists of the two **cerebellar hemispheres** and a median part—the **vermis** [see Figs. 24.1, 24.2; Fig. 29.1]. It surrounds the posterior surface of the brainstem [Fig. 29.2]. The two cerebellar hemispheres lie inferior to the posterior part of the cerebrum and are separated from it by the tentorium cerebelli. The cerebellum has a superior [Fig. 29.2] and an antero-inferior surface [Fig. 29.3]. The superior aspect of the vermis is the median ridge on the superior surface [Fig. 29.2]. The vermis is more clearly separated from the cerebellar hemispheres on the antero-inferior surface, as it lies in a deep median hollow between the two cerebellar hemispheres (the **vallecula of the cerebellum**) [Fig. 29.3]. Each part of the vermis is continuous with a part of the hemispheres—a feature which is more obvious on the superior surface.

The general features of the cerebellum can be understood from its development. The cerebellum develops from a ridge of tissue which lies transversely in the thin roof of the fourth ventricle, opposite the pons. This ridge expands a great deal posteriorly but remains attached to the brainstem over a narrow area. The roof of the fourth ventricle is drawn posteriorly into the expanding cerebellum and forms a tent-like recess [Fig. 29.1]. The thin roof of the fourth ventricle is formed by the **superior and inferior medullary vela**

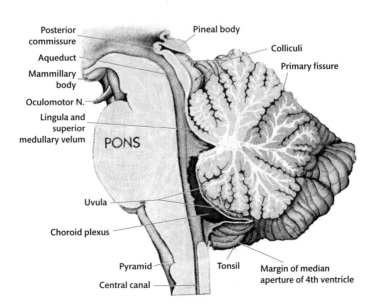

Fig. 29.1 Median section through the brainstem and cerebellum.

Labels: Posterior commissure; Aqueduct; Mammillary body; Oculomotor N.; Lingula and superior medullary velum; PONS; Uvula; Choroid plexus; Pyramid; Central canal; Pineal body; Colliculi; Primary fissure; Tonsil; Margin of median aperture of 4th ventricle

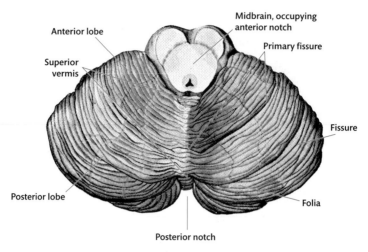

Anterior lobe

Superior vermis

Midbrain, occupying anterior notch

Primary fissure

Fissure

Folia

Posterior lobe

Posterior notch

Fig. 29.2 Superior surface of the cerebellum.

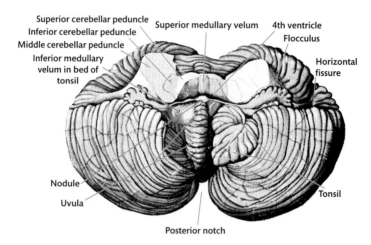

Superior cerebellar peduncle
Inferior cerebellar peduncle
Middle cerebellar peduncle
Inferior medullary velum in bed of tonsil

Superior medullary velum

4th ventricle

Flocculus

Horizontal fissure

Nodule

Uvula

Tonsil

Posterior notch

Fig. 29.3 Antero-inferior surface of the cerebellum. The right tonsil has been removed so as to display more fully the inferior medullary velum.

[Figs. 29.1, 29.4] which sweep superiorly and inferiorly from the apex of the cerebellar recess.

The cerebellum becomes greatly folded during development, so that the surface is irregular with transversely running **fissures** and **folia** (the cortex between the fissures) [Fig. 29.2]. Of the great number of fissures formed in the cerebellum, three are of particular importance: (1) **primary fissure** [Figs. 29.1, 29.2]—this deep fissure cuts across the superior surface of the cerebellum and separates the anterior and posterior lobes; (2) **horizontal** (or intercrural) **fissure** which extends from one middle cerebellar peduncle to the other and lies

close to the junction of the superior and antero-inferior surfaces of the cerebellum [Fig. 29.3]; and (3) **posterolateral fissure** on the antero-inferior surface of the cerebellum [Fig. 29.3].

The vermis and cerebellar hemispheres are subdivided into three lobes by the three fissures. The **anterior lobe** lies in front of the primary fissure. The **posterior lobe** lies between the primary and posterolateral fissures [Fig. 29.2]. The **flocculonodular lobe** lies beyond the posterolateral fissure. It is made up of the nodule of the vermis and the flocculus of the cerebellar hemisphere [Fig. 29.3]. The lobes are further subdivided into ten lobules,

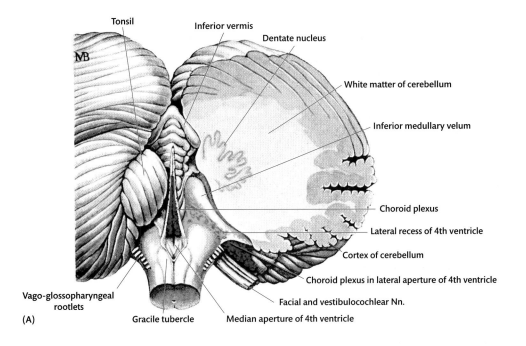

(A)

- Tonsil
- Inferior vermis
- Dentate nucleus
- White matter of cerebellum
- Inferior medullary velum
- Choroid plexus
- Lateral recess of 4th ventricle
- Cortex of cerebellum
- Choroid plexus in lateral aperture of 4th ventricle
- Facial and vestibulocochlear Nn.
- Median aperture of 4th ventricle
- Gracile tubercle
- Vago-glossopharyngeal rootlets

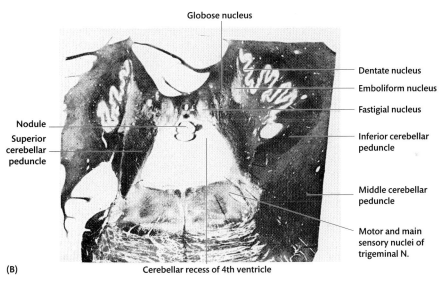

(B)

- Globose nucleus
- Dentate nucleus
- Emboliform nucleus
- Fastigial nucleus
- Inferior cerebellar peduncle
- Middle cerebellar peduncle
- Motor and main sensory nuclei of trigeminal N.
- Cerebellar recess of 4th ventricle
- Nodule
- Superior cerebellar peduncle

Fig. 29.4 (A) Dissection of the left inferior surface of the cerebellum to show the median and lateral apertures of the fourth ventricle. The medulla oblongata has been displaced anteriorly so as to open up the median aperture. Note the choroid plexus which is visible at both apertures and can also be seen through the thin roof of the fourth ventricle. (B) Oblique transverse section, parallel to the cerebellar recess of the fourth ventricle, to show the cerebellar nuclei. [Compare with Fig. 13.11.]

the detailed description of which is beyond the scope of this book. However, you should note the position of the: (1) lingula, a part of the vermis which lies on the superior medullary velum [Fig. 29.1]; (2) uvula, a part of the inferior vermis; and (3) tonsils. The paired tonsils are part of the cerebellar hemispheres and lie in continuity with the uvula on the antero-inferior aspect [Fig. 29.3]. ➲ The tonsils lie close to the foramen magnum and are forced down into the vertebral canal when there is a sudden increase in intracranial pressure—a condition known as **tonsillar herniation**.

Using the instructions given in Dissection 29.1, identify the main parts of the cerebellum.

Objective

I. To identify the main parts of the cerebellum.

Instructions

1. Remove the meninges from the superior and posterior surfaces of the cerebellum, but avoid depressing the cerebellum too strongly to expose all of its superior surface.

2. With the assistance of Figs. 29.2 and 29.3, identify its main parts, including the primary fissure, horizontal fissure, superior and inferior vermis, the hemispheres, tonsils, and the flocculonodular lobe.

Cerebellar peduncles

Three pairs of compact bundles of nerve fibres— the **inferior**, **middle**, and **superior cerebellar peduncles**—connect the cerebellum with the brainstem. Note the relative positions of these, as they enter the cerebellum, in Fig. 28.3. The superior cerebellar peduncle lies medially, the middle laterally, and the inferior between the two.

Inferior cerebellar peduncle

The inferior cerebellar peduncle forms on the posterolateral surface of the medulla oblongata [see Fig. 28.2]. It ascends between the superior and middle cerebellar peduncles and passes posteromedially into the vermis of the cerebellum. (Some of its fibres enter the cerebellar hemispheres.) The inferior cerebellar peduncle contains mainly afferent fibres to the cerebellum: the posterior spinocerebellar tract (from the spinal cord), cuneocerebellar fibres from the accessory cuneate nucleus, olivocerebellar fibres from the inferior olivary nucleus, vestibulocerebellar fibres from the vestibular nuclei and nerve, and fibres from the reticular system. It also transmits efferent cerebellar fibres to the vestibular nuclei and the reticular formation of the medulla oblongata [see Fig. 28.3].

Middle cerebellar peduncle

This is the largest and most lateral of the three peduncles. It is formed by pontocerebellar fibres which arise in the opposite half of the pons from the pontine nuclei and pass to the cerebellum. They transmit impulses which reach the pons from the cerebral cortex through the corticopontine fibres. The peduncle enters the cerebellum through the anterior end of the horizontal fissure [see Figs. 28.1, 28.2, 28.3].

Superior cerebellar peduncle

The superior cerebellar peduncle is the principal efferent pathway from the cerebellum. It contains the dentato-thalamic and dentato-rubro-thalamic tracts. Its fibres arise mainly from the dentate nucleus. Each of these peduncles begins in the roof of the fourth ventricle and passes anteriorly as it ascends, forming the lateral wall of the superior part of the fourth ventricle. The fibres of the superior cerebellar peduncle decussate in the tegmentum of the inferior part of the midbrain and pass to the thalamus and to the red nucleus of the opposite side. Some fibres descend into the pons in the central tegmental fasciculus [see Figs. 28.9A, 28.9B; see also Fig. 29.7]. The anterior spinocerebellar tract enters the cerebellum in the superior cerebellar peduncle.

Interior of the cerebellum

The surface of the cerebellum is covered by a thin layer of grey matter—the **cerebellar cortex**— which overlies the deeper **white matter**. The **deep nuclei of the cerebellum** are situated deep in the white matter of the cerebellum. They are the **dentate**, **globose**, **fastigial**, and **emboliform** nuclei [Fig. 29.4].

Using the instructions given in Dissection 29.2, cut the cerebellum to expose the white matter and deep nuclei.

Deep nuclei of the cerebellum

The **dentate nucleus** is the largest and most lateral of a group of four nuclei which lie in the white matter of the cerebellum. It lies close to the cerebellar recess of the fourth ventricle. It has the shape of a thin, crinkled lamina of grey matter, very similar in appearance to the inferior olivary nucleus in gross section. Like the inferior olivary nucleus, it has a wide mouth, or hilus, which faces anterosuperiorly. The other three deep nuclei—the **emboliform**, **globose**, and **fastigial**—lie between the dentate nucleus and the midline.

Objectives

I. To remove the right half of the cerebellum and examine the cut surface of the vermis. **II.** To make a horizontal section through the cerebellar hemisphere and identify the dentate nucleus.

Instructions

1. Split the cerebellum into two equal parts by a median sagittal section through the vermis. Make this incision carefully, separating the two parts as the incision is deepened.

2. Note that approximately halfway between the superior and inferior margins of the cerebellum, a narrow slit is opened into. This is the **cerebellar recess of the fourth ventricle**.

3. Identify the cerebellar peduncles of the right side, and make a vertical incision through them, just posterior to the brainstem.

4. Remove the right half of the cerebellum from the remainder of the brain.

5. Examine the mid-sagittal section of the vermis, and note the folded grey matter of the cortex and the white matter deep to it. The white matter fits the complex folds of the cortex and has the appearance of a branching tree—the **arbor vitae cerebelli** [Fig. 29.1].

6. Make a transverse incision midway through the right half of the cerebellum.

7. Identify the **dentate nucleus**, a crinkled bag of grey matter within the central mass of white matter. It lies relatively close to the midline. It is the largest of the deep nuclei of the cerebellum [Fig. 29.4; see Fig. 29.9].

8. Remove the remains of the membranes from the surface of the midbrain, avoiding, if possible, damage to the trochlear nerves.

9. Identify the pineal body between the superior colliculi [see Fig. 28.3], and note that it is attached to the dorsal surface of the brain at the junction of the midbrain and diencephalon, inferior to the splenium of the corpus callosum.

Cerebellar cortex

The cerebellar cortex has a uniform structure throughout and consists of three layers: (1) the deepest layer of small granule cells—this is the **granular layer**; the axons of the granule cells go superficially to the molecular layer; (2) the middle layer—the **Purkinje cell layer**—which has a single row of large cell bodies of the **Purkinje cells**; they send their axons into the white matter and their branching dendrites superficially where they spread out in a plane at right angles to the folia; and (3) a surface layer—the **molecular layer**—which has stellate and basket cells; this layer also has the dendrites of the Purkinje cells, and the axons of the granule cells pass running parallel to the folia [Fig. 29.5].

Afferent fibres

The cerebellum receives sensory impulses from the spinal cord and vestibular nuclei, and motor information from the cerebral cortex and basal ganglia [Chapter 31]. All afferent fibres end in the cerebellar cortex. There are two types of afferent fibres—the mossy fibres and climbing fibres. The fibres from the inferior olivary nucleus (the olivocerebellar fibres) are the **climbing fibres**. They ascend through the deeper layers and end by synapsing in the molecular layer with the dendrites of the Purkinje cell. All other fibres (spinocerebellar, pontocerebellar, and others) are **mossy fibres**. They end in the molecular layer by synapsing with the granule cells [Fig. 29.5].

Cerebellar circuitry

All the afferents to the cerebellum end in the cerebellar cortex, though they give collateral branches to the deep nuclei. The mossy fibres end by synapsing with the granule cells in the granular layer, and the axons of the granule cells synapse with the dendrites of the Purkinje cells in the molecular layer. The climbing fibres end by synapsing with the dendrites of the Purkinje cells in the molecular layer. (All the afferents to the cerebellum send their impulses directly or indirectly to the Purkinje cell dendrites in the molecular layer.)

All the output from the cerebellar cortex is through the axons of the Purkinje cells, which project to the deep nuclei. The deep nuclei give rise to all the efferent fibres of the cerebellum [Fig. 29.5].

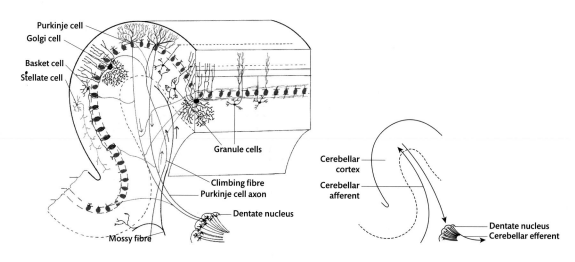

Fig. 29.5 A diagram of the main nerve cells and their processes in the cerebellar cortex. A single folium is shown cut longitudinally (right) and transversely (left). Both mossy and climbing fibres send collaterals to the cerebellar nuclei. Inset: cerebellar circuitry in brief.

Efferent fibres

The deep nuclei give rise to the efferents of the cerebellum.

Functional subdivisions of the cerebellum

Based on the functions and connections, the cerebellum is divided into three parallel sagittal regions [Fig. 29.6]. Each of these regions includes an area of cortex and an underlying deep nucleus. The vermis and paravermal cerebellar cortex, along with the globose and emboliform nuclei, form the **spinocerebellum**. The remaining lateral area of the cortex and the dentate nucleus form the **pontocerebellum** or the **neocerebellum**. The flocculonodular lobe with the fastigial nucleus forms the **vestibulocerebellum**.

Connections of the vestibulocerebellum

The afferent fibres from the vestibular nuclei pass to the cortex of the flocculonodular lobe—the vestibulocerebellum. Purkinje fibres from this cortex project to the fastigial nucleus, and efferents of the fastigial nuclei hook over the superior cerebellar peduncle and descend in the inferior cerebellar peduncle to the vestibular nuclei and the reticular formation of the medulla oblongata.

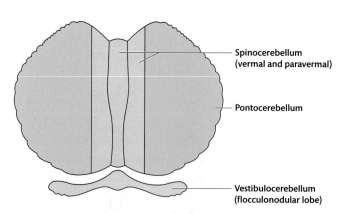

Fig. 29.6 Schematic representation of the functions areas of the cerebellum. The cerebellum is shown 'opened out'. The superior surface on the upper half, and the antero-inferior surface on the lower half of the image.

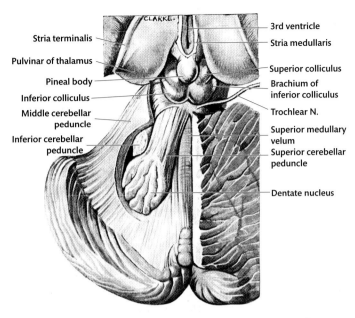

Labels on figure (clockwise):
Stria terminalis
Pulvinar of thalamus
Pineal body
Inferior colliculus
Middle cerebellar peduncle
Inferior cerebellar peduncle

CLARKE.

3rd ventricle
Stria medullaris
Superior colliculus
Brachium of inferior colliculus
Trochlear N.
Superior medullary velum
Superior cerebellar peduncle
Dentate nucleus

Fig. 29.7 Dissection to show the dentate nucleus, cerebellar peduncles, tectum of the midbrain, and superior surface of the diencephalon.

Connections of the spinocerebellum

The spinocerebellar and cuneocerebellar fibres pass to the vermis and paravermal regions—the spinocerebellum. The spinocerebellum projects to the reticular formation and vestibular nuclei through the globose and emboliform nuclei.

Connections of the pontocerebellum

The pontocerebellar fibres ascend to the cerebellar cortex of the lateral sides of the hemisphere. The pontocerebellum projects through the dentate nucleus. The axons of the dentate nucleus emerge from its medial side to form the superior cerebellar peduncle [Fig. 29.7]. The fibres of the superior cerebellar peduncle go to the red nucleus and thalamus. The major output from the cerebellum is from the pontocerebellum.

Connections of the cerebellum

The main afferent and efferent pathways of the cerebellum are shown in Fig. 29.8.

Overview of the spinocerebellar tracts

The spinocerebellar tracts extend from the spinal cord through parts of the brainstem into the cerebellum [Fig. 29.8]. The following is a quick review of the main features of the tracts.

Posterior spinocerebellar tracts

The **posterior spinocerebellar tract** arises from the cells of the thoracic nucleus (lamina VII) and ascends in the posterolateral part of the lateral column of the same side [see Figs. 27.4, 27.6]. In the medulla oblongata, the posterior spinocerebellar tract lies anterior to the spinal tract of the trigeminal nerve. It then passes posteriorly over the lateral surface of the spinal tract of the trigeminal and enters the inferior cerebellar peduncle [see Figs. 28.2, 28.6B]. This tract transmits to the cerebellum proprioceptive information from the inferior half of the same side of the body [Fig. 29.8].

Anterior spinocerebellar tracts

Fibres of the **anterior spinocerebellar tract** arise from laminae V to VII of the lumbosacral spinal cord and carry information from the lower limb. The fibres cross the midline in the spinal cord, ascend in the lateral column immediately anterior to the posterior spinocerebellar tract [see Figs. 27.4, 27.6], pass through the medulla oblongata and pons anterior to the spinal tract of the trigeminal nerve, and turn posteriorly into the cerebellum over the superior cerebellar peduncle [see Fig. 28.2]. They cross the midline a second time to enter the cerebellar hemisphere on the same side as the origin of the fibres [Fig. 29.8].

See Clinical Application 29.1 for the practical implications of the anatomy discussed in this chapter.

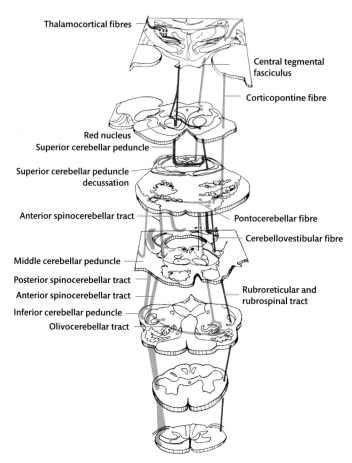

Thalamocortical fibres

Central tegmental fasciculus

Corticopontine fibre

Red nucleus
Superior cerebellar peduncle

Superior cerebellar peduncle decussation

Anterior spinocerebellar tract

Pontocerebellar fibre

Cerebellovestibular fibre

Middle cerebellar peduncle
Posterior spinocerebellar tract
Anterior spinocerebellar tract

Rubroreticular and rubrospinal tract

Inferior cerebellar peduncle
Olivocerebellar tract

Fig. 29.8 A diagram to show the main afferent (pontocerebellar, olivocerebellar, and anterior and posterior spinocerebellar pathways = blue) and efferent (to the red nucleus and thalamus = red) connections of the cerebellum. Serial sections are shown through the spinal cord, lower medulla, upper medulla, medulla–pons junction, pons, midbrain, and thalamus.

CLINICAL APPLICATION 29.1 Cerebellar lesions

The vestibulocerebellum consists of the flocculonodular lobe and has two-way connections with the vestibular nuclei. Lesions in this part of the cerebellum would result in loss of balance, dizziness, and nystagmus (a condition where the eyes make involuntary repetitive movements from side to side).

The spinocerebellum consists of the vermis and paravermal region. Lesions in the vermis result in truncal ataxia—an inability to stand without support.

Diseases of the pontocerebellum (neocerebellum) result in problems with planning movements and ipsilateral inco-ordination. When fine, purposeful movements are attempted, the hand trembles as the target is approached. This is known as **intention tremor** and is due to lack of

co-ordination between the agonists and antagonists acting on the elbow and wrist. For the same reason, the hand may go past the target object—**overshoot**. Another sign of inability to plan movements accurately and inco-ordination is **dysdiadochokinesis**—an inability to perform alternating movements, such as pronation and supination, smoothly. Co-ordination is tested using the 'finger to nose' test where the patient is asked to alternately touch their nose and the physician's outstretched finger; and the 'heel to knee' test where the patient is asked to lie supine, place the heel of one foot on the opposite knee, and move it down the shin. An inability to execute these movements smoothly is a sign of cerebellar disease.

CHAPTER 30
The diencephalon

Diencephalon

The diencephalon develops from the primitive forebrain vesicle and encloses the third ventricle [see Table 24.1]. It is made up of the thalamus, epithalamus, hypothalamus, and subthalamus.

Epithalamus

The epithalamus consists of the **pineal gland**, a small structure which is attached to the habenular and posterior commissures by its stalk, and the habenular nuclei [Fig. 30.1]. The pineal gland

secretes melatonin, a hormone implicated in the sleep–wake cycle.

The habenular nuclei

The **habenular nuclei** lie in the habenular triangle. These are small triangular areas which lie between the medial aspect of the thalamus, the pineal stalk, and the superior colliculus [Fig. 30.2]. The nuclei receive fibres from the septal nuclei through the stria medullaris thalami [Fig. 30.2]. They give rise to a small bundle of fibres—the fasciculus retroflexus—which runs through the upper part of the tegmentum of the midbrain and ends in the interpeduncular nucleus, a small collection of cells in the posterior perforated substance [see Fig. 30.7].

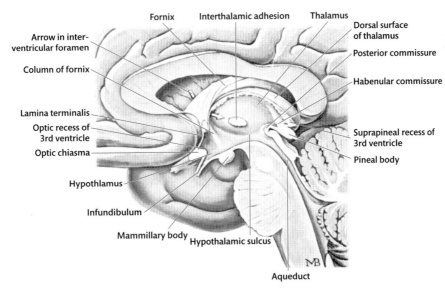

Fig. 30.1 Median section through the brain to show parts of the diencephalon.

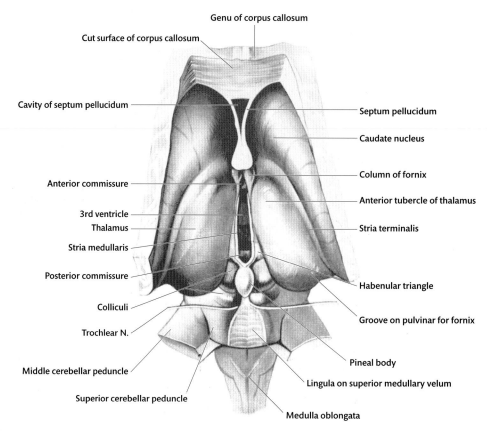

Genu of corpus callosum

Cut surface of corpus callosum

Cavity of septum pellucidum

Septum pellucidum

Caudate nucleus

Column of fornix

Anterior commissure

Anterior tubercle of thalamus

3rd ventricle

Thalamus

Stria terminalis

Stria medullaris

Posterior commissure

Habenular triangle

Colliculi

Groove on pulvinar for fornix

Trochlear N.

Middle cerebellar peduncle

Pineal body

Superior cerebellar peduncle

Lingula on superior medullary velum

Medulla oblongata

Fig. 30.2 The thalami and third ventricle seen from above after removal of the overlying tela choroidea. [Compare with Fig. 32.7.]

Thalamus

The thalamus is a large mass of grey matter on the dorsal part of the diencephalon. It is concerned with the processing of sensory information. Many of its cells transmit impulses to the sensory areas of the cortex, but it also has reciprocal connections with most parts of the cerebral cortex and with a number of subcortical masses of grey matter [see Fig. 30.6A].

Surfaces of the thalamus

The thalamus has four surfaces—medial, lateral, superior, and inferior surfaces; and two ends—anterior and posterior ends.

The anterior two-thirds of the **medial surface** of the two thalami are covered with ependyma. They form the lateral walls of the third ventricle, superior to the hypothalamic sulcus [Fig. 30.1]. The two thalami are frequently fused across the cavity of the third ventricle by the **interthalamic adhesion**. The posterior thirds are widely separated from each

other and abut medially on the superior part of the midbrain [see Fig. 28.3].

The **posterior end** of the thalamus (the **pulvinar**) is wide and overhangs the superior part of the midbrain [Fig. 30.2].

The **superior surface** is limited laterally by the stria terminalis and the thalamostriate vein [Fig. 30.2]. It tapers anteriorly to end in the rounded **anterior tubercle** of the thalamus, just posterior to the interventricular foramen and the column of the fornix. The groove for the fornix courses obliquely across the superior surface. The area lateral to the groove is covered with the ependyma of the floor of the lateral ventricle. The groove and the area medial to it are covered by the tela choroidea of the lateral ventricle. Where the superior and medial surfaces meet, a delicate ridge of white matter runs anteroposteriorly on the thalamus. This is the **stria medullaris thalami** [Fig. 30.2]. It is made up of fibres which arise in the septal nuclei (in the frontal lobe, anterior to the lamina terminalis) and ends in the habenular nucleus. The

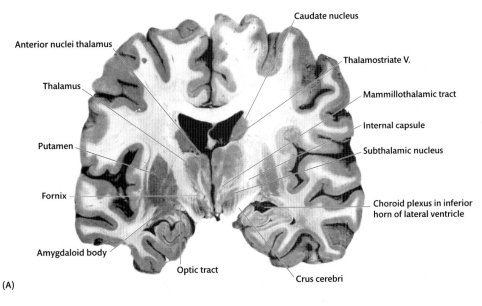

(A)

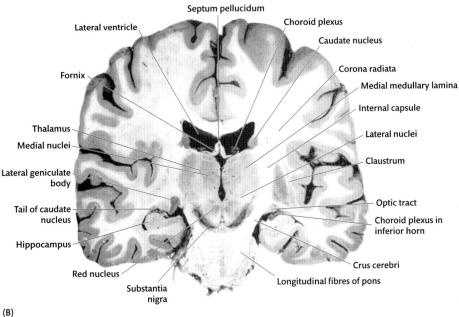

(B)

Fig. 30.3 (A) Coronal section through the brain at the level of the mammillary bodies. (B) Coronal section through the brain, passing through the basilar part of the pons. Note the division of the thalamus into medial and lateral nuclei.

stria has the ependymal roof of the third ventricle attached to its medial margin, posterior to the interventricular foramen [Fig. 30.2].

The **lateral surface** of the thalamus is hidden at present, but it lies in contact with the internal capsule [Fig. 30.3].

The **inferior surface** is mostly hidden from view, as it rests on the hypothalamus. The posterior part of this surface (the pulvinar) is free and exhibits two rounded swellings—the medial and lateral geniculate bodies [see Fig. 28.2].

Nuclei of the thalamus

The thalamus is divided into a number of separate cell groups or nuclei by two layers of white matter which run approximately in the sagittal plane. These are the medial and lateral medullary laminae. The **lateral medullary lamina** lies close to the internal capsule. A thin, broken lamina of grey matter—the **reticular nucleus** of the thalamus—lies lateral to the lateral medullary lamina between it and the internal capsule [Fig. 30.3].

The **medial medullary lamina** lies midway between the third ventricle and the internal capsule. It divides the thalamus into **medial** and **lateral nuclei** [Fig. 30.4]. The **medial nuclei** (mediodorsal nuclei) lie close to the third ventricle. The lateral mass of nuclei is further subdivided into **lateral nuclei** (lateral posterior and dorsal lateral) and **ventral nuclei** (ventral anterior, ventral lateral, ventroposterior lateral, and ventroposterior medial). Inferiorly, the medial medullary lamina curves medially and separates the medial nucleus of the thalamus from the ventral nuclei. There is no clear line of demarcation between the lateral nucleus and the ventral nuclei.

Anteriorly, the medial medullary lamina splits into two to enclose the **anterior nucleus** [Fig. 30.3]. Posteriorly, the medial medullary lamina encloses the **centromedian nucleus** [Fig. 30.4] and a number of other small **intralaminar nuclei**.

The **pulvinar** lies behind the ventral nucleus, lateral to the medial medullary lamina. It is best seen on the inferior and lateral aspects of the thalamus [Fig. 30.2]. The **medial geniculate** and **lateral geniculate bodies** lie on the inferior surface of the pulvinar.

The **medial geniculate body** is a well-defined oval mass [Fig. 30.4]. The **lateral geniculate body** lies anterolateral to the medial geniculate body [Figs. 30.3B, 30.4, 30.5] and is directly continuous anteriorly with the **optic tract**.

Connections of the thalamus

The main afferent to the thalamus are: (1) the **spinothalamic tract**, **medial lemniscus**, and fibres from the **trigeminal nuclei**; (2) visual fibres of the **optic tract**; (3) **acoustic fibres** from the inferior colliculus; (4) the **mammillothalamic tract** from the mammillary body of the hypothalamus; (5) **cerebellar fibres**, either directly from the dentate nucleus or through the red nucleus; and (6) fibres from the **globus pallidus** of the corpus striatum. In addition to these, most of the thalamic nuclei receive: (7) fibres from the area of the cerebral cortex to which they project; and (8) many intrathalamic connections.

The thalamus sends efferent fibres to almost all parts of the cerebral cortex [Fig. 30.6]. In addition, it sends fibres to the hypothalamus, corpus striatum, and reticular formation of the brainstem.

Anterior nucleus

The anterior nucleus of the thalamus receives the **mammillothalamic tract** from the mammillary nuclei in the hypothalamus [see Fig. 32.5]. It sends efferent fibres to the cingulate gyrus. The anterior nucleus is part of the limbic system which connects the hippocampus, hypothalamus, thalamus, and other parts of the limbic lobe [Chapter 32].

Ventral posterior nucleus

Fibres of the **spinothalamic tract**, **medial lemniscus**, and **trigeminothalamic tract** (from the sensory nuclei of the trigeminal nerve) end in the ventral posterior nucleus. The spinothalamic tract and medial lemniscus convey sensory impulses from the opposite side of the body and end in the **ventroposterior lateral** nucleus of the thalamus. The trigeminothalamic tract conveys sensory impulses from the opposite half of the face

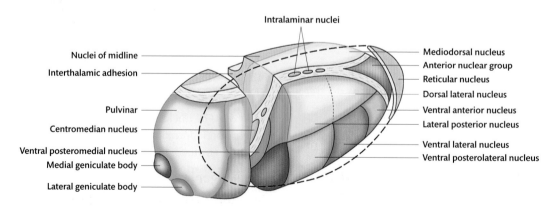

Intralaminar nuclei

Nuclei of midline
Interthalamic adhesion
Pulvinar
Centromedian nucleus
Ventral posteromedial nucleus
Medial geniculate body
Lateral geniculate body

Mediodorsal nucleus
Anterior nuclear group
Reticular nucleus
Dorsal lateral nucleus
Ventral anterior nucleus
Lateral posterior nucleus
Ventral lateral nucleus
Ventral posterolateral nucleus

Fig. 30.4 Main nuclear masses of the thalamus, viewed from the lateral side. (Only the anterior extent of the reticular nucleus is shown; its full extent is depicted by the interrupted black line.)

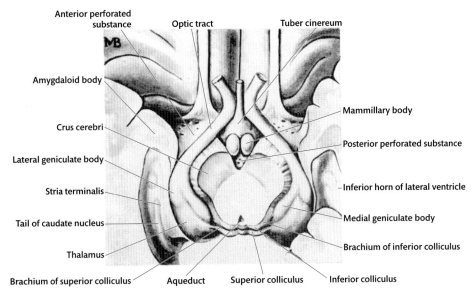

Fig. 30.5 Base of the brain seen from below to show the optic tracts.

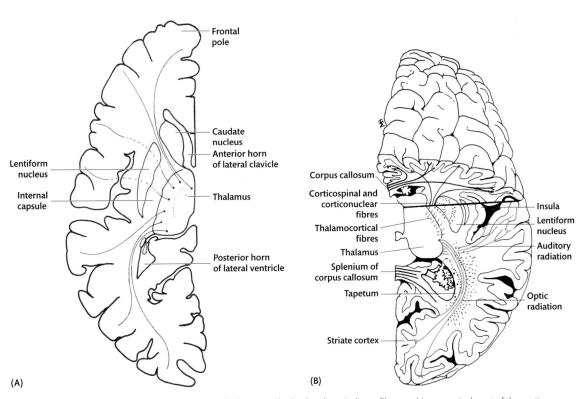

(A)

(B)

Fig. 30.6 (A) Thalamocortical radiations to the cerebral cortex. The broken lines indicate fibres arching superiorly out of the section over the lentiform nucleus. (B) Diagrammatic representation of projection fibres. Pink = descending 'motor' fibres; blue = ascending sensory fibres; black = commissural fibres of the corpus callosum.

and ends in the **ventroposterior medial** nucleus of the thalamus [see Fig. 31.28]. Efferents from these two nuclei project to the sensory cortex of the cerebrum through the thalamocortical radiations (see General sensory radiations, p. 342).

Medial geniculate body

The medial geniculate body is part of the auditory pathway. It receives the **brachium of the inferior colliculus**, which carries auditory impulses from the inferior colliculus [see Fig. 29.2], and sends efferent fibres to the transverse temporal gyrus through the **auditory radiation** [see Fig. 24.5; Figs. 30.5, 30.6].

Lateral geniculate body

The lateral geniculate body is part of the visual pathway. Each lateral geniculate body receives fibres from the contralateral visual field through the optic tract. It gives rise to the fibres of the **optic radiation** which convey visual impulses to the occipital lobe of the cerebral cortex [see Figs. 30.6, 31.33].

Other connections of the thalamus

The thalamus receives fibres from the cerebellum—the dentato-thalamic and dentato-rubro-thalamic tracts [see Fig. 29.8], the globus pallidus (part of the deep nuclei of the cerebrum), the subthalamic nucleus in the diencephalon, and all parts of the cerebral cortex and the reticular formation of the brainstem.

General sensory radiations

The **thalamocortical fibres** are those fibres which transmit sensory information from the thalamus to the cerebral cortex. They form the **sensory radiations**, and fibres reach the cerebral cortex through the internal capsule and corona radiata [Fig. 30.6].

Hypothalamus

The hypothalamus forms the lateral wall of the third ventricle, inferior to the hypothalamic sulcus [Fig. 30.1]. Parts of the hypothalamus—the mammillary bodies and infundibulum—appear on the inferior surface of the brain in the interpeduncular fossa. Laterally, the hypothalamus extends to the lower part of the internal capsule. Inferiorly, it is continuous with the tegmentum of the midbrain, without any line of demarcation.

Nuclei of the hypothalamus

The hypothalamus contains numerous nuclei in groups, which are arbitrarily divided into three groups anteroposteriorly—the **chiasmatic** or **supraoptic nuclei** (in the region above the optic chiasma), **tuberal nuclei** (above the infundibulum), and posterior or **mammillary nuclei** (above the mammillary bodies). These groups are further divided, from medial to lateral, into a most medial or **periventricular group**, **medial**

group, and **lateral group**. The connections of only a few important nuclei are discussed.

Connections of the hypothalamus

The connections of the hypothalamus are complex, and only a few important ones are mentioned here. The hypothalamus receives input from the hippocampus, thalamus, and brainstem. It gives efferent fibres to other parts of the brain and to the pituitary.

Connections of the mammillary body

The mammillary body is part of the limbic system. It receives input from the hippocampal formation through the fornix. It gives fibres to the anterior nucleus of the thalamus through the **mammillothalamic tract** [Fig. 30.7] and to the tegmentum of the midbrain through the **mammillotegmental tract** [Fig. 30.7].

Connections of the supraoptic and paraventricular nuclei

Cells in the supraoptic and paraventricular nuclei have axons extending into the posterior pituitary to end in relation to vascular sinusoids there. They carry neurosecretions produced in these nuclei to the blood vessels of the posterior pituitary. They form the hypothalamohypophyseal tract.

Vascular connections

The hypothalamus and hypophysis are also connected by the hypothalamohypophyseal portal system. Through this vascular system, secretions of the arcuate, preoptic, and other nuclei of the hypothalamus reach the anterior pituitary and influence secretion of hormones produced in it.

Functions of the hypothalamus

The hypothalamus is concerned with a number of visceral functions. It controls the autonomic nervous system, regulates temperature, and regulates eating, drinking, sleeping and waking, sexual arousal, fear, and rage.

Subthalamus

The subthalamus lies just rostral to the tegmentum of the midbrain, lateral to the hypothalamus [Fig. 30.3B]. It receives fibres from the globus pallidus through the subthalamic fasciculus. Most of its efferent fibres pass back to the globus pallidus, but some probably descend into the midbrain.

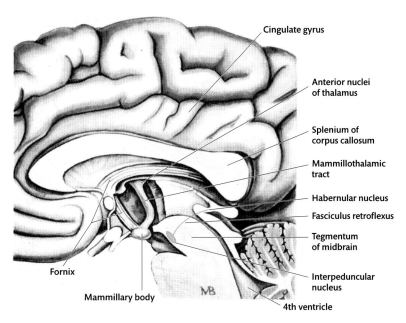

Cingulate gyrus

Anterior nuclei
of thalamus

Splenium of
corpus callosum

Mammillothalamic
tract

Habernular nucleus

Fasciculus retroflexus

Tegmentum
of midbrain

Interpeduncular
nucleus

4th ventricle

Fornix

Mammillary body

MB

Fig. 30.7 Dissection to show the fornix and mammillothalamic tract.

➲ Lesions of the subthalamic nucleus give rise to hemiballism, a condition marked by abrupt onset of wild, flailing movement of the opposite upper limb.

See Clinical Applications 30.1 and 30.2 for the practical implications of the anatomy discussed in this chapter.

CLINICAL APPLICATION 30.1 Thalamic infarct

A 72-year-old woman presented in the Neurology clinic with a two-day history of numbness on the right side of her face, decreased sensation in her right arm, and loss of sensation in her right foot. A computerized tomogram (CT scan) revealed a small lacunar infarct in the left thalamus.

Study question 1: which nucleus in the thalamus receives sensory input from the right side of the face? (Answer: the left ventroposterior medial (VPM) nucleus.)

Study question 2: trace the pathway from the right side of the face to the left VPM nucleus. (Answer: right side of face > trigeminal nerve > main sensory and spinal nuclei of trigeminal > trigeminothalamic tract on left side > ascends in pons and midbrain > ends in VPM nucleus of thalamus [see Fig. 28.5B].)

Study question 3: which nucleus in the thalamus receives sensory input from the right leg? (Answer: the left ventroposterior lateral (VPL) nucleus.)

Study question 4: trace the pathway from the right leg to the left VPL nucleus. (Answer: (1) pathway for crude touch, vibration, and position sense: sensory nerves of leg > dorsal root ganglion > fasciculus gracilis > nucleus gracilis > internal arcuate fibres > medial lemniscus on left side > VPL nucleus of thalamus; (2) pathway for pain and temperature: sensory nerves of leg > dorsal root ganglion > cells in posterior grey horn > spinothalamic tract of left side > VPL nucleus of thalamus.)

CLINICAL APPLICATION 30.2 Role of geniculate bodies

The geniculate bodies are thalamic nuclei concerned with the auditory and visual pathways. They differ from each other in that the lateral geniculate body is the only route through which impulses generated in the opposite half of the field of vision can reach the cerebral cortex, while each

medial geniculate body carries auditory impulses originating in both cochleae. Thus, destruction of one lateral geniculate body produces blindness in the opposite half of the field of vision, but destruction of one medial geniculate body has little effect on hearing.

CHAPTER 31
The cerebrum

Introduction to the cerebrum

Begin your study of this region by reviewing the relationship between the skull and brain, with the help of a dry skull. Note the relationship of the parts of the brain to the folds of the dura mater (the falx cerebri and the tentorium cerebelli) in a cadaver where the brain has been removed. Also review the external features of the cerebrum described in Chapter 24.

The **longitudinal fissure** is the narrow cleft between the two cerebral hemispheres. It is occupied by: (1) the falx cerebri; (2) the fold of the arachnoid which follows the surface of the falx; (3) the pia mater covering the medial surfaces of the hemispheres; and (4) the arteries and veins which lie in the subarachnoid space. (The falx was removed when the brain was taken from the skull, but the other structures are still *in situ*.)

Each cerebral hemisphere has three surfaces: (1) the convex **superolateral surface** [Fig. 31.1]; (2) the **medial** surface; and (3) the **inferior surface** [Fig. 31.2]; and three borders: the (1) **superomedial**; (2) **inferolateral**; and (3) **medial** borders. The inferior surface has an anterior orbital part which rests on the floor of the anterior cranial fossa, and a posterior tentorial part which rests on the floor of the middle cranial fossa and the tentorium cerebelli. The medial surface is flat and vertical and lies against the falx cerebri.

The **superomedial border** is self-explanatory. The **superciliary border** (part of the

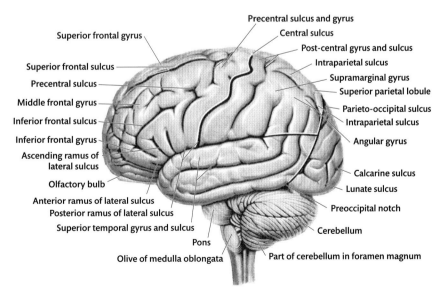

Fig. 31.1 Lateral surface of the brain to show the main sulci and gyri. The division of the superolateral surface into lobes by the central sulcus and two arbitrary lines is shown.

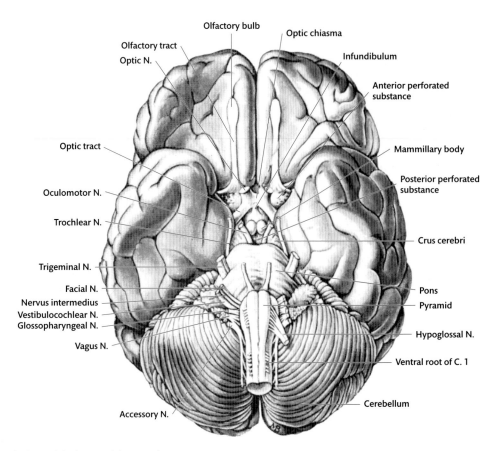

Fig. 31.2 The base of the brain and the cranial nerves.

inferolateral border) lies at the junction of the superolateral and orbital surfaces. About 3 cm from the occipital pole, the inferolateral border exhibits a notch—the preoccipital notch [Fig. 31.1]—where the inferior anastomotic vein enters the transverse sinus. The border at the junction of the medial and orbital surfaces is the **medial orbital border**, and that at the junction of the medial and tentorial surfaces is the **medial occipital border**.

Using the instructions given in Dissection 31.1, section the cerebrum in the midline.

DISSECTION 31.1 Hemisection of the cerebrum

Objectives

I. To remove the right half of the cerebral hemisphere.
II. To identify the features seen on the medial side of the cerebral hemisphere.

Instructions

1. Separate the two cerebral hemispheres at the longitudinal fissure, and expose the mass of white matter which joins them deep in the fissure. This is the **corpus callosum**, the posterior part of which (**splenium**) has already been seen as a thick, rounded mass superior to the pineal body.

2. At the splenium of the corpus callosum, identify the **great cerebral vein** emerging between the pineal body and the splenium of the corpus callosum.

3. Divide the corpus callosum in the midline, starting at the splenium. Proceed carefully, noting that the corpus callosum is much thinner immediately anterior to the splenium and that a thin layer of pia mater lies inferior to the corpus callosum in this part.

4. Divide the right posterior cerebral artery close to its origin from the basilar artery.

5. Turn to the right side of the brain, and make a transverse cut through the upper part of the right half of the midbrain so as to join the two ends of the median cut. Now lift away the right hemisphere.

6. Examine the medial aspect of the hemisphere.

7. Pass a fine probe through the cerebral aqueduct from the posterosuperior part of the third ventricle to the fourth ventricle.

8. Identify the features on the medial surface of the cerebrum, using Fig. 31.3. The cut surface of the corpus callosum is seen near the middle. Identify its parts: the rostrum, genu, body, and splenium.

9. The third ventricle lies inferior to the body of the corpus callosum.

10. The fornix—an arch of white matter—lies in close apposition to the corpus callosum posteriorly. Anteriorly, it curves downwards as the column of the fornix.

11. The septum pellucidum is a thin vertical sheet of white matter which stretches from the corpus callosum to the fornix. The septum is made up of two laminae (the **laminae of the septum pellucidum**) which enclose a narrow space—the **cavum septi pellucidi**—between them [see Fig. 30.2].

12. Follow the rostrum of the corpus callosum downwards. At its lower extremity, a round bundle of fibres will be seen in the midline, immediately anterior to the columns of the fornix. This is the **anterior commissure** [see Fig. 31.7].

13. Identify the thin lamina terminalis which extends inferiorly from the anterior commissure and forms the anterior wall of the third ventricle.

14. Trace the lamina terminalis down to the cut end of the optic chiasma.

15. Turn to the inferior surface of the brain, and identify the optic chiasma and the cut end of the anterior communicating artery which unites the two anterior cerebral arteries above the chiasma.

16. Identify the interventricular foramen, as it lies inferior to the fornix, and pass a probe through it into the lateral ventricle.

17. Identify the choroid plexus in the roof of the third ventricle.

18. Identify the thalamus on the lateral wall of the third ventricle and the bridge of tissue crossing the third ventricle—the interthalamic adhesion.

19. Identify the infundibulum and mammillary bodies on the inferior aspect of the third ventricle.

Septum pellucidum

The septum pellucidum is made up of neural tissue. It consists of two thin parallel laminae, each of which connects the fornix to the corpus callosum and fills the interval in the concavity of its genu. Its two laminae may be separated by the **cavity of the septum pellucidum**.

Cerebral cortex

Start your study of the cerebral cortex by removing the arachnoid mater from the surface and identifying the named sulci and gyri.

Remove the arachnoid mater of the brain, following the instructions provided in Dissection 31.2.

Cerebral sulci and gyri

The cerebral cortex extends as an uninterrupted sheet over the whole surface of the hemisphere and consists of nerve cells which are arranged in six layers parallel to the surface [Fig. 31.4]. These layers are differentiated from each other in a microscopic section by their different cell contents. In general, the cerebral cortex varies both in thickness and microscopic structure in its various parts. The cortex is thicker on the summits of the gyri than in the depths of the sulci.

There are great individual variations in the details of the sulci and gyri, so attention should be given mainly to the major sulci and gyri. These can be identified with the help of Figs. 31.5, 31.6, 31.7, 31.8, and 31.9.

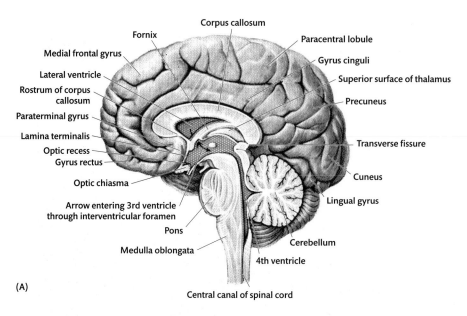

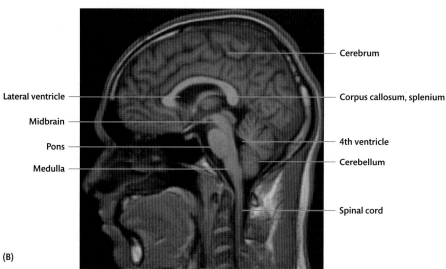

Fig. 31.3 (A) Medial surface of the right hemisphere. The septum pellucidum has been removed to expose the lateral ventricle. The arrow passes through the interventricular foramen from the lateral to the third ventricle. Ependymal lining of ventricles = blue. (B) T1-weighed sagittal magnetic resonance imaging (MRI) of the brain.

DISSECTION 31.2 Removal of the arachnoid mater

Objectives

I. To remove the arachnoid from the surface of the cerebrum. **II.** To identify and trace the middle cerebral artery and its branches.

Instructions

1. Review the vessels on the surfaces of the cerebral hemisphere, and then proceed to strip the arachnoid from its surface.

2. On the superolateral surface of the brain, strip the arachnoid towards the lateral sulcus [Fig. 31.1], pulling it off along the line of the other sulci.

3. Note the large branches of the middle cerebral artery which arise from the lateral sulcus.

4. Remove the arachnoid mater from the medial and inferolateral surfaces.

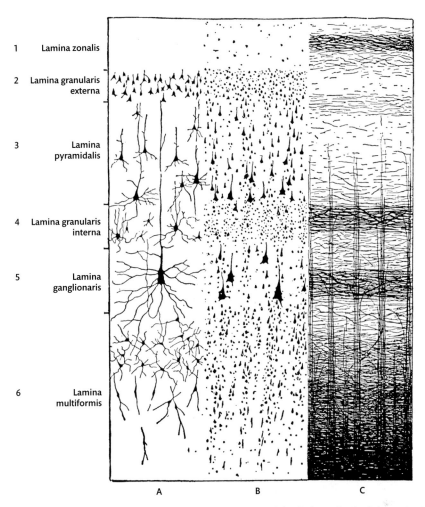

1   Lamina zonalis

2   Lamina granularis externa

3   Lamina pyramidalis

4   Lamina granularis interna

5   Lamina ganglionaris

6   Lamina multiformis

A   B   C

Fig. 31.4 Arrangement of cells and myelinated nerve fibres in the cerebral cortex. (A) cells shown by the Golgi method; (B) cells shown by the Nissl method; (C) nerve fibres shown by the Weigert method.

Reprinted from *An Introduction to Neurology*, 5th edition, Herrick, CJ. W.B. Saunders (Elsevier) 1938.

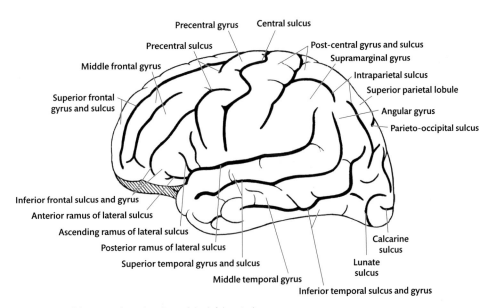

Precentral gyrus   Central sulcus

Precentral sulcus   Post-central gyrus and sulcus

Middle frontal gyrus   Supramarginal gyrus

Intraparietal sulcus

Superior frontal gyrus and sulcus   Superior parietal lobule

Angular gyrus

Parieto-occipital sulcus

Inferior frontal sulcus and gyrus

Anterior ramus of lateral sulcus

Ascending ramus of lateral sulcus

Posterior ramus of lateral sulcus   Calcarine sulcus

Superior temporal gyrus and sulcus   Lunate sulcus

Middle temporal gyrus

Inferior temporal sulcus and gyrus

Fig. 31.5 Sulci and gyri of the superolateral surface of the left hemisphere.

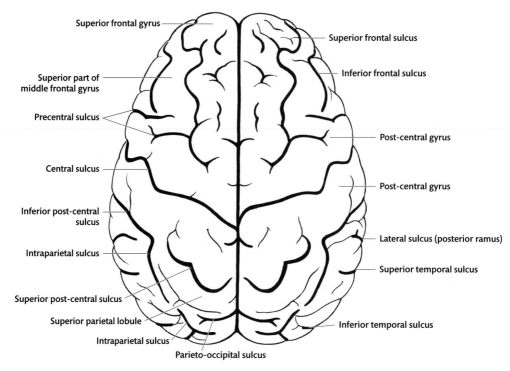

Fig. 31.6 Sulci and gyri of the superior surface of the cerebral hemispheres.

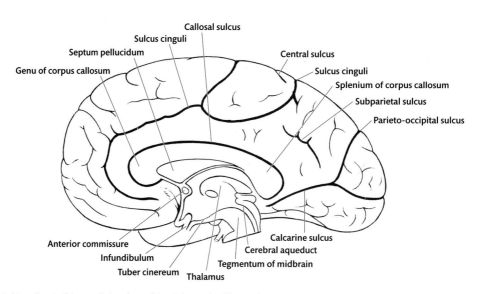

Fig. 31.7 Sulci and gyri of the medial surface of the right cerebral hemisphere.

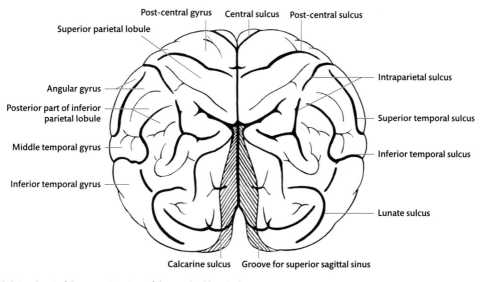

Fig. 31.8 Sulci and gyri of the posterior view of the cerebral hemispheres.

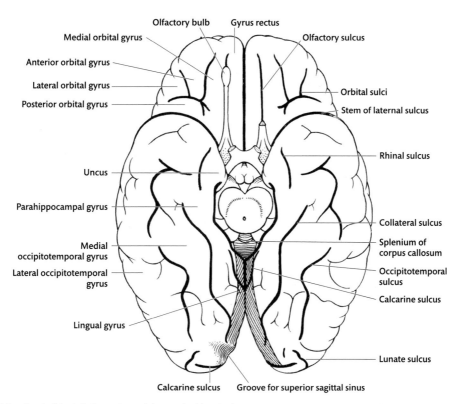

Fig. 31.9 Sulci and gyri of the inferior surface of the cerebral hemispheres.

The **sulci** vary in depth, from slight grooves to deep fissures. Some sulci—calcarine and collateral sulci [Figs. 31.7, 31.9]—are sufficiently deep to indent the wall of the lateral ventricle. The **gyri** consist of a central core of white matter (nerve fibres running to and from the overlying cortex), covered by a layer of grey matter—the **cerebral cortex**.

Lateral sulcus

The various parts of the deep and complex **lateral sulcus** are formed by the meeting of the folds of the cortex around the insular cortex that is buried deeply [Figs. 31.3, 31.9]. The **stem of the lateral sulcus** lies in the depression which runs laterally between the temporal pole and the posterior part of the orbital surface of the hemisphere [Fig. 31.9]. It contains the middle cerebral artery and veins. The stem ends on the superolateral surface of the cerebrum by dividing into **anterior**, **ascending**, and **posterior rami** [Fig. 31.5]. The anterior and ascending rami extend into the inferior frontal gyrus. The posterior ramus runs backwards and separates the frontal and parietal lobes of the brain from the temporal lobe inferiorly. The terminal part of the posterior ramus curves upwards into the parietal lobe. When the lips of the lateral sulcus are pulled apart, the insula is exposed. The main branches of the middle cerebral artery can be seen running over it before emerging from the sulcus on to the superolateral surface of the hemisphere.

Central sulcus

This important sulcus begins superiorly on the medial surface of the hemisphere, approximately

midway between the frontal and occipital poles [Fig. 31.7]. It crosses the superomedial border and extends antero-inferiorly on the superolateral surface to end just above the posterior ramus of the lateral sulcus, 2–3 cm behind its origin. The central sulcus separates the frontal and parietal lobes of the hemisphere. It is of special importance because it separates the main '**motor**' and '**sensory**' **areas** of the cerebral cortex [Fig. 31.10].

Parieto-occipital and calcarine sulci

These two deep sulci form a Y-shaped depression on the medial aspect of the posterior part of the hemisphere [Fig. 31.7]. The superior end of the **parieto-occipital sulcus** reaches the superolateral surface, and the posterior end of the calcarine may extend round the occipital pole on to the superolateral surface [Fig. 31.4]. When the **calcarine sulcus** extends to the superolateral surface, the end is surrounded by the **lunate sulcus** [Figs. 31.5, 31.8]. An imaginary line joining the superior end of the parieto-occipital sulcus to the preoccipital notch separates the occipital lobe from the parietal and temporal lobes [Fig. 31.1].

The **calcarine sulcus** is of considerable functional significance, for the nerve fibres conveying visual impulses to the cerebral cortex end in the cortex which lines its walls and extends on to the medial surface [Fig. 31.11].

Lobes of hemispheres

The arbitrary division of the hemisphere into lobes is completed on the superolateral surface by: (1) extending the central sulcus down to meet the

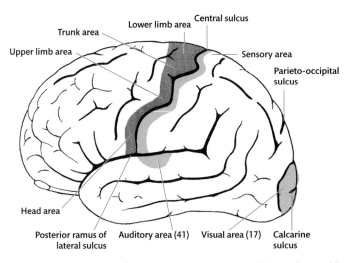

Fig. 31.10 Diagram of the superolateral surface of the left hemisphere. 'Motor' area = red; 'sensory' area = blue.

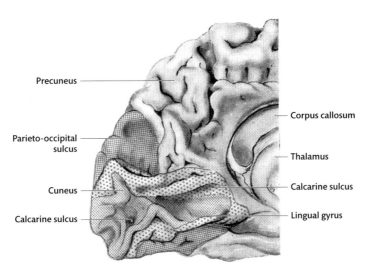

Fig. 31.11 Posterior part of the medial surface of the left hemisphere. The calcarine sulcus has been forced open to expose the cortex lying in its depths. Fine blue dots = visual receptive area; coarse blue dots = visual association area; upper and lower dark blue areas have long association connections with other parts of the cortex.

posterior ramus of the lateral sulcus; and (2) extending the horizontal part of the posterior ramus of the lateral sulcus posteriorly to meet an imaginary line joining the parieto-occipital sulcus and the preoccipital notch [Fig. 31.1]. The **frontal lobe** lies in front of the central sulcus. The **occipital lobe** lies behind the imaginary line joining the parieto-occipital sulcus to the preoccipital notch. The **temporal lobe** lies below the posterior ramus of the lateral sulcus, and the **parietal lobe** lies between the central sulcus, the posterior ramus of the lateral sulcus, and the imaginary line joining the parieto-occipital sulcus to the preoccipital notch.

Sulci and gyri on the superolateral surface

On the frontal lobe, in front of, and parallel to, the central sulcus is the **precentral sulcus**, with the **precentral gyrus** between the two [Fig. 31.5]. The '**motor**' area, the area responsible for movement of skeletal muscles of the opposite side of the body, lies in the anterior wall of the central sulcus and the adjacent part of the precentral gyrus. Most of the corticospinal and corticonuclear fibres arise from the motor cortex. Within the motor cortex, there is a further functional subdivision—movements of the opposite side of the head and neck are brought about by neurons lying in the inferior precentral region; and neurons controlling movements of the upper limb, trunk, lower limb,

and perineum follow in sequence superiorly. The area for the lower limbs and genitalia lies in the part of the post-central gyrus on the medial surface of the cerebrum [Fig. 31.7].

⊃ The frontal branch of the **middle meningeal artery** runs on the dura mater, parallel to, and a short distance anterior to, the central sulcus [see Fig. 8.17]. Haemorrhage from this artery is likely to press on this region of the brain and interfere with the voluntary movements in the opposite half of the body.

The anterior part of the frontal lobe has the **superior** and **inferior frontal sulci**, which divide the cortex of this area into **superior**, **middle**, and **inferior frontal gyri** [see Fig. 34.1]. The '**motor speech area**' lies in the inferior frontal gyrus [Figs. 31.5, 31.10]. This region is intimately connected with the control of movements of the larynx and tongue through connections with the motor area immediately posterior to it. The complex mechanism which subserves speech involves many other regions of the brain, most commonly in the left hemisphere.

The **post-central gyrus** and **post-central sulcus** lie immediately behind the central sulcus in the parietal lobe. The '**sensory**' area lies in the posterior wall of the central sulcus and the adjacent part of the post-central gyrus. It receives sensory stimuli from the opposite side of the body through the thalamic radiations. Similar to the arrangement of motor neurons in the motor cortex, sensory fibres from the opposite side of the head end in the inferior post-central region, and the other regions of the body are represented in sequence superiorly [Figs. 31.5, 31.7, 31.10].

The **intraparietal sulcus** in the posterior part of the parietal lobe divides this area into **superior** and **inferior parietal lobules** [Fig. 31.5]. The posterior ramus of the lateral sulcus and the superior and inferior temporal sulci sweep superiorly into the inferior parietal lobule and divide it into three parts arranged around the ends of these sulci. The two anterior parts are the **supramarginal** and **angular gyri** and are important in the recognition of structures and symbols, and body image.

The superolateral surface of the temporal lobe is divided into the **superior**, **middle**, and **inferior temporal gyri** by the **superior** and **inferior temporal sulci** [Fig. 31.1]. The **auditory area** is the cortical area to which auditory impulses are primarily relayed. It lies on the middle of the superior surface of the superior temporal gyrus—the **transverse temporal gyrus**—and extends on to the lateral surface, inferior to the post-central gyrus [Fig. 31.10]. If the superior temporal gyrus is pulled inferiorly, the transverse temporal gyrus will be seen running across its superior surface.

The terminal part of the **calcarine sulcus** curves around the superomedial border of the cerebrum and appears on the superolateral surface of the occipital lobe. The short **lunate sulcus** surrounds the end of the calcarine sulcus. The cerebral cortex enclosed by the lunate sulcus is part of the visual cortex [Figs. 31.5, 31.10].

Sulci and gyri on the inferior surface

The H-shaped **orbital sulcus** on the orbital surface of the frontal lobe divides the major part of this surface into the **anterior, medial, posterior**, and **lateral orbital gyri** [Fig. 31.9]. The **olfactory sulcus** lies on the medial side of the medial orbital gyrus and separates it from the **gyrus rectus**. The **olfactory bulb** and **tract** lie in the **olfactory sulcus**.

The **uncus** is a raised area on the inferior surface of the temporal lobe. It is separated from the remainder of the temporal lobe by the **rhinal sulcus** [Fig. 31.9]. The uncus is continuous posteriorly with the **parahippocampal gyrus**, which is separated from the remainder of the temporal lobe by the **collateral sulcus**. The collateral sulcus is often continuous with the rhinal sulcus. The uncus

and parahippocampal gyrus form the **inferomedial border** of the hemisphere and lie close to the free margin of the tentorium. The remainder of the inferior surface of the temporal lobe is divided into the **medial** and **lateral occipitotemporal gyrus** by the **occipitotemporal sulcus**.

Sulci and gyri on the medial surface

The **callosal sulcus** lies immediately adjacent to the corpus callosum. The **cingulate sulcus** lies parallel to the callosal sulcus. It begins inferior to the genu of the corpus callosum and curves forwards, upwards, and backwards to run posteriorly in the frontal lobe. At its posterior end, it curves upwards towards the superomedial border [Fig. 31.7]. The **cingulate gyrus** lies between the callosal and cingulate sulci. The **medial frontal gyrus** lies in front of, and superior to, the cingulate sulcus as it curves [Figs. 31.3, 31.7]. The cortex on either side of the central sulcus on the medial surface of the brain is the **paracentral lobule**, and contains the parts of the sensory and motor cortices of the lower limbs.

Review the position of the parieto-occipital and calcarine sulci. The cerebral cortex in front of the parieto-occipital sulcus is the **precuneus**, and the area between the parieto-occipital and calcarine sulcus is the **cuneus**. The **lingual gyrus** lies inferior to the calcarine sulcus and extends onto the inferior surface of the cerebrum [Fig. 31.7]. The visual cortex lies on the banks of the calcarine sulcus, in the cuneus and lingual gyrus [Figs. 31.11]. This cortex has a very well-defined white stria running through it and is called the **striate cortex**.

Using the instructions given in Dissection 31.3, incise the visual cortex and inspect it.

DISSECTION 31.3 Examination of the visual cortex

Objective

I. To examine the visual cortex.

Instructions

1. Cut a slice through the calcarine sulcus, posterior to its junction with the parieto-occipital sulcus, and examine the cortex for the presence of the stria.

Insular cortex

The insula is that part of the cerebral cortex which is submerged in the lateral sulcus. It is roughly triangular in shape, and its margin is formed by the **circular sulcus**. The cortex of the insula is continuous with the cortex on the deep surfaces of the **opercula**—the folds of the hemisphere which hide the insula from view. The apex of the insula is known as the **limen insulae** [Fig. 31.12]. The surface of the insula is marked by a number of sulci and gyri radiating superiorly from the stem of the lateral sulcus, which lies at the apex. The middle cerebral artery lies on the limen insulae, as it passes laterally on to the surface of the insula. Medial to the limen insulae is the **anterior perforated substance** through which the central branches of the middle and anterior cerebral arteries pass into the substance of the brain [Fig. 31.9].

Dissection 31.4 provides instructions on dissection of the insula.

Olfactory pathway

The olfactory bulb and tract lie in the olfactory sulcus on the inferior aspect of the frontal lobe [Fig. 31.13]. The **olfactory bulb** is a narrow, oval body

DISSECTION 31.4 The insula

Objective

I. To remove the opercula and expose the insula.

Instructions

1. Expose the insula on the right cerebral hemisphere by removing the frontal, frontoparietal, and temporal opercula.

2. The greater part of the insula and the posterior part of the **superior longitudinal bundle** are now seen in the root of the operculum [see Fig. 31.22A].

which lies on the dura mater, immediately above the cribriform plate of the ethmoid. It receives the 12–20 olfactory nerves from the olfactory mucosa in the nasal cavity. ➲ Fractures of the anterior cranial fossa are therefore liable to damage the olfactory bulb and lead to anosmia.

The olfactory tract extends posteriorly in the olfactory sulcus [Fig. 31.13]. Posteriorly, it splits into the **medial** and **lateral olfactory striae** at the anterior margin of the anterior perforated substance. Between the two striae, there is a small grey elevation—the **olfactory trigone**. The medial stria curves round the posterior end of the gyrus rectus

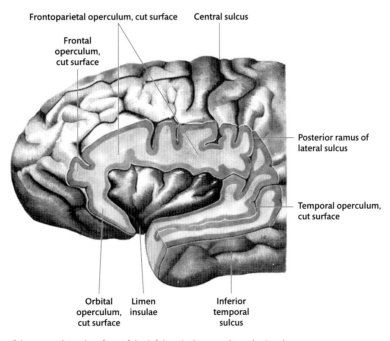

Frontoparietal operculum, cut surface

Central sulcus

Frontal operculum, cut surface

Posterior ramus of lateral sulcus

Temporal operculum, cut surface

Orbital operculum, cut surface

Limen insulae

Inferior temporal sulcus

Fig. 31.12 Dissection of the superolateral surface of the left hemisphere to show the insula.

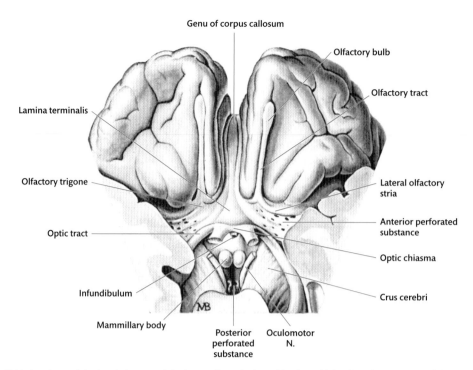

Fig. 31.13 Orbital surfaces of the hemispheres and the interpeduncular fossa. The frontal lobes have been separated slightly to show the genu of the corpus callosum, and the optic chiasma has been pulled inferiorly to uncover the lamina terminalis.

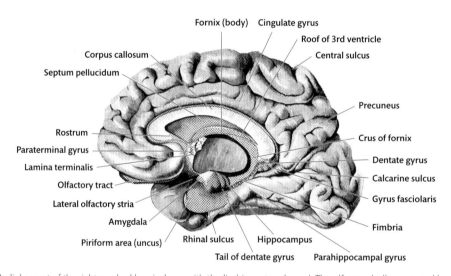

Fig. 31.14 Medial aspect of the right cerebral hemisphere, with the limbic parts coloured. The olfactory bulb, tract, and lateral stria, the uncus, and the dentate gyrus are shown in red. The hippocampus, indusium griseum, paraterminal gyrus, septum pellucidum, and medial olfactory stria are shown in blue.

to the medial side of the hemisphere and ends in the region of the **paraterminal gyrus** [Fig. 31.3, 31.14]. The lateral stria runs posterolaterally on the margin of the anterior perforated substance, curves round the stem of the lateral sulcus, and enters the uncus and anterior part of the parahippocampal gyrus. The uncus and anterior part of the parahippocampal gyrus constitute the piriform lobe.

Limbic lobe

A rim of the cerebral cortex adjacent to the corpus callosum and diencephalon is known as the limbic lobe. (The term limbic system includes the limbic cortex, as well as related subcortical nuclei.) The limbic lobe is made up of the cingulate gyrus, parahippocampal gyrus, hippocampus, dentate gyrus, paraterminal gyrus, and uncus. (The hippocampus and dentate gyrus are seen deep within the parahippocampal gyrus.)

Hippocampus

The hippocampus lies deep within the parahippocampal gyrus in the floor of the inferior horn of the lateral ventricle [Fig. 31.14]. Anteriorly, it turns medially near the tip of the inferior horn and becomes continuous with the uncus. This part of the hippocampus is ridged and known as the pes hippocampi [see Fig. 32.12]. The hippocampus tapers posteriorly and is continuous with a small ridge—the gyrus fasciolaris—which curves round the inferior surface of the splenium [Fig. 31.14].

Dentate gyrus

The **dentate gyrus** lies in the depths of the hippocampal sulcus—the sulcus lying medial to the parahippocampal gyrus [Fig. 31.14]. It is a small gyrus, transversely ridged to give the appearance of 'teeth'. It continues anteriorly with the uncus. Posteriorly, the dentate gyrus is continuous with the gyrus fasciolaris and, through it, with the thin layer of grey matter on the superior surface of the corpus callosum—the **indusium**

griseum. The indusium griseum follows the curve of the corpus callosum to the paraterminal gyrus, inferior to the rostrum of the corpus callosum [Fig. 31.14].

Alveus, fimbria, and fornix

The alveus, fimbria, and fornix together form the efferent pathway for the hippocampus. Start your study of the fornix by noting the continuity of the fimbria, crus, body, and column of the fornix with one another, using Figs. 31.14 and 31.15. Each fornix is composed of fibres which enter it from the fimbria and, together with the fimbria, the fornix forms almost one complete turn of a spiral. (The fimbria and fornix together connect the hippocampus to the mammillary body.) There is one fornix in each hemisphere, but the two are so closely fused beneath the middle of the trunk of the corpus callosum that they are usually described as a single structure.

The efferent fibres arising from the hippocampus run across the floor of the inferior horn of the lateral ventricle to form the **alveus**. The alveus continues as the **fimbria** of the hippocampus—a narrow strip of white matter on the medial margin of the hippocampus. It is continuous posteriorly with the **crus of the fornix** [Fig. 31.15]. The crus of the

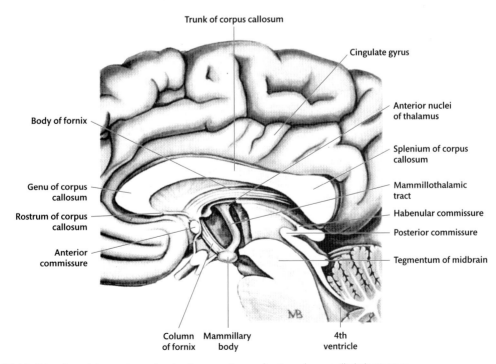

Fig. 31.15 Medial surface of the cerebrum showing the commissures, fornix, and mammillothalamic tract.

fornix is a flattened strip which arches upwards, medially, and forwards under the splenium of the corpus callosum to become continuous with that of the other side to form the **body of the fornix**. Anteriorly, the body becomes more cylindrical and separates to form the **columns of the fornix**. The columns run inferiorly between the anterior commissure and the interventricular foramen, curve posteriorly through the anterior hypothalamus, and end in the mammillary body [Fig. 31.15].

The fibres in the fornix pass to: (1) the opposite hippocampus through the **commissure of the fornix**, which is situated where the two crura meet, inferior to the corpus callosum [see Fig. 32.5]; (2) the septal and anterior hypothalamic regions; and (3) the mammillary body. In addition, (4) a few of its fibres may pass directly to the anterior nuclei of the thalamus. The fornix also contains fibres which pass from the cells in the region of the anterior commissure—the septal nuclei—to the hippocampus.

The fornix forms the margin of the **choroid fissure** between the beginning of the fimbria and the interventricular foramen. It therefore has the ependyma of the choroid plexus attached to its sharp lateral margin throughout this length [see Fig. 32.9].

The crura and body of the fornix groove the posterior and superior surfaces of the thalamus, respectively, and lie in the medial part of the floor of the lateral ventricle [see Fig. 30.2]. The columns of the fornix form slight ridges on the lateral wall of the third ventricle, inferior to the interventricular foramen [see Fig. 30.1].

Impulses from the hippocampus reach the mammillary body, anterior nucleus of the thalamus, and cingulate gyrus in series. Some fibres which arise in the cingulate gyrus pass through the cingulum to the parahippocampal gyrus and the hippocampus, thus producing feedback to the hippocampus. This entire circuit on the margin of the hemisphere (including parts of the hypothalamus) has been called the **limbic lobe**.

In addition to the specific connections mentioned earlier, all parts of the cerebral cortex are connected to the thalamus, striatum, brainstem reticular formation, and claustrum.

Arterial supply to the cerebral cortex

Review the details of the arterial supply to the cerebral cortex described in Chapter 26. The cortex is supplied by the anterior, middle, and posterior cerebral arteries [see Figs. 26.4, 26.5, 26.6]. All three arteries supply parts of the three surfaces. The superolateral surface is mainly supplied by the middle cerebral artery [see Fig. 26.6], the medial surface by the anterior cerebral artery [see Fig. 26.5], and the inferior surface by the posterior cerebral artery [see Fig. 26.4].

White matter of the cerebrum

The white matter of the cerebrum consists of the nerve fibres which lie deep to the cerebral cortex. They connect the various parts of the cortex with each other and with the other parts of the central nervous system. The white matter is classified as: (1) **association fibres**, which connect parts of the cerebral cortex within one hemisphere; (2) **commissural fibres**, which cross the midline and connect corresponding parts of the two cerebral cortices; and (3) **projection fibres**, which connect the cerebral cortex with other regions of the central nervous system. All three types of fibre bundles contain fibres passing in both directions.

Association fibres

Association fibres are of different lengths. **Short association fibres** pass from one part of a gyrus to another part of the same gyrus, or loop around one sulcus to an adjacent gyrus [Fig. 31.16]. **Long association fibres** connect distant parts of the cortex. The long association fibre bundles are: (1) the **cingulum** on the medial aspect of the brain [Fig. 31.17]; (2) the **superior longitudinal bundle** or **fasciculus** on the superolateral aspect [Fig. 31.16]; (3) the **fasciculus uncinatus** on the superolateral and orbital aspects [Fig. 31.16]; and (4) the **inferior longitudinal bundle** on the tentorial aspect.

Cingulum

Dissection 31.5 provides instructions on dissection of the cingulum and superior longitudinal bundle.

The cingulum is a thick bundle of long association fibres which connects all parts of the cerebral cortex on the medial aspect of the hemisphere. It extends from the region of the paraterminal gyrus to the uncus and forms an almost complete circle (cingulum means a girdle) [Fig. 31.16].

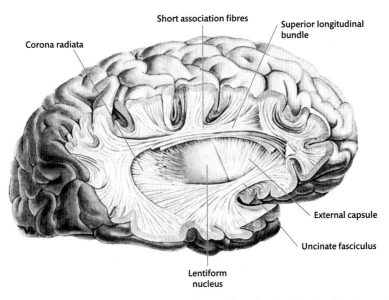

Short association fibres

Superior longitudinal bundle

Corona radiata

External capsule

Uncinate fasciculus

Lentiform nucleus

Fig. 31.16 Dissection of the superolateral surface of the right hemisphere to show the white fibre bundles deep to the cortex.

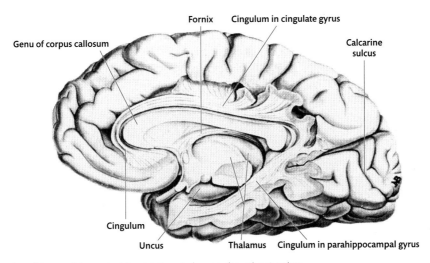

Fornix   Cingulum in cingulate gyrus

Genu of corpus callosum

Calcarine sulcus

Cingulum

Uncus   Thalamus   Cingulum in parahippocampal gyrus

Fig. 31.17 Dissection of the medial aspect of the right hemisphere to show the cingulum.

DISSECTION 31.5 The cingulum and superior longitudinal bundle

Objectives

I. To expose the cingulum.   **II.** To expose the superior longitudinal bundle.

Instructions

1. On the right hemisphere, scrape away the grey matter of the cingulate gyrus, and expose a rounded bundle of white matter lying longitudinally within it. It is simplest to determine the edge of the cingulum by removing the cortex between it and the superior surface of the corpus callosum, and then extending the removal superiorly.

2. Tear away the parts of the frontal lobe which still cover the anterior parts of the insula, and uncover the anterior part of the superior longitudinal bundle. This part is less clearly seen than the posterior part because it is traversed by many fibres of the corona radiata passing laterally through it.

3. (In the interest of time, the remaining white matter will not be dissected.) The structures revealed sequentially as the hemisphere is dissected, from lateral to medial, are shown in a series of figures [see Fig. 31.22].

Fasciculus uncinatus

The fasciculus uncinatus is a thick bundle of association fibres which passes between the frontal and temporal lobes of the brain [Fig. 31.16]. Its inferior fibres hook round the stem of the lateral sulcus into the anterior part of the temporal lobe. The superior fibres pass directly backwards and downwards towards the posterior part of the temporal lobe. It is narrow in the middle, but at both ends, the fibres spread out, giving it the shape of a bent bundle [Fig. 31.16].

Superior longitudinal bundle

The superior longitudinal bundle is a thick bundle of longitudinal association fibres. It lies immediately external to the circular sulcus of the insula [Fig. 31.16]. It extends around the insula from the frontal pole to the tip of the temporal pole and is thickest superior to the posterior half of the insula. Fibres enter and leave its external surface throughout its length, and it occupies approximately the same position on the lateral surface of the brain as the cingulum does on the medial surface. It connects the various parts of the cerebral cortex on the superolateral surface of the cerebral hemisphere.

Inferior longitudinal bundle

The inferior longitudinal bundle is a bundle of association fibres which runs horizontally through the temporal and occipital lobes, near their inferior surfaces. It connects the various parts of the cerebral cortex on the tentorial surface of the hemisphere.

Commissural fibres

The commissural fibres connect corresponding parts of the brain across the midline. The largest commissure is the **corpus callosum**. Other commissures of the forebrain are: (1) the **anterior commissure**; (2) **posterior commissure**; (3) **habenular commissure**; and (4) the **commissure of the fornix**.

Corpus callosum

Relations and parts of the corpus callosum

The corpus callosum unites the medial surfaces of the two cerebral hemispheres. Its upper surface forms the floor of part of the longitudinal fissure. The anterior cerebral vessels lie on the pia mater covering it, and the falx cerebri touches it posteriorly. It is covered on each side by the cingulate gyrus. Attached to the inferior surface of the corpus callosum in each hemisphere is the septum pellucidum, with the fornix attached to its inferior margin. In the midline, the corpus callosum overlies a thin sheet of pia mater—the **tela choroidea of the third** and **lateral ventricles** above the roof of the median, slit-like third ventricle [see Fig. 32.7].

The main part, or **trunk**, of the corpus callosum is thinner than the extremities [Fig. 31.15]. The posterior end, or **splenium**, is thick and rounded because of the large number of fibres which it transmits from the parietal, occipital, and temporal lobes. It overlies the upper part of the midbrain and extends posteriorly to the highest part of the cerebellum [Fig. 31.15]. Anteriorly, the corpus callosum is folded back on itself to form the **genu**, the lower, recurved portion of which, the **rostrum**, thins rapidly as it passes posteriorly. The tip of the rostrum is usually connected by neuroglia to the superior end of the lamina terminalis, anterior to the anterior commissure [Fig. 31.7].

The corpus callosum is formed by cortical fibres which converge in the midline and then fan out into the opposite hemisphere [Fig. 31.18]. Fibres of the corpus callosum radiate into the part of the hemisphere which lies adjacent to it. Fibres in the rostrum extend inferiorly to the orbital surface of the frontal lobe. Fibres from the genu pass to the anterior part of the frontal lobe, forming the **forceps minor**. Fibres from the trunk go to the remainder of the frontal lobe and to the parietal lobe, and fibres from the splenium radiate to the posterior parts of the parietal lobe and to the occipital and temporal lobes. Fibres connecting the medial surface of the two occipital lobes form the **forceps major**. Fibres connecting the inferior parts of the temporal and occipital lobes form a sheet of white matter on the roof and lateral wall of the posterior horn of the lateral ventricle—the **tapetum** [Figs. 31.18, 31.19]. The individual fibres retain the same relationship to each other throughout their course and connect similar parts of the two hemispheres. Fibres from the medial surface of the hemisphere form U-shaped bundles hooking through the superficial part of the commissure, while fibres from the lateral aspect of the hemisphere lie more deeply and run a more horizontal course [see Fig. 8.18; Figs. 31.3, 31.18].

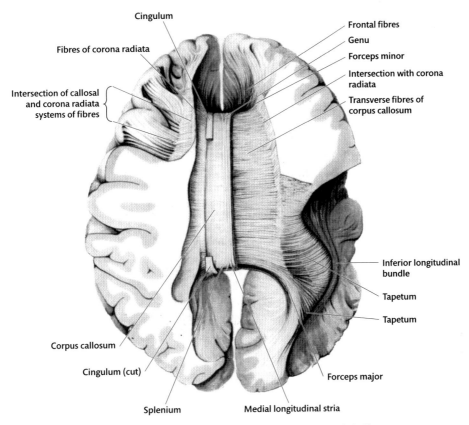

Fig. 31.18 The corpus callosum exposed from above. The course of its fibres is seen in the right half.

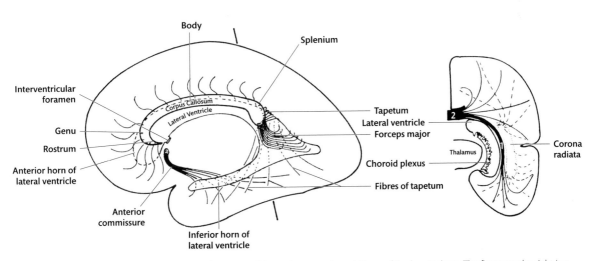

Fig. 31.19 Diagram to illustrate the course and position of the major commissural fibres of the hemisphere. The figure on the right is a coronal section along the line in the left figure. 1 = the tapetum; 2 = the splenium of the corpus callosum.

Anterior commissure

The anterior commissure is a bundle of fibres which crosses the midline in the superior part of the lamina terminalis, immediately anterior to the column of the fornix and the interventricular foramen [Figs. 31.15, 31.19]. The fibres in this commissure arise mainly in the temporal lobe and olfactory bulbs.

Posterior commissure

The slender posterior commissure crosses the midline, immediately dorsal to the upper part of the aqueduct and inferior to the root of the pineal body. It is composed mainly of fibres from the superior colliculi, the medial longitudinal bundle, and a number of nuclei associated with the superior part of that bundle [Fig. 31.15].

Habenular commissure

The habenular commissure lies at the root of the pineal body and is separated from the posterior commissure by the small pineal recess of the third ventricle. The commissure unites the two habenular nuclei [see Fig. 30.2; Fig. 31.15].

Deep structures of the cerebrum

Lying deep within the hemisphere are the deep nuclei and the projection fibres. The deep nuclei of the cerebrum lie deep in the white matter. They are: (1) the corpus striatum, consisting of the caudate nucleus and putamen; (2) the globus pallidus; (3) the claustrum [Fig. 31.21]; and (4) the amygdala. The putamen and globus pallidus together make up the lentiform nucleus.

The deep structures are best studied by examining horizontal and coronal sections through them. It is important at this stage to identify the main parts of the lateral ventricle, and the location of these parts within the lobes of the hemisphere [Fig. 31.20].

Horizontal section of the brain

A horizontal section of the brain is made following the instructions given in Dissection 31.6.

Projection fibres

The relationship between the corona radiata, internal capsule, and lentiform nucleus is best understood by studying Figs. 31.22A, 31.22B, 31.22 C, and 31.22D, a series of diagrams based on dissection of the cerebrum from the lateral side. Note the relationship of the internal and external capsules to the lentiform nucleus and the continuity of the corona radiata, internal capsule, and crus cerebri.

External capsule

This thin layer of white matter lies on the lateral surface of the lentiform nucleus and separates it from the claustrum and the white matter of the insula [Fig. 31.22B; see also Fig. 31.28].

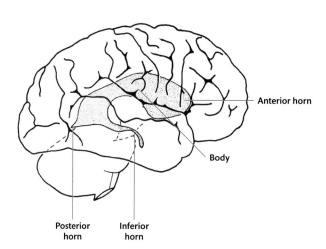

Fig. 31.20 Drawing to show the parts and position of the lateral ventricle (shaded) in the cerebral hemisphere. The posterior horn in this case is particularly small.

Objective

I. To cut the brain horizontally and identify the deep nuclei and white matter on the section.

Instructions

Sections of the hemisphere can be carried out on the left side which is nearly intact. It is desirable to have both horizontal and coronal sections for study. For this purpose, groups of students should combine their specimens.

1. Make a horizontal cut through the left hemisphere, passing through the interventricular foramen and the inferior half of the splenium of the corpus callosum. This is best carried out with a long knife pulled through the brain in a single sweep.

2. Examine the cut surface of the cerebrum, and identify the structures shown in Fig. 31.21. Start by identifying the grey matter: (1) the cortex; (2) the **lentiform nucleus** which is divided into its three segments by the **medial** and **lateral medullary laminae**—the outermost segment is the **putamen**, and the inner two segments are the **globus pallidus**; (3) the head of the **caudate nucleus**; (4) the **claustrum** (a thin layer of grey matter with a slightly scalloped lateral surface); and (5) the **thalamus**.

3. Identify the parts of the **lateral ventricle** which have been opened—the **anterior horn** and **posterior horn**.

4. Identify the V-shaped **internal capsule** lying medial to the lentiform nucleus. It is divisible into **anterior** and **posterior limbs** which meet at the **genu**.

5. Identify the **external capsule** (white matter) between the putamen and claustrum.

6. Medial to the **anterior limb of the internal capsule**, identify the **head of the caudate nucleus** in relation to the anterior horn of the lateral ventricle. Medial to the **posterior limb of the internal capsule**, identify the thalamus, and further posteriorly the tail of the caudate nucleus. Note that, in the posterior limb, the fibres are cut transversely and appear darker in colour than the fibres of the anterior limb which are cut longitudinally.

7. Identify the **optic radiation** passing towards the occipital lobe. It is lighter in colour than the tapetum which separates it from the posterior horn of the lateral ventricle [see Fig. 31.31].

8. Identify the **genu** and **splenium** of the **corpus callosum**.

9. Note the position and extent of the **striate cortex**.

Corona radiata

The corona radiata is a collection of projection fibres passing from the cerebral cortex to other parts of the central nervous system [Figs. 31.16, 31.19, 31.22, 31.23]. It consists of fibres passing inferiorly from the cortex and fibres passing superiorly to the cortex. Fibres of the corona radiata are continuous with the internal capsule around the periphery of the lentiform nucleus, and spread out in a fan-like fashion into the cerebral cortex [Figs. 31.22, 31.23].

Internal capsule

Certain gross features of the internal capsule are obvious from the study of Figs. 31.21, 31.22, 31.23, and 31.24. (1) It has an anterior limb, a posterior limb, and a genu, which lie medial to the lentiform nucleus. These parts are best seen in Fig. 31.21. The anterior limb lies between the head of the caudate nucleus and lentiform nucleus, and the posterior limb between the lentiform nucleus and thalamus. The genu is the part where the anterior and posterior limbs meet. (2) The internal capsule is continuous superiorly with the corona radiata, and inferiorly with the crus cerebri [Figs. 31.22D, 31.23, 31.24]. (3) Its fibres radiate in a fan-shaped manner, so that fibres from the frontal lobe enter its anterior limb, run a long course in it, and enter the medial part of the crus cerebri. The temporal fibres enter it posteriorly, just superior to the optic tract, run a very short distance in it, and enter the posterolateral part of the crus with the occipital fibres. It follows from this that the position of the various groups of fibres in the internal capsule and crus is determined by their point of origin in the hemisphere. Motor fibres which arise in the precentral gyrus

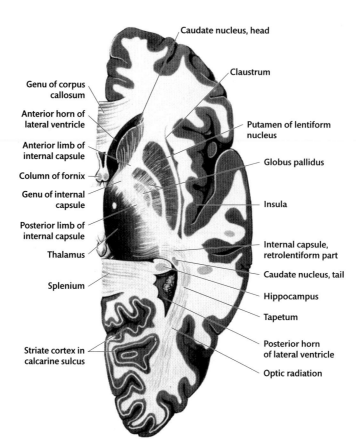

Caudate nucleus, head

Claustrum

Genu of corpus callosum

Anterior horn of lateral ventricle

Anterior limb of internal capsule

Putamen of lentiform nucleus

Globus pallidus

Column of fornix

Genu of internal capsule

Insula

Posterior limb of internal capsule

Thalamus

Internal capsule, retrolentiform part

Caudate nucleus, tail

Splenium

Hippocampus

Tapetum

Posterior horn of lateral ventricle

Striate cortex in calcarine sulcus

Optic radiation

Fig. 31.21 Horizontal section through the cerebral hemisphere at the level of the interventricular foramen.

(**corticonuclear** and **corticospinal fibres**), near the midpoint between the frontal and occipital poles, will enter the middle of the internal capsule and crus [Fig. 31.21].

Fibres of the internal capsule which emerge posterior to the lentiform nucleus (**retrolentiform part**) pass to and from the occipital lobe [Figs. 31.21, 31.24]. Fibres which emerge beneath the posterior end of the lentiform nucleus (**sublentiform part**) pass to and from the temporal lobe [Fig. 31.24].

Optic radiation

The optic radiation is made up of fibres which arise from the **lateral geniculate body** [Fig. 31.21]. They sweep forwards into the retrolentiform part of the internal capsule, spread out into a broad sheet

which turns around the lateral surface of the lateral ventricle, and pass towards the occipital lobe, lateral to the tapetum and the posterior horn of the lateral ventricle. The inferior fibres sweep far forwards on the superior surface of the inferior horn of the lateral ventricle (close to the optic tract) before turning backwards [Figs. 31.21, 31.25].

Auditory radiation

Fibres of the auditory radiation arise in the medial geniculate body. They pass anterolaterally into the sublentiform part of the internal capsule, between the roof of the inferior horn of the lateral ventricle and the lentiform nucleus. They end on the transverse temporal gyrus and, to a small extent, on its lateral surface [see Fig. 30.6B; Figs. 31.10A, 31.24].

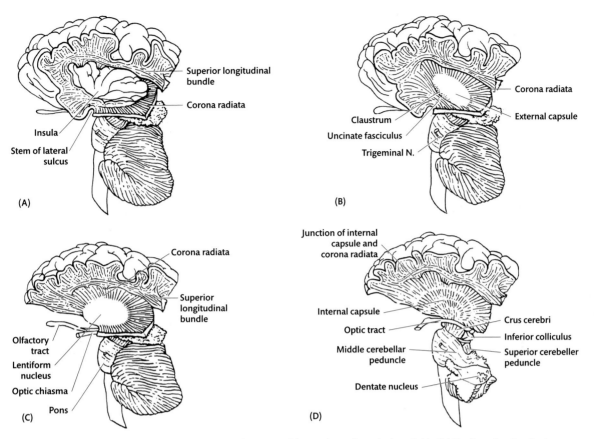

Fig. 31.22 Diagrammatic representations of the deep dissection of the cerebrum from the lateral side. (A) The frontal and parietal parts of the operculum have been removed to expose the insula and superior longitudinal bundle. (B) The insula has been removed, and the external capsule, claustrum, and fasciculus uncinatus are shown. (C) The structures exposed in (B) are removed to expose the lentiform nucleus. The fibres of the corona radiata (around the lentiform nucleus) are seen. (D) The lentiform nucleus has been removed to expose the internal capsule. The continuity of the internal capsule with the crus cerebri and corona radiata is seen.

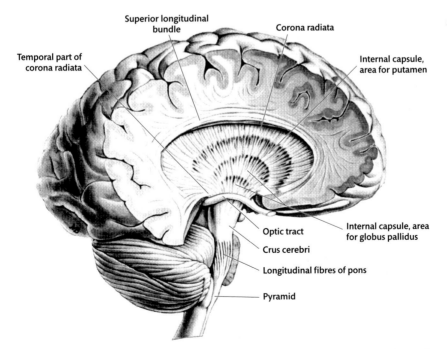

Fig. 31.23 Dissection to show the continuity of the corona radiata, internal capsule, crus celebri, longitudinal fibres of the pons, and the pyramid.

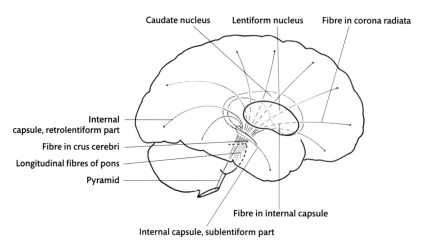

Fig. 31.24 Diagram to show the arrangement of fibres in the corona radiata, internal capsule, crus cerebri, pons, and pyramid.

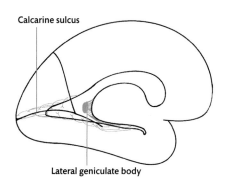

Fig. 31.25 Medial view of the left cerebral hemisphere showing the relation of the optic radiation to the lateral ventricle and calcarine sulcus.

Deep nuclei of the cerebrum

The deep nuclei of the cerebrum are also known as the basal ganglion. They include the: (1) caudate nucleus; (2) putamen; (3) globus pallidus; (4) claustrum; and (5) amygdala. Identify the parts of the caudate nucleus, globus pallidus, putamen, and claustrum in Fig. 31.21.

Before studying the deep nuclei, complete Dissection 31.7 on coronal sections through the brain.

DISSECTION 31.7 Coronal sections of the brain

Objective

I. To cut the brain in coronal slices to see the arrangement of the deep nuclei and white matter around the ventricles.

Instructions

1. Make a series of coronal sections as follows: (1) through the posterior part of the genu of the corpus callosum [Fig. 31.26]; (2) through the anterior perforated substance [Fig. 31.27]; (3) immediately anterior to the infundibulum [Fig. 31.28]; (4) immediately anterior to the mammillary bodies [Fig. 31.29]; (5) obliquely downwards through the crus cerebri and pons (if present) [Fig. 31.30]; and (6) through the splenium of the corpus callosum [Fig. 31.31].

2. With the assistance of Figs. 31.26, 31.27, 31.28, 31.29, 31.30, and 31.31, identify the structures seen in the coronal sections. These are the head and body of the caudate nucleus, putamen, globus pallidus, thalamus, parts of the corpus callosum, parts of the internal capsule, internal and external medullary laminae of the lentiform nucleus, and anterior horn, body, and posterior horn of the lateral ventricle. Relate the position of these structures to those seen in the horizontal section. In this manner, try to build a mental three-dimensional picture of the internal structures of the cerebral hemisphere. (Place the sections together to reconstruct the hemisphere, and take them apart several times to familiarize yourself with the internal arrangement.)

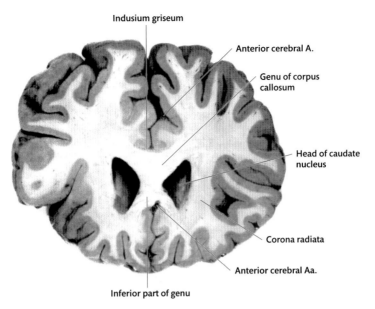

Indusium griseum

Anterior cerebral A.

Genu of corpus callosum

Head of caudate nucleus

Corona radiata

Anterior cerebral Aa.

Inferior part of genu

Fig. 31.26 Coronal section through the genu of the corpus callosum and the anterior horns of the lateral ventricles, anterior view.

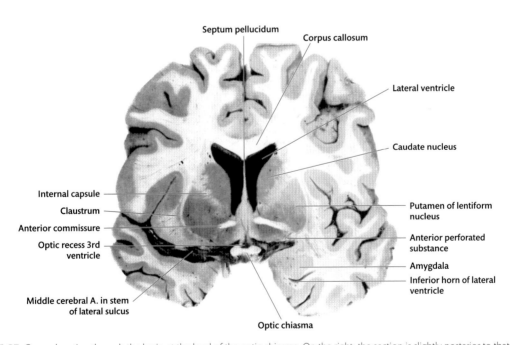

Septum pellucidum

Corpus callosum

Lateral ventricle

Caudate nucleus

Internal capsule

Claustrum

Anterior commissure

Optic recess 3rd ventricle

Putamen of lentiform nucleus

Anterior perforated substance

Amygdala

Inferior horn of lateral ventricle

Middle cerebral A. in stem of lateral sulcus

Optic chiasma

Fig. 31.27 Coronal section through the brain at the level of the optic chiasma. On the right, the section is slightly posterior to that on the left half.

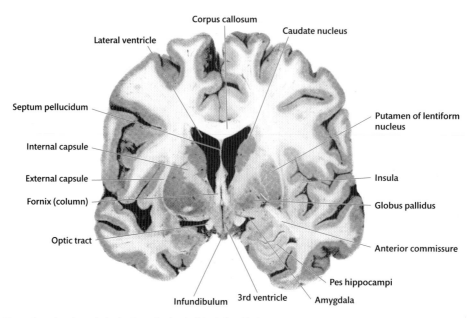

Corpus callosum

Caudate nucleus

Lateral ventricle

Septum pellucidum

Internal capsule

External capsule

Fornix (column)

Optic tract

Putamen of lentiform nucleus

Insula

Globus pallidus

Anterior commissure

Pes hippocampi

Infundibulum   3rd ventricle   Amygdala

Fig. 31.28 Coronal section through the brain at the level of the infundibulum.

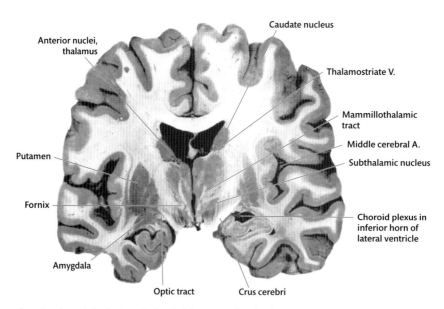

Anterior nuclei, thalamus

Caudate nucleus

Thalamostriate V.

Mammillothalamic tract

Middle cerebral A.

Subthalamic nucleus

Putamen

Fornix

Choroid plexus in inferior horn of lateral ventricle

Amygdala

Optic tract   Crus cerebri

Fig. 31.29 Coronal section through the brain at the level of the mammillary bodies.

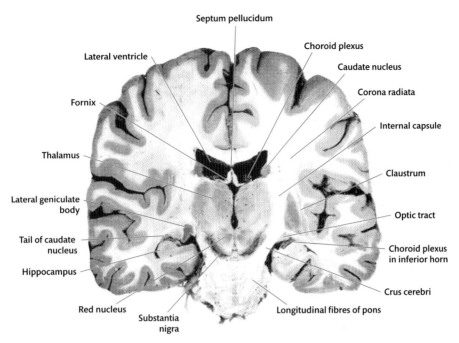

Septum pellucidum

Choroid plexus

Caudate nucleus

Corona radiata

Internal capsule

Claustrum

Optic tract

Choroid plexus
in inferior horn

Crus cerebri

Longitudinal fibres of pons

Lateral ventricle

Fornix

Thalamus

Lateral geniculate
body

Tail of caudate
nucleus

Hippocampus

Red nucleus

Substantia
nigra

Fig. 31.30 Coronal section through the brain passing through the basilar part of the pons. Note the division of the thalamus into anterior, medial, lateral, and centromedian nuclei on the left.

369

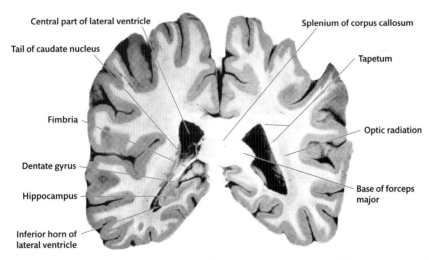

Central part of lateral ventricle

Tail of caudate nucleus

Fimbria

Dentate gyrus

Hippocampus

Inferior horn of
lateral ventricle

Splenium of corpus callosum

Tapetum

Optic radiation

Base of forceps
major

Fig. 31.31 Coronal section through the splenium of the corpus callosum to show the continuity of the central part and inferior horn of the lateral ventricle. Note how the fibres of the splenium and its tapetum virtually surround the posterior part of the lateral ventricle, as the fibres of the genu surround the anterior horn. Compare with Fig. 31.26.

Corpus striatum or basal ganglia

The corpus striatum consists of the **caudate nucleus**, **putamen**, and **globus pallidus**. The putamen and globus pallidus together form the **lentiform nucleus**. The caudate nucleus and putamen together are known as the **striatum**. The corpus striatum can be considered as one mass, partially separated by the fibres of the internal capsule. The head of the caudate nucleus is fused to the putamen, below the anterior limb of the internal capsule. The body and tail of the caudate nucleus are connected to the putamen by strands of grey matter between the bundles of the internal capsule [see Fig. 34.4A]. The caudate nucleus and putamen are identical in histological structure and have similar connections, in contrast to the putamen and globus pallidus which are very different.

Caudate nucleus

The caudate nucleus is comma-shaped [Fig. 31.24]. It has a wide, thick **head** anteriorly, followed by a short **body** and long thin **tail**. The head lies in the lateral wall of the anterior horn of the lateral ventricle [Figs. 31.24, 31.26, 31.27]. It is fused with the anterior end of the lentiform nucleus, inferior to the anterior limb of the internal capsule. This part of the head is also fused with the anterior perforated substance, and the striate branches of the middle and anterior cerebral arteries enter it [Fig. 31.27]. The head tapers rapidly to the narrow **body**, which runs posteriorly in the lateral part of the floor of the central portion of the lateral ventricle [Figs. 31.24, 31.28, 31.29]. The **tail of the caudate nucleus** is narrow and flat, and continues posteriorly from the body. It turns inferiorly and runs anteriorly in the roof of the inferior horn of the lateral ventricle to end in relation to the amygdala [Figs. 31.24, 31.30, 31.31].

The ventricular surface of the caudate nucleus is covered with ependyma. The deep surface of the head is fused anteriorly with the putamen. Posteriorly, it is applied to the anterior limb of the internal capsule. The deep surfaces of the body and tail lie on the internal capsule.

Lentiform nucleus

The lentiform nucleus is a large, lens-shaped mass of grey matter which lies lateral to the internal capsule. It is divided into three parts by two vertical sheets of white matter—the **lateral** and **medial medullary laminae**. The lateral, darker part of the lentiform nucleus is the **putamen**; the two paler medial parts are the segments of the **globus pallidus**. The lentiform nucleus has three surfaces—lateral, medial, and inferior surfaces.

The **lateral surface** is smooth and convex, and is grooved by the lateral striate vessels. It is separated from the claustrum by the external capsule [Fig. 31.21].

The **medial surface** projects medially and comes to a point opposite the interventricular foramen [Fig. 31.21]. This point lies on the genu of the internal capsule, between the head of the caudate nucleus anteriorly and the thalamus posteriorly. The striate arteries traverse and supply the lentiform nucleus and continue through the internal capsule, to supply the caudate nucleus and the lateral part of the thalamus.

The **inferior surface** is fused anteriorly with the anterior perforated substance and, through it is continuous with the amygdala [Fig. 31.28]. In this part, the lentiform nucleus is pierced by the anterior commissure [Fig. 31.27]). Posteriorly, the lentiform nucleus lies on the white matter which passes laterally into the temporal lobe. This white matter contains the **sublentiform part of the internal capsule** (auditory radiation) and separates the lentiform nucleus from the tail of the caudate nucleus, the optic tract, and the inferior horn of the lateral ventricle [Fig. 30.30].

Connections and functions of the corpus striatum (basal ganglion)

The following are the main connections of the corpus striatum.

1. The caudate nucleus and putamen receive a considerable number of fibres from the cerebral cortex, thalamus, and substantia nigra.
2. The efferent fibres of both these nuclei pass to the globus pallidus and substantia nigra.
3. The main efferent fibre from the globus pallidus—the **ansa lenticularis**—passes medially through and around the inferior part of the internal capsule to the thalamus. Other fibres pass to the subthalamus and the tegmentum of the midbrain [Fig. 31.32].
4. From the thalamus, impulses are conveyed to the posterior part of the frontal lobe (motor area).

The corpus striatum is concerned with the regulation of muscle tone and control of associated

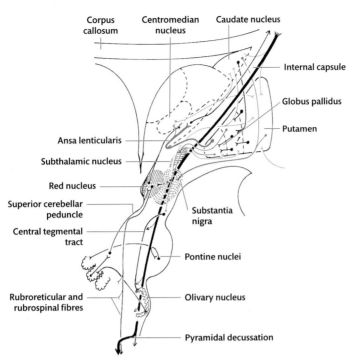

Corpus callosum

Centromedian nucleus

Caudate nucleus

Internal capsule

Globus pallidus

Putamen

Ansa lenticularis

Subthalamic nucleus

Red nucleus

Superior cerebellar peduncle

Central tegmental tract

Substantia nigra

Pontine nuclei

Rubroreticular and rubrospinal fibres

Olivary nucleus

Pyramidal decussation

Fig. 31.32 Diagram to show some of the principal connections of the basal ganglia. Afferent fibres to the striatum from the thalamus and cortex = blue; efferent fibres from the globus pallidus to the thalamus, substantia nigra, and reticular formation = red; internal capsule and connections between the putamen and globus pallidus = black.

movements, and has a part in the control of voluntary movements. ⤷ Damage to the corpus striatum leads to a state of increased muscle tone, the disappearance of associated movements like swinging of the arms in walking, and tremor at rest.

Claustrum

The **claustrum** is a thin sheet of grey matter which lies between the external capsule and the white matter of the insula. It belongs to the deep nuclei of the forebrain [Figs. 31.21, 31.27, 31.28, 31.29, 31.30].

Amygdala

The **amygdala** is a group of nuclei which lies at the tip of the inferior horn of the lateral ventricle. It is continuous with the tail of the caudate nucleus posteriorly, and with the cortex of the uncus medially. It receives afferent fibres from the thalamus, hypothalamus, and various parts of the cerebral

cortex. Its main efferent is the stria terminalis. The **stria terminalis** is a delicate bundle of fibres which arises in the amygdala, follows the curve of the caudate nucleus with the thalamostriate vein, and ends in the anterior hypothalamus and septal nuclei [Fig. 31.29; see also Fig. 32.6].

Blood supply of deep structures

The **lateral striate arteries** (also known as lenticulostriate arteries) are branches of the middle cerebral artery. They enter the brain through the anterior perforated substance. The **medial striate arteries** arise from the anterior cerebral artery, usually near the anterior communicating artery, and run a recurrent course to the anterior perforated substance [see Fig. 26.3]. Both sets of arteries ascend through the anterior perforated substance to enter and supply the caudate nucleus, lentiform nucleus, and internal capsule which runs between them [Fig. 31.28]. They also pierce the internal capsule and supply the lateral surface of the thalamus. The **recurrent artery** also arises from the anterior cerebral artery and supplies parts of the head of the caudate nucleus, putamen, globus pallidus, and internal capsule. Small central branches of the posterior cerebral artery (**thalamoperforate arteries**) supply the thalamus and some parts of the posterior limb of the internal capsule.

Visual pathway

The visual pathway from the retina to the visual cortex in the occipital lobe consists of the optic nerve, optic chiasma, optic tract, lateral geniculate body, and optic radiation. Visual impulses received in the retina of both eyes are transmitted to the brain through the **optic nerve** [Chapter 12]. The optic nerve leaves the orbit in the optic canal and enters the middle cranial fossa. At the **optic chiasma**, optic nerve fibres from the nasal half of each retina cross the midline and join the **optic tract** of the opposite side. Fibres from the temporal half of the retina continue in the optic tract of the same side. Thus, each optic tract contains fibres from the temporal half of the ipsilateral retina and nasal half from the contralateral retina [Fig. 31.33]. Most of the fibres of the optic tract end in the lateral geniculate body. From the lateral geniculate body, fibres project to the visual cortex through the optic radiation. In the optic radiation, fibres from the superior quadrants of the retina sweep superiorly to reach the visual cortex above the calcarine sulcus, and fibres from the inferior quadrants of the retina reach the visual cortex below the calcarine sulcus. Fibres from the inferior quadrant take an indirect course. They run anteriorly in the temporal lobe, curve around the inferior horn of the lateral ventricle, and then reach the cerebral cortex [Fig. 31.25].

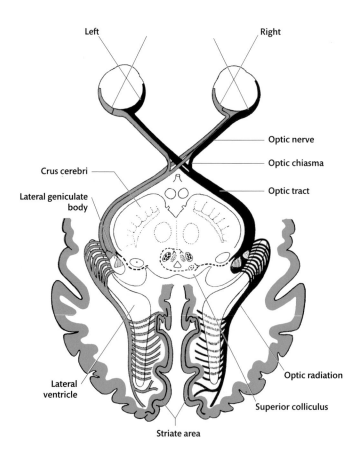

Fig. 31.33 Composite diagram to show the projection of the visual field upon the retinae, and the visual pathway.

Some fibres in the optic tract bypass the lateral geniculate body and enter the superior colliculus. These fibres form the **brachium of the superior colliculus** and are concerned with the production of visual reflexes such as turning of the head and eyes towards a sudden flash of light, and constriction of the pupil when light is shone into the eye [Figs. 30.5, 31.33].

Corticospinal tracts

The corona radiata, internal capsule, crus cerebri, longitudinal fibres of the ventral part of the pons, pyramid, and the corticospinal tracts form one continuous bundle of fibres [Fig. 31.34]. Only those fibres which enter the corticospinal tracts run through the whole extent of this pathway. It is through this 'motor' pathway that the cerebral cortex acts on the spinal cord.

The majority of fibres in the corticospinal tract arise in the motor cortex [Figs. 31.10, 31.34]. In the ventral part of the upper medulla, they form the pyramids. The majority of fibres decussate in the pyramidal decussation to form the lateral corticospinal tract in the lateral column of the spinal cord. The corticospinal tract ends in the grey matter of the spinal cord on the anterior horn cells, and controls the movement of skeletal muscles of the trunk and limbs. Some pyramidal fibres do not decussate in the medulla but continue as the anterior corticospinal tract in the spinal cord [see Figs. 27.4, 28.10]. The anterior corticospinal tracts extend down to the thoracic region of the spinal cord. Its fibres cross at every level superior to this and end in the grey matter of the opposite side [Fig. 31.35]. ➲ Damage to the corticospinal tract anywhere along its course will cause an upper motor neuron type of paralysis of the muscles supplied by it.

Dorsal column–medial lemniscus pathway

The dorsal column–medial lemniscus pathway is concerned with appreciation of crude touch, two-point discrimination, and proprioception. The first-order neurons are located in the dorsal root ganglion, from which the fibres enter the spinal cord at the dorsal root entry zone and ascend in the posterior column [see Fig. 27.3]. These fibres end in the nuclei gracilis and cuneatus in the lower part of the medulla [see Figs. 28.3, 28.7; Fig. 31.36]. Second-order neurons arise from the nuclei gracilis and cuneatus, cross the midline as internal arcuate fibres, and ascend in the medial lemniscus through the upper medulla, pons, and midbrain. They end in the ventroposterior lateral (VPL) nucleus of the

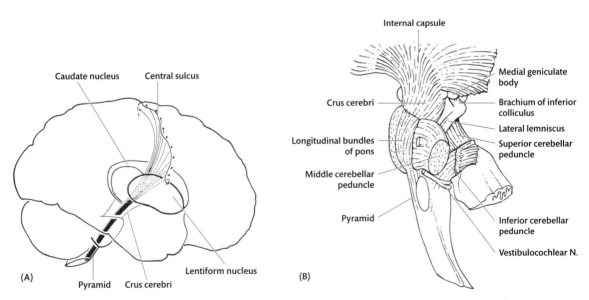

Fig. 31.34 (A) Diagram to show the course of fibres arising in the precentral gyrus (motor cortex) and passing through the corona radiata, internal capsule, crus cerebri, pons, and pyramid. (B) Deep dissection of the brainstem. The left half of the pons has been removed to show the longitudinal fibres passing through it to become continuous with the pyramid in the medulla oblongata.

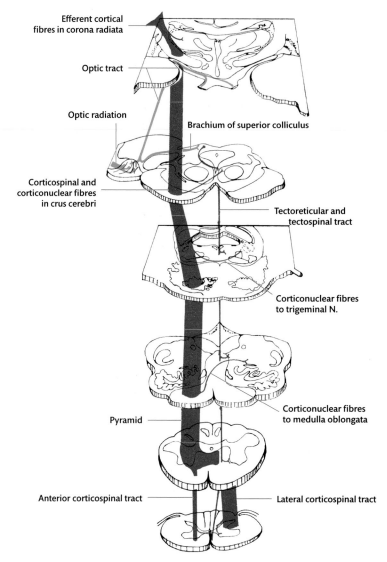

Efferent cortical
fibres in corona radiata

Optic tract

Optic radiation

Brachium of superior colliculus

Corticospinal and
corticonuclear fibres
in crus cerebri

Tectoreticular and
tectospinal tract

Corticonuclear fibres
to trigeminal N.

Corticonuclear fibres
to medulla oblongata

Pyramid

Anterior corticospinal tract

Lateral corticospinal tract

Fig. 31.35 A diagram to show the course of the corticonuclear and corticospinal fibres (red) through the brainstem. Serial sections are shown through the spinal cord, lower medulla, upper medulla, pons, midbrain, and thalamus.

thalamus. Third-order neurons from the VPL nucleus ascend to the sensory cortex in the thalamo-cortical or sensory radiations [see Fig. 30.6B; Fig. 31.10].

Spinothalamic tract

The spinothalamic tract carries sensation of fine touch and pain from the body, to the thalamus. The first-order neurons are located in the dorsal root ganglion. Their fibres end in the posterior grey horn of the spinal cord. The second-order neurons arise from the posterior horn cells, cross the midline in the white commissure, and ascend in the anterolateral column of the spinal cord [see

Fig. 27.6] and through the brainstem [Fig. 31.36]. They end in the VPL nucleus of the thalamus. The third-order neurons from the thalamus ascend to the sensory cortex through the sensory radiation. (Note: the thalamic nuclei of termination and the final pathway for the dorsal column–medial lemniscus pathway and spinothalamic tract are the same.)

Auditory pathway

The auditory impulses from the internal ear reach the cochlear nucleus which lies on either side of the inferior cerebellar peduncle at the junction of the medulla and pons [see Fig. 28.9]. Some fibres

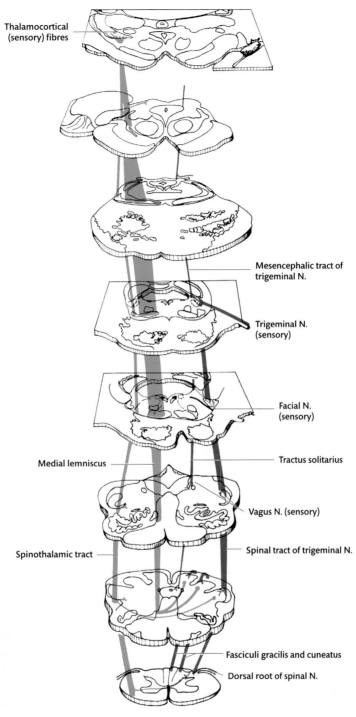

Thalamocortical (sensory) fibres

Mesencephalic tract of trigeminal N.

Trigeminal N. (sensory)

Facial N. (sensory)

Medial lemniscus

Tractus solitarius

Vagus N. (sensory)

Spinothalamic tract

Spinal tract of trigeminal N.

Fasciculi gracilis and cuneatus

Dorsal root of spinal N.

Fig. 31.36 An outline diagram to show the spinothalamic and dorsal column–medial lemniscus pathway. Serial sections are shown through the spinal cord, mid-medulla, upper medulla, lower and upper pons, lower and upper midbrain, and thalamus.

from the cochlear nucleus cross the midline in the trapezoid body [see Fig. 28.12]. They form the lateral lemniscus at the lateral end of the trapezoid body and are joined by uncrossed fibres from the cochlear nucleus of that side. The lateral meniscus

ascends with the medial lemniscus and spinothalamic tract. The ascending fibres in the lateral lemniscus are therefore from the cochlear nucleus of the same side—uncrossed fibres, and the cochlear nucleus of the opposite side, having crossed in the

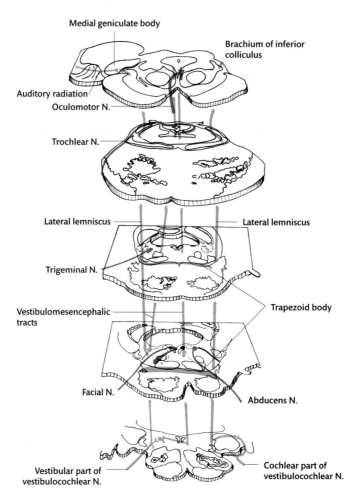

Medial geniculate body

Brachium of inferior colliculus

Auditory radiation

Oculomotor N.

Trochlear N.

Lateral lemniscus — — Lateral lemniscus

Trigeminal N.

Vestibulomesencephalic tracts

Trapezoid body

Facial N.

Abducens N.

Vestibular part of vestibulocochlear N.

Cochlear part of vestibulocochlear N.

Fig. 31.37 An outline diagram to show the ascending connections of the cochlear part of the vestibulocochlear nerve (blue). Serial sections are shown through the upper medulla, lower and upper pons, lower midbrain, and junction of the midbrain and thalamus.

trapezoid body. The lateral lemniscus ends in the inferior colliculus. The inferior colliculus sends impulses through the **brachium of the inferior colliculus** to the medial geniculate body. From the medial geniculate body, the auditory impulses reach the transverse temporal gyrus through the auditory radiation [Fig. 31.37].

➲ From the above description, it is clear that each lateral lemniscus and the other parts of the auditory pathway superior to it carry impulses from both

ears. This arrangement enables the appreciation of time difference in the arrival of sounds at the two ears and sound localization. It also explains why damage to this pathway on one side does not cause hearing loss on one side. By contrast, injury to the vestibulocochlear nerve would result in hearing loss on that side.

See Clinical Applications 31.1, 31.2, 31.3, 31.4, and 31.5 for the practical implications of the anatomy discussed in this chapter.

CLINICAL APPLICATION 31.1 Middle cerebral artery stroke

A 60-year-old woman on irregular treatment for diabetes mellitus, hypertension, and hypercholesterolaemia was taking her regular evening walk when she suddenly developed right-sided hemiparesis, hemianaesthesia, loss of consciousness, and seizures. On awakening, she had severe weakness of the right arm and right leg, and an inability to express herself verbally (motor aphasia). Imaging studies showed features of a stroke caused by a middle cerebral artery (MCA) territory infarct [Fig. 31.38].

Study question 1: what is an infarct? (Answer: an infarct is an acute shortage of blood supply to tissue or an organ, resulting in focal death of tissue, in this case, to the region of the brain supplied by the MCA.)

Study question 2: what is the cause for a cerebral stroke? (Answer: there are two main causes for strokes, and strokes are classified accordingly as: (1) ischaemic strokes; and (2) haemorrhagic strokes. Ischaemic strokes are more common and caused by obstruction of blood vessels, either by a thrombus within a cerebral blood vessel or an embolus (dislodged thrombus) from another vessel outside the cranial cavity. Haemorrhagic strokes are caused by rupture of cerebral blood vessels.)

Study question 3: on which side is the lesion? (Answer: sensory and motor fibres cross in the spinal cord or medulla oblongata. To cause signs in the right side of the body, as seen in this case, the MCA infarct would have to be on the left. Also the motor speech centre situated in the left cerebral hemisphere (dominant hemisphere) is affected in this patient.) Motor aphasia suggests that the anterior branch of the MCA is probably affected in this patient. Posterior branch lesions would cause sensory aphasia with deficits in reception of verbal commands. Main trunk lesions would cause extensive sensorimotor deficit and global aphasia.

Study question 4: what symptoms would be seen in a stroke affecting the right MCA territory? (Answer: a right MCA stroke would cause left-sided hemiparesis, hemianaesthesia, and other specific deficits such as inattention to a sensory stimulus on the left side, dressing apraxia (an inability to use familiar items of clothing to dress oneself), constructional apraxia (an inability to draw or construct simple configurations), and topographic memory deficit where an individual gets lost in familiar surroundings. These are all functions of the right (non-dominant) hemisphere.)

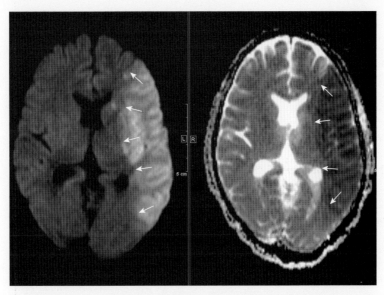

Fig. 31.38 Diffusion-weighted magnetic resonance image showing an infarct in the middle cerebral artery. Arrows indicate the boundary of the infarcted area.

CLINICAL APPLICATION 31.2 Brain tumour

A 48-year-old man presented with complaints of persistent headache, vomiting, and loss of appetite. Magnetic resonance imaging revealed an astrocytoma in the medial part of the parietal lobe [Fig. 31.39].

Study question 1: given the location of the tumour, which part of the body is likely to exhibit a sensory loss? (Answer: the right lower limbs and perineum.)

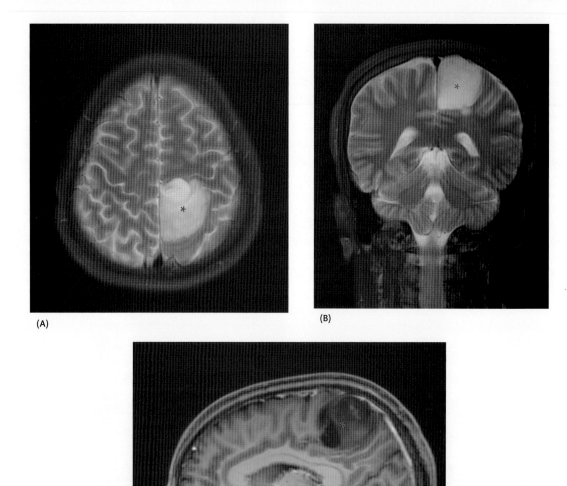

(A)

(B)

(C)

Fig. 31.39 A brain tumour—astrocytoma—in the parietal lobe (asterisk). (A) T2-weighted axial magnetic resonance imaging (MRI). (B) T2-weighted coronal MRI. (C) T1-weighted sagittal post-contrast MRI.

CLINICAL APPLICATION 31.3 Visual field defects

The visual field is divided into four quadrants—right upper, right lower, left upper, and left lower quadrants. Impulses from the visual field pass through the eye and fall on a segment of the retina. (1) Visual impulses from the left half of the field of vision fall on the right half of the retinae (the temporal half of the right retina and the nasal half of the left retina). (2) Visual impulses from the right half of the field of vision fall on the left half of the retinae (the temporal half of the left retina and the nasal half of the right retina). (3) Visual impulses from the upper half of the field of vision fall on the lower half of retinae. (4) Visual impulses from the lower half of the field of vision fall on the upper half of retinae.

Damage to any part of the visual pathway will lead to a defect in the field of vision. The type of visual field defect will depend on the site and size of the lesion. Fig. 31.40A shows the location of six lesions in the visual pathway, indicated by letters A–E. Fig. 31.40B shows the visual field defect in each of these lesions.

Lesion A: damage to a small part of the right retina on the temporal side. Visual field defect: monocular scotoma (focal loss of vision) in the right eye, affecting part of the left field of vision.

Lesion B: damage to the right optic nerve. Visual field defect: blindness in the right eye.

Lesion C: damage to the optic chiasma. Visual field defect: bitemporal hemianopia. Severing of fibres from the nasal halves of both retinae will lead to loss of the temporal half of the field of vision in both eyes. Further fibres from parts of the retinae cross in the upper part of the chiasma. Therefore, damage to the upper part of the chiasma will result in a lower bitemporal visual field defect, and damage to the lower part of the chiasma will result in an upper bitemporal visual field defect.

Lesion D: damage to the optic tract. Visual field defect: contralateral homonymous hemianopia. Each optic tract contains fibres from the temporal half of the ipsilateral retina and the nasal half of the contralateral retina—parts of the retinae receiving impulses from the opposite half of the visual field. As such, destruction of one optic tract will result in loss of the opposite half of the field of vision—contralateral homonymous hemianopia.

Lesion F: damage to the entire optic radiation. Visual field defect: contralateral homonymous hemianopia—same as the result of damage to the optic tract.

Lesion E: damage confined to the optic radiation fibres which curve around the inferior horn of the lateral ventricle. Visual field defect: contralateral homonymous superior quadrantanopia—due to damage to fibres carrying impulses from the superior quadrants of the opposite visual fields.

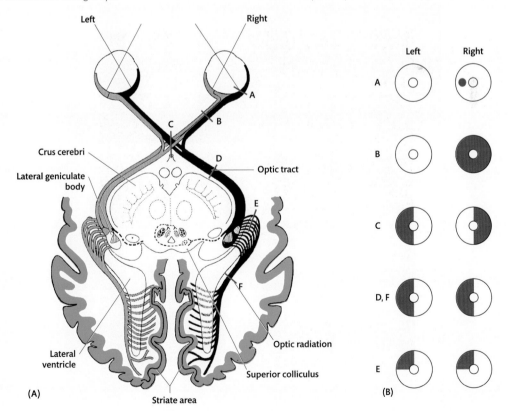

Fig. 31.40 (A) Visual pathway with lesions at different sites. (B) Visual field defects arising from visual pathway lesions.

CLINICAL APPLICATION 31.4 Scotomata

Fibres carrying impulses from corresponding points of the two retinae lie together in the optic radiation. Hence a small injury in the radiation produces a blind spot (*scotoma*) in the contralateral half of the field of vision in the corresponding area of both eyes. It is more obvious to the patient than a scotoma produced by a small retinal lesion in one eye, as the latter is covered by the image on the intact retina of the other eye.

Scotomata produced by injuries of the upper part of the radiation or striate cortex are seen in the lower half of the field of vision, and vice versa, but both are in the contralateral field.

CLINICAL APPLICATION 31.5 Basal ganglia infarct

The head of the caudate nucleus, putamen, and globus pallidus are supplied mainly by the deep branches of the middle cerebral artery. Fig. 31.41 is a diffusion-weighted magnetic resonance (MR) image of an acute infarct of the left basal ganglia. Such cases may be asymptomatic. Signs of contralateral upper motor neuron type of hemiparesis, due to involvement of corticospinal and corticonuclear tracts, and sensory loss due to involvement of thalamocortical fibres may be present.

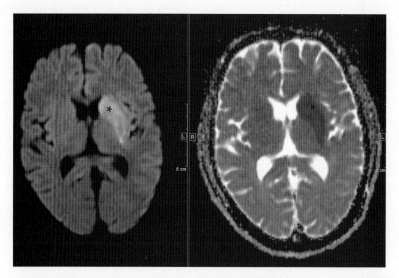

Fig. 31.41 Diffusion-weighted MRI showing an acute infarct in the left basal ganglia (asterisk).

CHAPTER 32
The ventricular system

Introduction

The ventricular system is a hollow, fluid-filled space derived from the cavities of the primitive brain vesicles. It is lined by ependyma. It consists of four ventricles: two lateral ventricles—one in each cerebral hemisphere—the third ventricle in the diencephalon, and the fourth ventricle between the pons, medulla, and cerebellum [Figs. 32.1, 32.2]. The ventricles contain cerebrospinal fluid (CSF) and the choroid plexus which produces it. The four ventricles are interconnected by the interventricular foramen between the two lateral ventricles and the third ventricle, and the cerebral aqueduct between the third and fourth ventricle. Inferiorly, the cavity of the fourth ventricle is continuous with the central canal in the inferior part of the medulla and, through that, with the central canal

of the spinal cord. The roof of the fourth ventricle has one median and two lateral apertures through which CSF leaves the ventricles and enters the sub-arachnoid space. From the subarachnoid space, the CSF drains into the superior sagittal sinus through the arachnoid villi and arachnoid granulations.

Formation of the choroid plexus

The choroid plexus lies within the ventricles and produces CSF. In specific locations of the developing brain, the pia mater covering the surface of the brain is invaginated into the ventricles and carries with it a covering of the ependymal lining of the ventricles. The invaginating pia mater is vascularized by a tuft of choroidal vessels and is known as the **tela choroidea**. The choroid plexus is formed by: (1) the invaginating vascularized pia mater; and (2) the ependymal covering [Fig. 32.3].

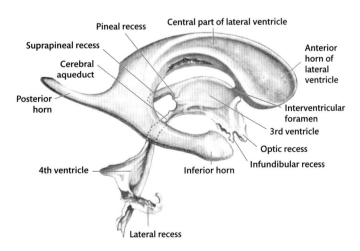

Fig. 32.1 Cast of the ventricles of the brain.

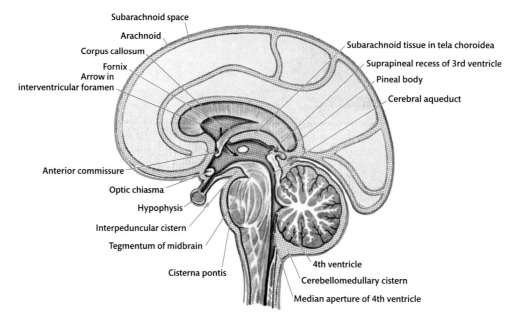

Subarachnoid space
Arachnoid
Corpus callosum
Fornix
Arrow in interventricular foramen
Anterior commissure
Optic chiasma
Hypophysis
Interpeduncular cistern
Tegmentum of midbrain
Cisterna pontis

Subarachnoid tissue in tela choroidea
Suprapineal recess of 3rd ventricle
Pineal body
Cerebral aqueduct
4th ventricle
Cerebellomedullary cistern
Median aperture of 4th ventricle

Fig. 32.2 Median section of the brain to show membranes and cisterns. Red = pia mater; blue stipple = subarachnoid space and ventricles; blue = arachnoid; pink = surface view of the shallow subarachnoid space. The lines of blue stipple running over the pink area indicate the places where the subarachnoid space is deeper around the branches of the anterior and posterior cerebral arteries.

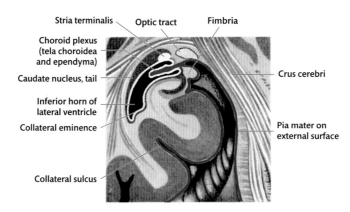

Stria terminalis
Optic tract
Fimbria
Choroid plexus (tela choroidea and ependyma)
Caudate nucleus, tail
Inferior horn of lateral ventricle
Collateral eminence
Collateral sulcus
Crus cerebri
Pia mater on external surface

Fig. 32.3 Coronal section through the inferior horn of the lateral ventricle.

Lateral ventricle

The lateral ventricle is a C-shaped cavity which lies in the cerebrum [Figs. 32.1, 32.4A]. It has an **anterior horn**, a **central part** or **body**, an **inferior horn**, and a **posterior horn**. The anterior end of the C—the anterior horn—extends into the frontal lobe and is continuous behind with the central part. The lower limb of the C runs forwards as the inferior horn in the temporal lobe. The posterior horn projects backwards from the convexity of the C into the occipital lobe [Fig. 32.1]. The size and shape of the lateral ventricle are very variable. ⮑ In young children, a prolonged increase in pressure in the ventricles causes the brain and skull to expand, as the sutures are not closed (hydrocephalus). In older children and adults, no such expansion is possible, and distension of the ventricle results in the loss of nervous tissue.

Using the instructions given in Dissection 32.1, divide the hemisphere to open the lateral ventricle.

DISSECTION 32.1 Opening of the lateral ventricle

Objective

I. To open into the lateral ventricle.

Instructions

Dissection 32.1 is illustrated in Fig. 32.4. It exposes the entire lateral ventricle by dividing the brain into two parts which may be readily fitted together again, so that the form and position of the ventricle and the choroid fissure may be appreciated.

1. Study Fig. 32.4A to gauge the approximate position of the lateral ventricle.

2. Place the point of a knife in the interventricular foramen, and make a vertical cut through the fornix, septum pellucidum, and medial aspect of the hemisphere, as shown in Fig. 32.4B.

3. Open the cut as it is made, and carry the point of the knife as far as the lateral edge of the lateral ventricle, but avoid cutting into its floor.

4. Now turn the knife, so that its edge faces posteriorly, and cut backwards and then downwards, following the curve of the lateral ventricle with the point of the knife. Extend the incision as far as the posterior ramus of the lateral sulcus [Fig. 32.4C], and open the cut as you proceed.

5. Note the ridge of the choroid plexus protruding into the ventricle from its floor [Fig. 32.5].

6. Depress the temporal lobe strongly, exposing the inferior part of the insula.

7. Keeping the knife in the ventricle and holding it as nearly vertical as possible, cut forwards through the medial part of the transverse temporal gyri on the superior surface of the temporal lobe, and enter the sulcus (circular sulcus) which separates the insula from the temporal lobe. This cut divides the white matter passing horizontally into the temporal lobe and opens into the roof of the inferior horn of the lateral ventricle.

8. Carry the cut anteriorly along the circular sulcus to the stem of the lateral sulcus [Fig. 32.4D], opening the cut and confirming that it enters the inferior horn of the lateral ventricle as you proceed.

9. The hemisphere is now separated into two parts which are held together by the ependyma which passes over the choroid plexus between them. The two parts are: (1) an anterior part, with the brainstem attached to it; and (2) a posterior part which includes parts of the frontal and parietal lobes, the arch of the fornix, the fimbria, the hippocampus, and the trunk and splenium of the corpus callosum.

10. Turn to the medial side, and lift the fornix away from the superior surface of the thalamus. Separate the choroid plexus from the fornix, and leave it attached to the thalamus.

11. Note the position of the choroid plexus of the lateral ventricle, and follow it from the interventricular foramen into the inferior horn of the ventricle.

12. Slowly separate the two parts of the cerebrum along the line of the choroid fissure, between the fornix and the thalamus, and note the posterior choroidal branches of the posterior cerebral artery passing to the choroid plexus. Divide these vessels to prevent them from pulling the choroid plexus from the surface of the thalamus.

13. When the two parts have been separated, they may be replaced as often as necessary to relate the internal appearances to the surface structures.

Transverse fissure, choroid fissure, and choroid plexus

The transverse fissure lies between the splenium of the corpus callosum and the dorsal surface of the thalamus [Fig. 32.2]. The tela choroidea common to the central part of the lateral ventricle and the third ventricle extends anteriorly through the transverse fissure below the fornix and superior to the roof of the third ventricle [Fig. 32.2]. It contains the internal cerebral veins and posterior choroidal branches of the posterior cerebral arteries [Fig. 32.6]. The tela choroidea narrows anteriorly, as the two lateral ventricles and their choroid plexuses approach one another, and ends in an apex at the interventricular foramen. The choroid plexus of the lateral ventricle becomes continuous with the corresponding choroid plexus of the third ventricle through the interventricular foramen [Figs. 32.6, 32.7]. These two strips of the choroid plexus in the third ventricle lie side by side on the inferior surface of the tela choroidea, close to the midline [Fig. 32.7].

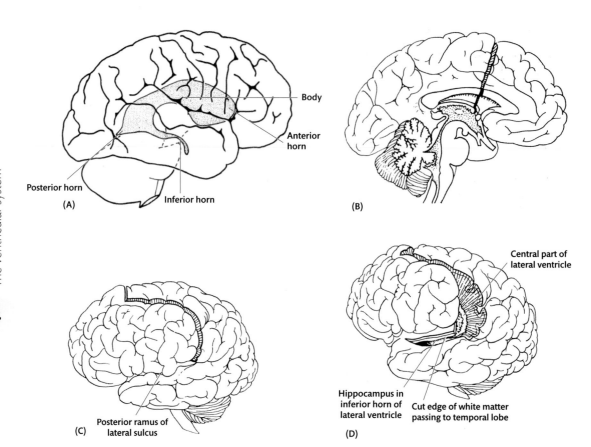

Fig. 32.4 (A) Drawing to show the parts and position of the lateral ventricle (shaded) in the cerebral hemisphere. (B), (C), and (D) Drawings to show the first, second, and third incisions to be made in Dissection 32.1.

The choroid fissure is the space along which the vascular pia mater enters into the lateral ventricle to form the choroid plexus of the lateral ventricle. No nervous tissue is developed in this narrow strip of the ventricular wall, so that the vascular pia mater is applied directly to the ependymal lining. The choroid fissure of the lateral ventricle follows the line of the C and lies in the concavity of the curve of the **fimbria** and **fornix**, between the fornix and the thalamus in the central part of the ventricle [Fig. 32.8] and below the fimbria in the inferior horn. (The choroid fissure should be distinguished from the transverse fissure [see Fig. 24.7], through which the tela choroidea of the third and central parts of the lateral ventricles is continuous with the pia mater on the surface of the midbrain.)

In the central part of each lateral ventricle, the choroid plexus of the lateral ventricle lies at the lateral extremity of a continuous sheet of the pia mater—**tela choroidea of the third and lateral ventricles**. This sheet covers the dorsal surface of the thalamus and the roof of the third

ventricle [Figs. 32.6, 32.7]. As the ventricles turn downwards, this pia mater is continuous with the pia mater on either side of the upper midbrain. In the inferior horn, each choroid fissure passes forwards to the posterior margin of the uncus, parallel to the optic tract and between it and the margin of the hemisphere [Figs. 32.3, 32.9].

Parts of the lateral ventricle

The **anterior horn** of the lateral ventricle curves inferiorly into the frontal lobe from the interventricular foramen. It is triangular-shaped in coronal section. The narrow floor is formed by the genu and rostrum, the roof by the trunk, and the anterior wall by the genu of the corpus callosum. The vertical medial wall is formed by the septum pellucidum and the column of the fornix, and the lateral wall by the bulging head of the caudate nucleus [see Figs. 31.21, 31.26, 31.27; Fig. 32.10].

The **central part** of the lateral ventricle is roofed by the trunk of the corpus callosum. The

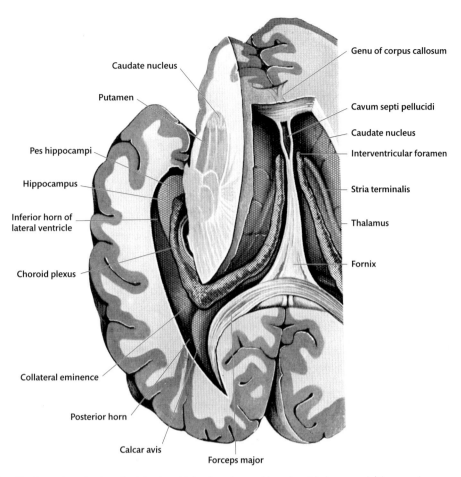

Caudate nucleus

Putamen

Pes hippocampi

Hippocampus

Inferior horn of
lateral ventricle

Choroid plexus

Collateral eminence

Posterior horn

Calcar avis

Forceps major

Genu of corpus callosum

Cavum septi pellucidi

Caudate nucleus

Interventricular foramen

Stria terminalis

Thalamus

Fornix

Fig. 32.5 Dissection from above to show the lateral ventricles. Ependyma = blue; choroid plexus = red. (The ependyma covering the choroid plexus is not shown.)

medial wall is formed by the fornix and septum pellucidum anteriorly, and the fornix posteriorly [see Figs. 31.29, 31.30]. The floor is made up of the following structures from lateral to medial: (1) the **caudate nucleus**, which lies in the angle between the floor and the roof and narrows rapidly as it is traced posteriorly [see Figs. 30.2, 31.28, 31.29, 31.30; Figs. 32.5, 32.6]; (2) the **thalamostriate vein**, which runs anteriorly in the groove between the thalamus and caudate nucleus and passes medially beneath the ependyma to join the internal cerebral vein at the interventricular foramen. A number of tributaries enter it from the centre of the hemisphere by running across the caudate nucleus, deep to the ependyma [see Fig. 32.6]; (3) the **stria terminalis**, which runs with the thalamostriate vein; it is a slender bundle of fibres running from the amygdala to the grey matter around the anterior commissure [see Fig. 30.2]; (4) a narrow strip of the dorsal surface of the thalamus; (5) the

choroid plexus [see Fig. 32.7]; and (6) the **fornix** [see Fig. 32.5].

The **posterior horn** begins inferior to the splenium of the corpus callosum and extends posteriorly into the occipital lobe. The roof, lateral wall, and floor are formed by a sheet of fibres from the splenium of the corpus callosum—the tapetum—which arches over it and passes inferiorly to the lower parts of the occipital lobe [see Fig. 31.19; Fig. 32.11]. The medial wall is invaginated by two ridges; the upper of these—the **bulb of the posterior horn**—is formed by the fibres of the forceps major. The lower ridge—the **calcar avis**—is produced by the calcarine sulcus which extends into it from the medial surface of the occipital lobe [Figs. 32.11, 32.12].

The **inferior horn** is the continuation of the ventricular cavity into the temporal lobe [see Figs. 32.1, 31.29, 31.30, 31.31]. It runs inferiorly, posterior to the thalamus, and then passes anteriorly,

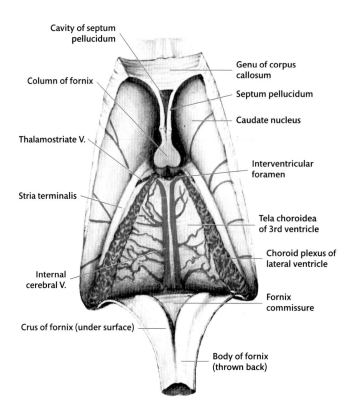

Fig. 32.6 Tela choroidea of the third and lateral ventricles exposed from above, by dividing the columns of the fornix and turning them backwards.

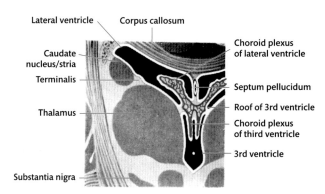

Fig. 32.7 Coronal section through the thalamus and associated structures, just posterior to the interventricular foramen. Note the choroid plexuses of the third and lateral ventricles.

curving medially to end at the uncus. The lateral wall is formed by the tapetum of the corpus callosum. The roof consists of the white matter which passes laterally into the temporal lobe (including the sublentiform part of the internal capsule), the stria terminalis, and the tail of the caudate nucleus [Fig. 32.9]. The stria terminalis and the caudate nucleus can be followed from the floor of the central part of the ventricle to the amygdala at the tip of the inferior horn. The floor is broad posteriorly where the inferior and posterior horns meet, and is often raised—the **collateral triangle**—by the collateral sulcus [Fig. 32.12]. Anteriorly the medial part is formed by the **hippocampus** covered by the **alveus**. The **amygdala** overlies the tip of the inferior horn of the lateral ventricle.

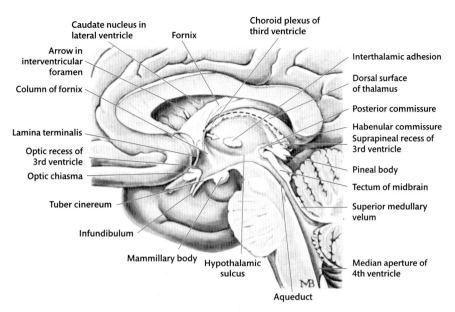

Fig. 32.8 Median section through the third and fourth ventricles of the brain. The septum pellucidum has been removed to expose the lateral ventricle. Red line = choroid fissure in the central part of the lateral ventricle.

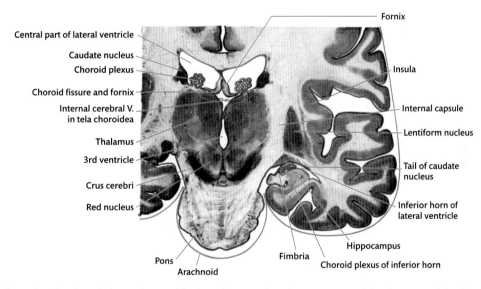

Fig. 32.9 Coronal section through the cerebrum, midbrain, and pons to show the arrangement of the pia mater and the choroid plexuses of the lateral ventricle. Pia mater = red; arachnoid mater, ependyma, and internal cerebral veins = blue.

The third ventricle

The narrow, slit-like third ventricle lies in the midline within the diencephalon. It extends from the lamina terminalis anteriorly to the superior end of the aqueduct and root of the pineal posteriorly [Fig. 32.13].

The **roof** of the third ventricle consists of a layer of ependyma, which is invaginated on each side by the overlying vascular pia mater to form the linear choroid plexus on either side [Fig. 32.8]. The roof is attached on both sides to the stria medullaris thalami. It extends from the interventricular foramen to the habenular commissure

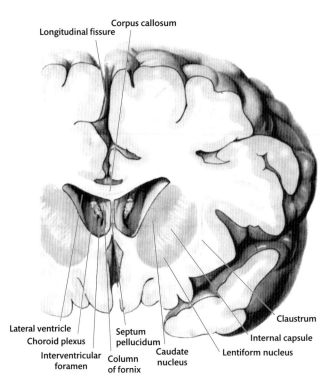

Fig. 32.10 Coronal section through the hemispheres behind the genu of the corpus callosum, seen from in front.

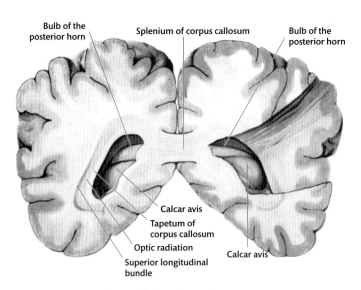

Fig. 32.11 Coronal section through the posterior horns of the lateral ventricles.

and curves over the superior surface of the pineal body to form the suprapineal recess of the ventricle [Figs. 32.2, 32.8].

The **floor** of the third ventricle extends posteriorly from the **optic recess** on the superior surface of the optic chiasma into the **infundibular recess**, and then passes above the mammillary bodies and the tegmentum of the midbrain to the aqueduct [Fig. 32.8].

The **anterior wall** is formed by the lamina terminalis. The anterior commissure lies at the superior end of this wall.

The **lateral wall** of the third ventricle is marked by a shallow groove—the **hypothalamic sulcus**—which extends from the interventricular foramen to the cerebral aqueduct. This sulcus separates the thalamus above from the hypothalamus below. Immediately above the sulcus, the two

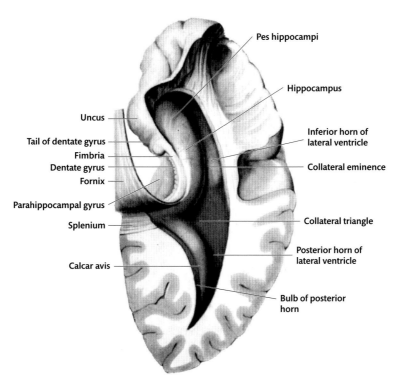

Fig. 32.12 Posterior and inferior horns of the right lateral ventricle, viewed from above.

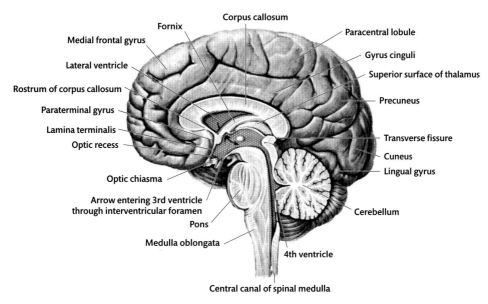

Fig. 32.13 Medial surface of the right half of a bisected brain. The septum pellucidum has been removed to expose the lateral ventricle. The arrow passes through the interventricular foramen from the lateral to the third ventricle. Ependymal lining of ventricles = blue.

thalami bulge towards each other and may fuse, forming the **interthalamic adhesion**. This adhesion has no functional significance, is variable in size, and is not a commissure. Immediately posterior to the anterior commissure, the column of the fornix forms a low ridge on the lateral wall. Posterior to the column of the fornix, and almost hidden by it, is a small, obliquely placed **interventricular foramen** which opens into the lateral ventricle. On each side, the narrow strip

The ventricular system

390

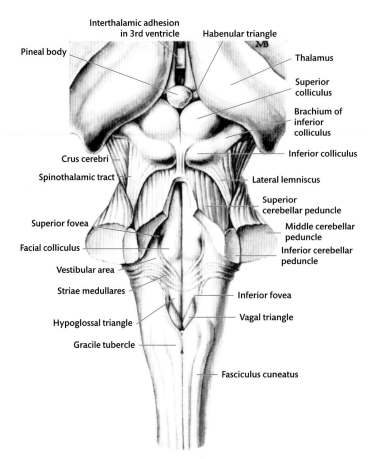

Pineal body

Interthalamic adhesion
in 3rd ventricle

Habenular triangle

Thalamus

Superior
colliculus

Brachium of
inferior
colliculus

Inferior colliculus

Crus cerebri

Spinothalamic tract

Lateral lemniscus

Superior
cerebellar peduncle

Superior fovea

Middle cerebellar
peduncle

Facial colliculus

Inferior cerebellar
peduncle

Vestibular area

Striae medullares

Inferior fovea

Vagal triangle

Hypoglossal triangle

Gracile tubercle

Fasciculus cuneatus

Fig. 32.14 Posterior view of the brainstem, showing the floor of the fourth ventricle.

of choroid plexus in the roof of the third ventricle becomes continuous with the choroid plexus of the corresponding lateral ventricle through the interventricular foramen. The foramen is often so narrow that it is nearly filled by the choroid plexus. ➲ Any hypertrophy of the plexus in this situation blocks the communication between the two ventricles, causing an increase in pressure in the lateral ventricle. If this is unilateral, it may be sufficient to cause compression of the opposite hemisphere and a shift of the midline structures towards that side.

The tela choroidea and choroid plexus of the third ventricle have been described earlier.

The fourth ventricle

The fourth ventricle is the cavity of the hindbrain. It extends from the superior border of the pons to the middle of the medulla oblongata. It lies behind the pons and the upper part of the medulla, and in front of the cerebellum and the medullary vela.

It narrows above to the superior angle where it becomes continuous with the cerebral aqueduct. Inferiorly, it continues with the small central canal of the inferior half of the medulla oblongata and spinal cord [Fig. 32.2].

The fourth ventricle is widest at the level of the junction of the pons and the medulla oblongata [see Fig. 28.3]. At this point, it extends laterally on each side to form a tubular **lateral recess**. The lateral recess curves over the posterior aspect of the inferior cerebellar peduncle, extends as far laterally as the tip of the flocculus, and opens into the subarachnoid space through the **lateral aperture** of the fourth ventricle. The lateral aperture lies posterior to the ninth and tenth cranial nerves [see Fig. 29.4A]. The deepest part of the ventricle is opposite the inferior part of the pons where the tent-like cerebellar recess extends posteriorly almost to the level of the dentate nuclei. Immediately inferior to this, the inferior medullary velum passes anteriorly, and the ventricle becomes a shallow slit. Its depth again increases towards the inferior angle, as the median part of the thin roof curves poste-riorly on the anterior surface of the cerebellum to the margin of the **median aperture** of the fourth ventricle [see Fig. 29.4A; Fig. 32.13].

⊃ Blockage of the median and lateral apertures by scar tissue following an injury or infection prevents the flow of cerebrospinal fluid into the subarachnoid space and causes it to accumulate in the cavities of the brain. This results in raised intracranial pressure. Similar scar tissue in the subarachnoid space can im-pede the flow of cerebrospinal fluid through it.

Roof of the fourth ventricle

Superior to the cerebellar recess, the superior med-ullary velum forms the greater part of the roof. This velum extends transversely between the two supe-rior cerebellar peduncles and gradually narrows as it approaches the tectum of the midbrain. Inferior to the cerebellar recess, the thin roof of the fourth ventricle extends in the midline from its cerebellar attachment to the margin of the median aperture [see Fig. 29.1] on the antero-inferior surface of the cerebellum. Laterally, the roof forms the bed of the tonsil (part of the cerebellum) and is attached to the posterior surface of the medulla oblongata. The lateral attachments converge towards the median aperture inferiorly, but superiorly they pass later-ally over the posterior surface of the inferior cer-ebellar peduncle to form the inferior limit of the lateral recess [see Fig. 29.4A].

Tela choroidea and choroid plexuses of the fourth ventricle

The pia mater on the surface of the brain passes be-tween the thin roof of the fourth ventricle and the cerebellum. It contains the posterior inferior cerebel-lar artery and forms the tela choroidea of the cho-roid plexus of the fourth ventricle. Each half of the choroid plexus is shaped like an inverted L. The two vertical limbs of the L lie on the roof of the fourth ventricle, on each side of the midline, from the mar-gin of the median aperture to the level of the lateral recess. From this point, the horizontal limbs of the L extend laterally into the roof of the corresponding lateral recess as far as the lateral aperture. At the lat-eral aperture, the extremities of the choroid plexus protrude as miniature cauliflower-like tufts, imme-diately inferior to the flocculus of the cerebellum. The extremities of both limbs of the L can be seen in the intact brain at the median and lateral apertures of the fourth ventricle [see Fig. 29.4].

Floor of the fourth ventricle

The floor of the fourth ventricle is diamond-shaped and covered by ependyma. It extends from the aqueduct superiorly to the central canal inferiorly. It is formed by the posterior surfaces of the pons and the superior half of the medulla oblongata. Its lateral boundaries are formed by the superior cerebellar peduncles, the inferior cerebellar peduncles, and the cuneate and gracile tubercles [Fig. 32.14]. For details on the other features of the floor of the fourth ventricle, see p. 309 and p. 310.

See Clinical Applications 32.1 and 32.2 for the practical implications of the anatomy discussed in this chapter.

CLINICAL APPLICATION 32.1 CSF rhinorrhoea

Fractures of the anterior cranial fossa could result in blood and cerebrospinal fluid leaking into the nose and/or the orbit. In addition, infection from the nose could spread to the meninges, and also into the frontal air sinus if the sinus invades the orbital part of the frontal bone.

CLINICAL APPLICATION 32.2 Hydrocephalus

Hydrocephalus literally means 'water in the head' and is due to excess fluid in the intracranial cavity. In infants with hydrocephalus, the fontanelles are bulged and the cranial cavity may expand to accommodate the excess fluid. The reasons for hydrocephalus are varied: (1) due to excess production of cerebrospinal fluid (CSF), as in the case of a choroid plexus papilloma—a rare tumour; (2) obstruction of CSF due to a mass or some congeni-tal malformation. Obstruction could be at the interven-tricular foramen, cerebral aqueduct, fourth ventricle, or in the subarachnoid space; and (3) decreased CSF absorption, due to damage or block of arachnoid gran-ulations.

Clinically, hydrocephalus is classified as: (1) commu-nicating hydrocephalus—when it is due to impaired CSF absorption or obstruction to flow in the subarachnoid space; and (2) non-communicating hydrocephalus when it is due to obstruction of flow in the ventricular system.

CHAPTER 33
MCQs for part 2: The brain and spinal cord

Each of the following questions have four options. Please choose the most correct answer.

1. **The lower extent of the spinal dura mater is at the level of the**

   A. L. 1 vertebra

   B. L. 3 vertebra

   C. S. 2 vertebra

   D. Coccyx

2. **Which of the following statements is NOT true about the thoracic nucleus of the spinal cord?**

   A. It extends through the thoracic and upper lumbar segments

   B. It is present in the ventral grey column

   C. It receives afferents from the fasciculus gracilis

   D. It sends axons to the cerebellum through the posterior spinocerebellar tract

3. **The nervus intermedius carries**

   A. Motor fibres

   B. Sensory fibres

   C. Parasympathetic fibres

   D. Both sensory and parasympathetic fibres

4. **Which one of the following is a branch of the vertebral artery?**

   A. Posterior inferior cerebellar artery

   B. Posterior cerebral artery

   C. Anterior inferior cerebellar artery

   D. Anterior cerebral artery

5. **The posterior external arcuate fibres arise from the**

   A. Arcuate nucleus

   B. Gracile nucleus

   C. Cuneate nucleus

   D. Accessory cuneate nucleus

6. **Fibres arising from pontine nuclei traverse the**

   A. Cerebral peduncle
   B. Superior cerebellar peduncle
   C. Middle cerebellar peduncle
   D. Inferior cerebellar peduncle

7. **The cranial nerve nucleus underlying the facial colliculus is the**

   A. Motor nucleus of the trigeminal nerve
   B. Chief sensory nucleus of the trigeminal nerve
   C. Abducens nucleus
   D. Motor nucleus of the facial nerve

8. **The climbing fibres are**

   A. Olivocerebellar fibres
   B. Cerebello-olivary fibres
   C. Pontocerebellar fibres
   D. Cerebellorubral fibres

9. **Which one of the following is a component of the tegmentum of the midbrain?**

   A. Red nucleus
   B. Substantia nigra
   C. Corticopontine fibres
   D. Corticonuclear fibres

10. **The artery that lies on the stem of the lateral sulcus is the**

    A. Anterior cerebral artery
    B. Middle cerebral artery
    C. Posterior cerebral artery
    D. Posterior communicating artery

11. **The name 'striate cortex' is given to the**

    A. Visual area
    B. Auditory area
    C. Motor area
    D. Broca's area

12. **The fibre bundle on the floor of the lateral ventricle between the thalamus and caudate nucleus is the**

    A. Stria medullaris thalami
    B. Stria medullaris
    C. Stria terminalis
    D. Linea terminalis

13. **Which one of the following is NOT true regarding the geniculate bodies?**

   A. The medial geniculate body receives the brachium of the inferior colliculus
   B. The lateral geniculate body is continuous anteriorly with the optic tract
   C. Destruction of the lateral geniculate body of one side will result in loss of vision in the same half of the field of vision
   D. Destruction of the medial geniculate body of one side has little effect on hearing

14. **Which one of the following is true regarding the uncinate fasciculus?**

   A. It is a commissure
   B. The fibre bundle passes between the temporal lobe and frontal lobe
   C. The fibre bundle passes between the temporal lobe and occipital lobe
   D. The fibre bundle passes between the frontal lobe and occipital lobe

15. **The afferent to the anterior nucleus of the thalamus is the**

   A. Mammillothalamic tract
   B. Medial lemniscus
   C. Spinal lemniscus
   D. Trigeminal lemniscus

Please go to the back of the book for the answers.

PART 3

Cross-sectional anatomy

397

CHAPTER 34

Cross-sectional anatomy of the head and neck

Cross-sectional anatomy of the head and neck

In this chapter, serial sections through the head and neck are presented alongside computerized to-mogram (CT) and magnetic resonance imaging (MRI) scans at approximately the same level. The relationship of the brain to the surrounding skull and soft tissue are shown. Fig. 34.1 is a sagittal section through the head on which the plane of Figs. 34.2, 34.3, 34.4, 34.5, 34.6, 34.7, 34.8, 34.9, 34.10, 34.11, and 34.12 are shown. Figs. 34.13, 34.14, and 34.15 are sections through the neck at sequentially lower levels. The CT and MRI scans are matched to the clos-est image available in the Visible Human Project.

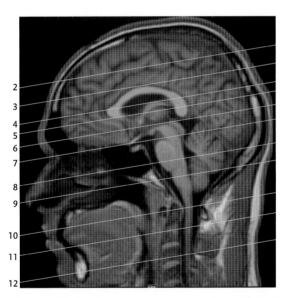

Fig. 34.1 Oblique lines on the sagittal section of the head to show the approximate plane of section for Figs. 34.2, 34.3, 34.4, 34.5, 34.6, 34.7, 34.8, 34.9, 34.10, 34.11, and 34.12.

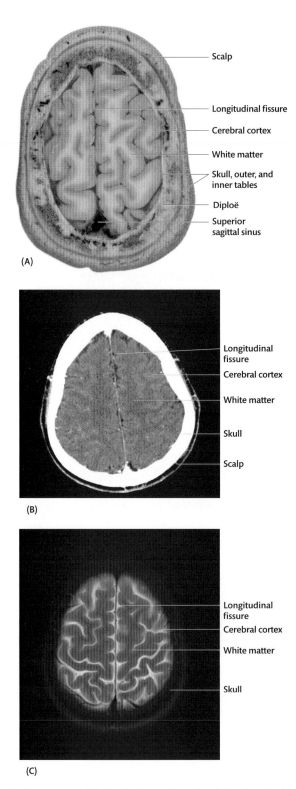

Fig. 34.2 (A) Cross-section through the upper part of the head, showing the scalp, skull, and cerebral hemisphere. (B) Post-contrast axial CT of the brain. (C) T2-weighted axial MRI.

Image A courtesy of the Visible Human Project of the US National Library of Medicine.

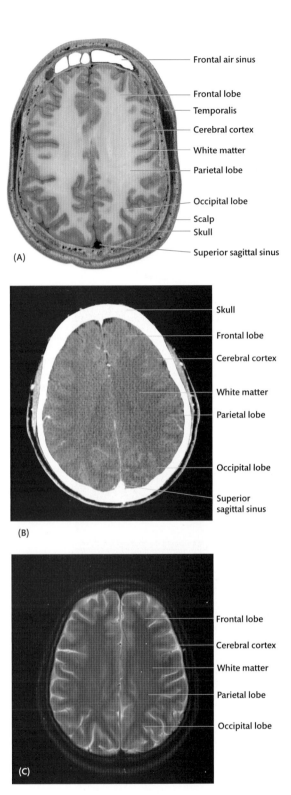

Fig. 34.3 (A) Cross-section through the upper part of the head at a slightly lower level than Fig. 34.2. The scalp, skull, and cerebral hemisphere are shown. (B) Post-contrast axial CT of the brain. (C) T2-weighted axial MRI.

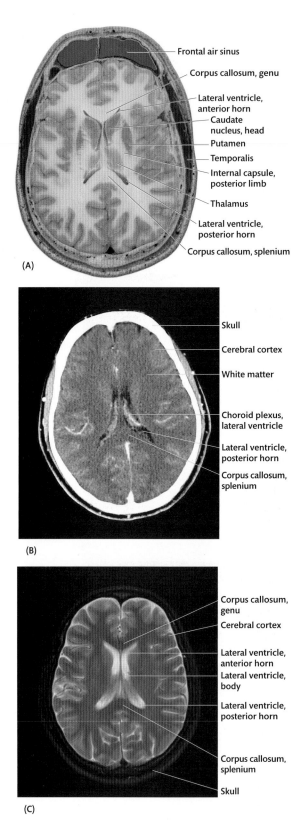

Frontal air sinus

Corpus callosum, genu

Lateral ventricle, anterior horn

Caudate nucleus, head

Putamen

Temporalis

Internal capsule, posterior limb

Thalamus

Lateral ventricle, posterior horn

Corpus callosum, splenium

(A)

Skull

Cerebral cortex

White matter

Choroid plexus, lateral ventricle

Lateral ventricle, posterior horn

Corpus callosum, splenium

(B)

Corpus callosum, genu

Cerebral cortex

Lateral ventricle, anterior horn

Lateral ventricle, body

Lateral ventricle, posterior horn

Corpus callosum, splenium

Skull

(C)

Fig. 34.4 (A) Cross-section through the head at a slightly lower level than Fig. 34.3. The cerebral hemispheres, lateral ventricles, and a small part of the thalamus are seen. (B) Post-contrast axial CT of the brain, showing parts of the lateral ventricle and the choroid plexus. (C) T2-weighted axial MRI. The lateral ventricle is seen clearly.

Image A courtesy of the Visible Human Project of the US National Library of Medicine.

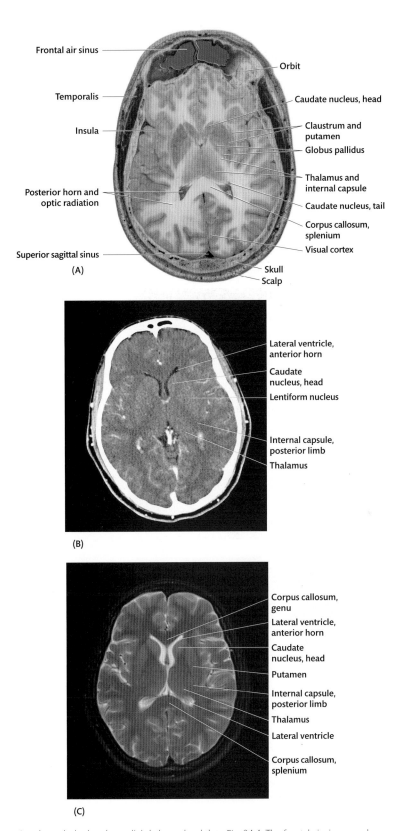

Frontal air sinus

Orbit

Temporalis

Caudate nucleus, head

Insula

Claustrum and putamen

Globus pallidus

Thalamus and internal capsule

Posterior horn and optic radiation

Caudate nucleus, tail

Corpus callosum, splenium

Superior sagittal sinus

Visual cortex

(A)

Skull
Scalp

Lateral ventricle, anterior horn

Caudate nucleus, head

Lentiform nucleus

Internal capsule, posterior limb

Thalamus

(B)

Corpus callosum, genu

Lateral ventricle, anterior horn

Caudate nucleus, head

Putamen

Internal capsule, posterior limb

Thalamus

Lateral ventricle

Corpus callosum, splenium

(C)

Fig. 34.5 (A) Cross-section through the head at a slightly lower level than Fig. 34.4. The frontal air sinus, cerebrum, and thalamus are seen. (B) Post-contrast axial CT. (C) T2-weighted axial MRI.

Image A courtesy of the Visible Human Project of the US National Library of Medicine.

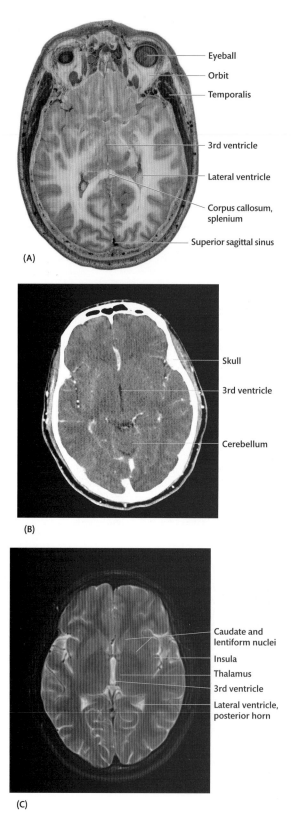

(A)

Eyeball

Orbit

Temporalis

3rd ventricle

Lateral ventricle

Corpus callosum, splenium

Superior sagittal sinus

(B)

Skull

3rd ventricle

Cerebellum

(C)

Caudate and lentiform nuclei

Insula

Thalamus

3rd ventricle

Lateral ventricle, posterior horn

Fig. 34.6 (A) Cross-section through the head at a slightly lower level than Fig. 34.5. The orbit, nasal cavity, and cerebral hemispheres are seen. (B) Post-contrast axial CT. (C) T2-weighted axial MRI. The CT and MRI images are taken above the orbit.

Image A courtesy of the Visible Human Project of the US National Library of Medicine.

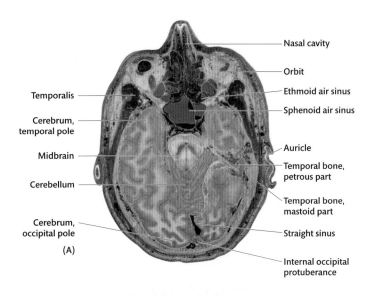

Nasal cavity

Orbit

Ethmoid air sinus

Sphenoid air sinus

Temporalis

Cerebrum, temporal pole

Midbrain

Cerebellum

Auricle

Temporal bone, petrous part

Temporal bone, mastoid part

Cerebrum, occipital pole

Straight sinus

(A)

Internal occipital protuberance

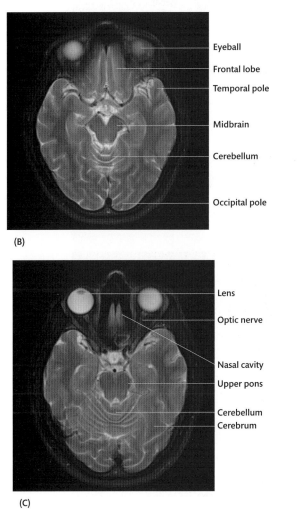

Eyeball

Frontal lobe

Temporal pole

Midbrain

Cerebellum

Occipital pole

(B)

Lens

Optic nerve

Nasal cavity

Upper pons

Cerebellum
Cerebrum

(C)

Fig. 34.7 (A) Cross-section through the head at a slightly lower level than Fig. 34.6. The nasal cavity, orbit, auricle, cerebrum, midbrain, and part of the cerebellum are seen. (B) T2-weighted axial MRI. (C) T2-weighted axial MRI at a slightly lower level than Fig. 34.7B. The upper pons and cerebellum are seen.

Image A courtesy of the Visible Human Project of the US National Library of Medicine.

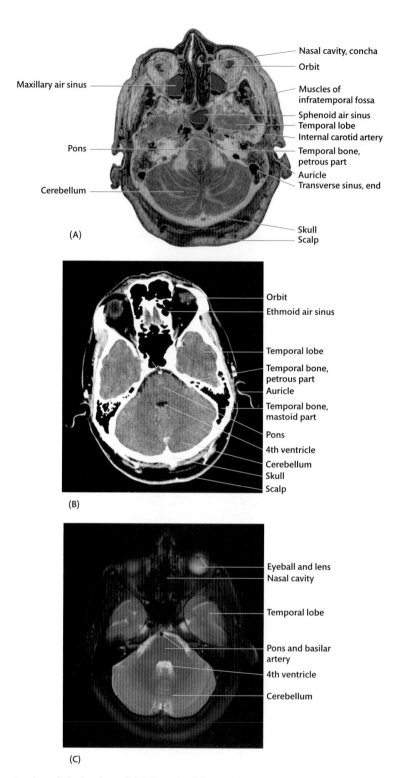

Nasal cavity, concha

Orbit

Maxillary air sinus

Muscles of
infratemporal fossa

Sphenoid air sinus

Temporal lobe

Internal carotid artery

Pons

Temporal bone,
petrous part

Auricle

Transverse sinus, end

Cerebellum

Skull

Scalp

(A)

Orbit

Ethmoid air sinus

Temporal lobe

Temporal bone,
petrous part

Auricle

Temporal bone,
mastoid part

Pons

4th ventricle

Cerebellum

Skull

Scalp

(B)

Eyeball and lens

Nasal cavity

Temporal lobe

Pons and basilar
artery

4th ventricle

Cerebellum

(C)

Fig. 34.8 (A) Cross-section through the head at a slightly lower level than Fig. 34.7. The lower part of the orbit, nasal cavity, upper part of the sphenoid and maxillary air sinus, infratemporal fossa, pons, and cerebellum are seen. (B) Post-contrast axial CT. Red arrow = basilar artery. (C) T2-weighted axial MRI.

Image A courtesy of the Visible Human Project of the US National Library of Medicine.

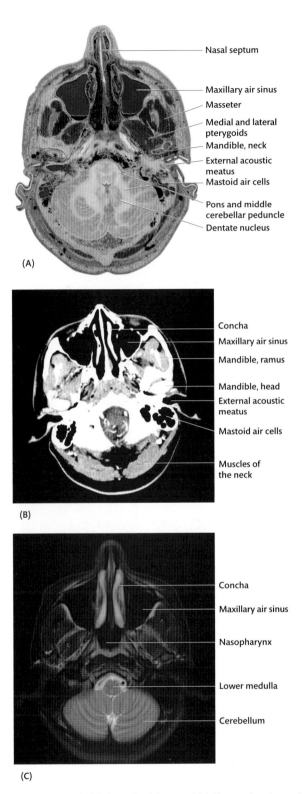

Fig. 34.9 (A) Cross-section through the head at a slightly lower level than Fig. 34.8. The nasal cavity, maxillary air sinus, right temporo-mandibular joint (= asterisk), muscles of mastication, external ear, mastoid air cells, pons, cerebellum, and middle cerebellar peduncle are seen. Red arrow = right internal carotid artery. (B) Post-contrast axial CT. (C) T2-weighted axial MRI. Asterisk = right lateral pterygoid.

Image A courtesy of the Visible Human Project of the US National Library of Medicine.

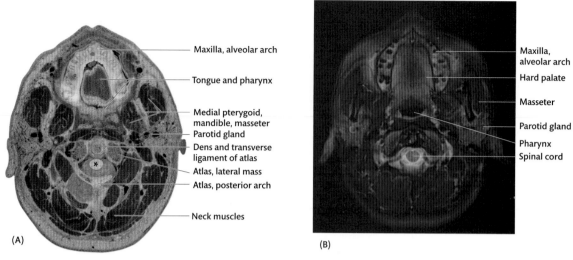

Fig. 34.10 (A) Cross-section through the head at a slightly lower level than Fig. 34.9. The alveolar arch of the maxilla, oral cavity, parotid gland, atlanto-axial joint, and neck muscles are seen. Asterisk = spinal cord. (B) T2-weighted axial MRI.

Image A courtesy of the Visible Human Project of the US National Library of Medicine.

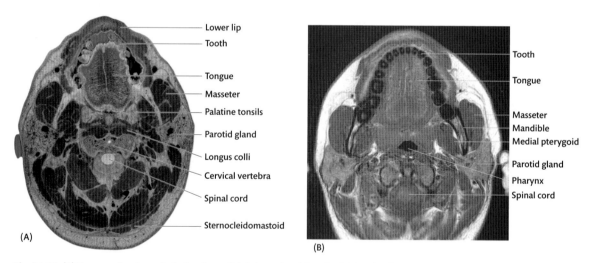

Fig. 34.11 (A) Cross-section through the head at a slightly lower level than Fig. 34.10. The alveolar arch of the mandible, oral cavity, and parotid gland are seen. (B) Axial MRI.

Image A courtesy of the Visible Human Project of the US National Library of Medicine.

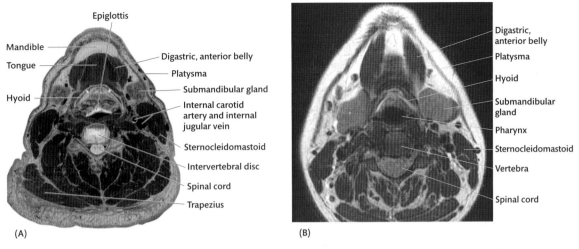

Fig. 34.12 (A) Cross-section through the head at the lower level of the chin, submandibular gland, and hyoid bone. (B) Axial MRI.
Image A courtesy of the Visible Human Project of the US National Library of Medicine.

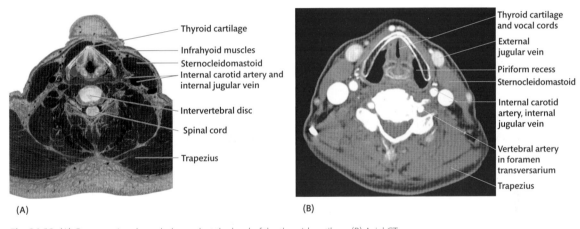

Fig. 34.13 (A) Cross-section through the neck at the level of the thyroid cartilage. (B) Axial CT.
Image A courtesy of the Visible Human Project of the US National Library of Medicine.

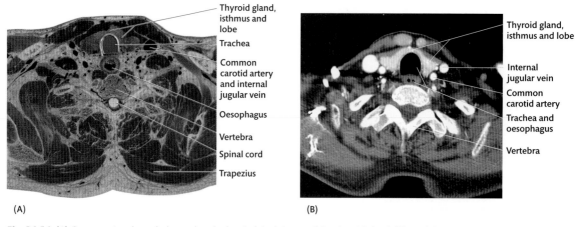

Fig. 34.14 (A) Cross-section through the neck at the level of the isthmus of the thyroid gland. (B) Axial CT.

Image A courtesy of the Visible Human Project of the US National Library of Medicine.

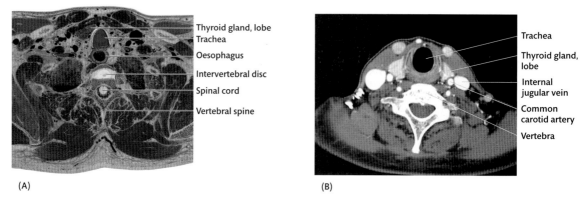

Fig. 34.15 (A) Cross-section through the neck at a level slightly lower than Fig. 34.14. (B) Axial CT.

Image A courtesy of the Visible Human Project of the US National Library of Medicine.

Answers to MCQs

Answers for part 1:
Head and neck

1. C
2. A
3. B
4. A
5. D
6. C
7. D
8. D
9. C
10. B
11. D
12. C
13. C
14. A
15. A

Answers for part 2:
The brain and spinal cord

1. C
2. B
3. D
4. A
5. A
6. C
7. C
8. A
9. A
10. B
11. A
12. C
13. C
14. B
15. A

Index

Note: references to figures and tables are indicated by *f* or *t* after the page number.

417